Pilates Applications for Health Conditions

of related interest

Fascia in Motion
Fascia-Focused Movement for Pilates
By Elizabeth Larkam
ISBN 978 1 90914 128 5
eISBN 978 1 91208 524 8

Centered, Second Edition
Organizing the Body through Kinesiology, Movement Theory and Pilates Techniques
Madeline Black
ISBN 978 1 91208 595 8
eISBN 978 1 91208 596 5

Pilates-Based Movement for Menopause A Guide for Teachers and Practitioners
Dinah Siman
Foreword by Elizabeth Larkam
ISBN 978 1 91342 667 5
eISBN 978 1 83997 647 6

A Movement Educator's Guide to Pregnancy and Childbirth
Jennifer Gianni
Forewords by Marie Jose Blom and Nora St John
ISBN 978 1 91342 653 8
eISBN 978 1 91342 654 5

Spinal Asymmetry and Scoliosis
Movement and Function Solutions for the Spine, Ribcage and Pelvis
Suzanne Clements Martin
ISBN 978 1 90914 172 8
eISBN 978 1 90914 173 5

Pilates Applications for Health Conditions

Volume 2

Locomotor system conditions

Edited by
Madeline Black and Elizabeth Larkam

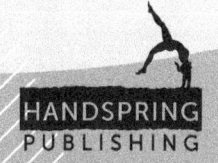

First published in Great Britain in 2025
by Handspring Publishing, an imprint of Jessica Kingsley Publishers
Part of John Murray Press

1

Copyright © Madeline Black and Elizabeth Larkam 2025, Chapter 1 © Suzanne Clements Martin, Chapter 2 © Lise Stolze, Chapter 3 © Christine Romani-Ruby, Chapter 4 © Kathleen McDonough, Chapter 5 © Glenn Withers, Chapter 6 © William Li, Chapter 7 © Ann McMillan, Chapter 8 © Stephanie Behrendt Comella, Chapter 9 © Christine Egan, Chapter 10 © Dawn-Marie Ickes, Chapter 11 © Rebekah Rotstein, Chapter 12 © Kelly Kane, Chapter 13 © Jo Strutt, Chapter 14 © Emilee Garfield, Chapter 15 © Dawn-Marie Ickes

The right of Madeline Black and Elizabeth Larkam to be identified as the Author of the Work has been asserted by them in accordance with the Copyright, Designs and Patents Act 1988.

All rights reserved. No part of this publication may be reproduced, stored in a retrieval system, or transmitted, in any form or by any means without the prior written permission of the publisher, nor be otherwise circulated in any form of binding or cover other than that in which it is published and without a similar condition being imposed on the subsequent purchaser.

A CIP catalogue record for this title is available from the British Library and the Library of Congress

ISBN 978 1 91208 597 2
eISBN 978 1 91208 598 9

Printed and bound in the Untited States by Integrated Books International

Jessica Kingsley Publishers' policy is to use papers that are natural, renewable and recyclable products and made from wood grown in sustainable forests. The logging and manufacturing processes are expected to conform to the environmental regulations of the country of origin.

Handspring Publishing
Carmelite House
50 Victoria Embankment
London EC4Y 0DZ

www.handspringpublishing.com

John Murray Press
Part of Hodder & Stoughton Limited
An Hachette UK Company

The authorised representative in the EEA is Hachette Ireland,
8 Castlecourt Centre, Dublin 15, D15 XTP3, Ireland (email: info@hbgi.ie)

Contents

	Foreword Diane Lee	11
	Foreword Kristi Cooper	13
	Preface	15
	Introduction Madeline Black and Elizabeth Larkam	17
	Timeline of the book	18
	How to use this book	18
	References	19
	Contributor Biographies	21
Chapter 1.	**Pilates and Spinal Asymmetry and Scoliosis: Effect on Gait** Suzanne Clements Martin	25
	Studio apparatus and props	26
	Methods and materials	26
	Session 2/12: Initial assessment	28
	Session 12/12: Post-assessment	28
	Session 3/12: Home program	32
	Session 11/12: Studio session	45
	The journey to Session 11	59
	References	65
Chapter 2.	**Pilates and Kyphosis: Effect on Gait** Lise Stolze	67
	Studio apparatus and props	68
	Methods and materials	68
	Session 2/12: Initial assessment	70
	Session 12/12: Post-assessment	70
	Session 3/12: Home program	73

	Session 11/12: Studio session	80
	The journey to Session 11	**90**
	References	94
Chapter 3.	**Pilates for Management of Central Lumbar Spinal Stenosis: Effect on Gait**	**97**
	Christine Romani-Ruby	
	Studio apparatus and props	**98**
	Methods and materials	**98**
	Session 2/12: Initial assessment	100
	Session 12/12: Post-assessment	100
	Session 3/12: Home program	103
	Session 11/12: Studio session	107
	The journey to Session 11	**122**
	References	126
Chapter 4.	**Pilates and Sacroiliac Joint Dysfunction: Effect on Gait**	**127**
	Kathleen McDonough	
	Studio apparatus and props	**128**
	Methods and materials	**128**
	Session 2/12: Initial assessment	130
	Session 12/12: Post-assessment	130
	Session 3/12: Home program	133
	Session 11/12: Studio session	142
	The journey to Session 11	**157**
	References	163
Chapter 5.	**Pilates and Hip Joint Dysfunction: Effect on Gait**	**165**
	Glenn Withers	
	Studio apparatus and props	**166**
	Methods and materials	**166**
	Session 2/12: Initial assessment	168
	Session 12/12: Post-assessment	168
	Session 3/12: Home program	171
	Session 11/12: Studio session	178
	The journey to Session 11	**187**
	References	192
Chapter 6.	**Pilates for Arthroscopic Knee Meniscus Repair Post-Surgery: Effect on Gait**	**193**
	William Li	
	Studio apparatus and props	**194**
	Methods and materials	**194**
	Session 2/12: Initial assessment	195

		Session 12/12: Post-assessment	195
		Session 3/12: Home program	197
		Session 11/12: Studio session	204
	The journey to Session 11		**219**
		References	222
Chapter 7.	**Pilates and Ankle Dysfunction: Effect on Gait**		**225**
	Ann McMillan		
	Studio apparatus and props		**226**
	Methods and materials		**226**
		Session 2/12: Initial assessment	228
		Session 12/12: Post-assessment	228
		Session 3/12: Home program	231
		Session 11/12: Studio session	241
	The journey to Session 11		**255**
		References	261
Chapter 8.	**Pilates and Spinal Cord Injury: Effect on Gait**		**263**
	Stephanie Behrendt Comella		
	Studio apparatus and props		**264**
	Methods and materials		**264**
		Session 2/12: Initial assessment	266
		Session 12/12: Post-assessment	266
		Session 3/12: Home program	269
		Session 11/12: Studio session	276
	The journey to Session 11		**287**
		References	292
Chapter 9.	**Pilates and Adolescence Congenital Muscular Torticollis: Effect on Gait**		**293**
	Christine Egan		
	Studio apparatus and props		**294**
	Methods and materials		**294**
		Session 2/12: Initial assessment	296
		Session 12/12: Post-assessment	296
		Session 3/12: Home program	300
		Session 11/12: Studio session	309
	The journey to Session 11		**320**
		References	324
Chapter 10.	**Pilates and Pregnancy-Related Diastasis Rectus Abdominus: Effect on Gait**		**325**
	Dawn-Marie Ickes		

	Studio apparatus and props	**327**
	Methods and materials	**327**
	Session 1/12	**327**
	Session 2/12: Initial assessment	328
	Session 12/12: Post-assessment	328
	Session 3/12: Home program	330
	Session 11/12: Studio session	339
	The journey to Session 11	**358**
	References	364
	Appendix: Diastasis Rectus Abdominus	**365**
	Special tests	365
	Assessment findings for Chapter 15: DRA special tests	366
Chapter 11.	**Pilates and Bone Health: Effect on Gait**	**367**
	Rebekah Rotstein	
	Studio apparatus and props	**368**
	Methods and materials	**369**
	Session 2/12: Initial assessment	370
	Session 12/12: Post-assessment	370
	Session 3/12: Home program	374
	Session 11/12: Studio session	382
	The journey to Session 11	**396**
	Acknowledgements	402
	References	402
Chapter 12.	**Pilates and Aging Well: Effect on Gait**	**403**
	Kelly Kane	
	Studio apparatus and props	**404**
	Methods and materials	**404**
	Session 2/12: Initial assessment	405
	Session 12/12: Post-assessment	405
	Session 3/12: Home program	408
	Session 11/12: Studio session	417
	The journey to Session 11	**429**
	References	436
Chapter 13.	**Pilates and Arrhythmogenic Right Ventricular Cardiomyopathy/Dysplasia: Effect on Gait**	**437**

Jo Strutt
- **Studio apparatus and props** — 438
- **Methods and materials** — 439
- **Session 1/12** — 439
  - Session 2/12: Initial assessment — 440
  - Session 12/12: Post-assessment — 440
  - Session 3/12: Home program — 443
  - Session 11/12: Studio session — 455
- **The journey to Session 11** — 469
  - References — 476

Chapter 14. Pilates for Recovery from Ovarian Cancer Post-Surgery: Effect on Gait — 477
Emilee Garfield
- **Studio apparatus and props** — 479
- **Methods and materials** — 479
  - Session 2/12: Initial assessment — 481
  - Session 12/12: Post-assessment — 481
  - Session 3/12: Home program — 484
  - Session 11/12: Studio session — 493
- **The journey to Session 11** — 504
- **Session 4/12** — 504
  - References — 508

Chapter 15. Pilates and Post-Robotic Nerve-Sparing Radical Prostatectomy: Effect on Gait — 509
Dawn-Marie Ickes
- **Studio apparatus and props** — 510
- **Methods and materials** — 510
  - Session 2/12: Initial assessment — 511
  - Session 12/12: Post-assessment — 511
  - Session 3/12: Home program — 514
  - Session 11/12: Studio session — 525
- **The journey to Session 11** — 538
  - References — 542

Abbreviations — 543

Glossary — 545

Foreword

Diane Lee

It is an honour to write a foreword for the publication of two volumes on the application of Pilates to health conditions by editors Madeline Black and Elizabeth Larkam; two Pilates professionals well known not only in their discipline but throughout the world of musculoskeletal therapy.

I am not an expert in Pilates. I have trained extensively as a client with Pilates practitioners and witnessed the benefits for my own conditions. I am a physical therapist who practices/teaches a whole person/whole body model known as The Integrated Systems Model (ISM). In this approach, clients with complex stories and multiple impairments often have many things they cannot do well; walk/run, sit, sleep, lift etc. They also have many impairments due to multiple past traumas. Where to begin? In ISM, we begin by prioritizing the goal, or task, the individual would like to work on – this is called the meaningful task. From that point, everything (assessment, treatment, training) is focused towards that goal. When that task is improved, we pick the next one. I have not had this prioritized task experience in any Pilates program I have attended, to date.

There are several features and concepts in these two volumes on Pilates for health conditions that complement the principles of ISM and that I truly appreciate about this work.

- It is meaningful task, and individual, focused. We know from much research that strategies for movement are individual and *task specific*. Therefore, if assessment and treatment/training are not directed toward the task that is sub-optimal, then relevant deficits may not be appreciated, nor changed, and goals not met. The task chosen for every contributor to this work was gait. Every health condition including Multiple Sclerosis, (MS), Ehlers-Danlos Syndrome (EDS), Postural Orthostatic Tachycardial Syndrome (POTS), Mast Cell Activation Syndrome (MCAS), long COVID, Pelvic Girdle Pain (PGP) Diastatis Rectus Abdominis (DRA), Bone Health, Aging Well etc. impacts movement and this is reflected in one's gait. Two more volumes could potentially be written if the meaningful task was sitting; another highly meaningful task and I'm sure the programs in those two volumes would look very different! Programs must be task specific and individual. The only way to demonstrate the uniqueness of each program is to choose a task and show through a case report the specificity to an individual. The bulk of these two volumes is filled with individual case reports. If the chapters were *condition or body region focused*, and not client-centered, the detail required for individualization would be lost.
- Each chapter contributor was required to complete a standardized whole body/person assessment form that is incredibly thorough and the findings from this assessment led to an individualized program. There are no recipes for specific conditions and/or body regions in these two volumes because every assessment is unique to the individual *even though the task goal (gait) is the same*. While the focus is on improving gait and addressing

mobility and control of the musculoskeletal system, the inclusion of cases that also have complex medical co-morbidities (such as those listed in #1 and more) allows us to see how the programs were adapted from the beginning, and on the fly, to accommodate the challenges these medical conditions present. Recovery, for most, is never linear and adding the self-report before every session allowed us to see how the program was paced/adapted.

- Many of the cases presented here would be excluded from a randomized controlled trial due to their multiple co-morbidities; yet, this is the practitioner's challenge. We see these individual's daily and it's extremely valuable for Pilates practitioners to now have these two volumes as a resource to provide guidance for assessment, treatment and training. While no two stories will ever be the same, there is enough convergence within the divergence presented here to find some help.

- Lastly, each chapter took us on a journey and revealed the progression of the program as well as the evolution of each individual's recovery. The concise theoretical information presented before each case and the clinical application of that knowledge in the Pilates program that followed reflects a high level of care – this work represents the state of the art/science of Pilates practice.

I'm sure these two volumes on Pilates Application for Health Conditions will be used by many for decades to come.

Diane Lee PT, South Surrey, BC, Canada

January 2025

Foreword

Kristi Cooper

Pilates is a practice that transforms lives. It extends beyond physical movement—it restores, strengthens, and empowers. Pilates Applications for Health Conditions represents a pivotal step in fulfilling Joseph H. Pilates' vision and establishing growing recognition of Pilates as a respected health and wellness practice.

I first met Madeline Black and Elizabeth Larkam about 15 years ago, at a pivotal time. I was in the early stages of launching Pilates Anytime, an online subscription platform dedicated to making Pilates accessible to all and preserving its oral history through the Pilates Legacy Project. They were established entities with prolific voices in preserving Pilates and sharing the application to individual health considerations.

I remember feeling nervous when I first approached each of them, hoping they would share my vision and contribute to what I was building. Thankfully, they both said yes! Thus began a longstanding personal and professional relationship with both. I have been in anatomical dissection courses with them at different times. You get to know a person in an anatomy lab! Through my business, I have also had the pleasure of working with and developing friendships with several of the contributors to this book.

I have witnessed Madeline and Elizabeth's unwavering individual commitment to honoring Pilates' legacy while continuously evolving its practice to meet the needs of diverse individuals and the industry. They never cease to inspire me and so many others. They constantly learn and always share the fruits of their efforts. I am a grateful recipient!

For those who have practiced Pilates, whether for fitness, rehabilitation, or as part of a journey to reclaim health, its impact is undeniable. Ask anyone with a regular practice—whether or not they have a diagnosed condition—and they will have their own story to tell. My journey with Pilates began over 40 years ago as a teenager. The reasons I practiced and became a teacher back then are vastly different from the reasons I returned after suffering a traumatic brain injury (TBI) in 2016. What I did know was that Pilates would be my path back to health, and I am forever grateful to those in this book—Elizabeth Larkam, Madeline Black, Dawn Marie-Ickes, Emilee Garfield, Rebekah Rotstein, and Jessie Lee—who supported me in my recovery.

This book is a treasure trove of expertise, offering practical applications and programs that give teachers confidence in their work. It is like having THE contact list of top professionals at your fingertips—what a gift!

This collection of wisdom, experience, and expertise will continue to shape the future of Pilates and its role in healthcare. It is an honor to witness this method's evolution and support the work of those who continue to use it.

The comprehensive scope of this book and meticulous attention to detail are a testament to the dedication of the co-editors and contributors. It is more than just a collection of knowledge—it is a guide, a resource, and an inspiration for those who seek to understand and apply Pilates in meaningful ways. Each exercise in every movement program is thoroughly documented in terms of its relationship to the vocabulary of JH Pilates, as recorded in the

Diane Lee

NCPT Study Guide. Exercises attributed to teachers designated by Mr. Pilates trace their origins. In recognition of Pilates Legacy, this book also includes the contributions of Eve Gentry, Kathy Grant, Romana Kryzanowska, and Carola Trier.

Times have changed! Historically, Pilates teachers relied on apprenticeship to learn. Now, it is easy to be distracted by re-created shapes and performance-based Pilates often displayed on various social media channels. This book, however, contrasts those fleeting images with solid information from leading contributors in the industry. In short, this book is the ultimate resource for accompanying your in-person and online training and workshops to take your practice to the next level.

Whether you are a teacher, practitioner, or simply someone curious about the profound impact of movement on well-being, this book will offer valuable insights that stand the test of time. I wholeheartedly recommend this book and encourage you to immerse yourself in the generously shared wisdom.

Kristi Cooper, Co-founder of Pilates Anytime

Preface

Handspring Publishing invited us to co-edit a book based on Pilates research. During our initial meetings in the Spring of 2018, we reviewed the available research and found limited applicability to the studio environment. Research design does not provide the Pilates teacher with the pedagogical detail needed to customize results for each client.

The privilege of longevity in studying, teaching, and writing in the movement field through four decades contributes to our unique perspective on human movement and Pilates. Given that we work in a movement lab (the studio), not a research lab, we have the responsibility of designing a book that enhances the daily work of Pilates teachers. We bring our combined experience to serve Pilates practitioners and their clients with this book: *Pilates Applications for Health Conditions.*

Health may be considered from a variety of perspectives. According to Gabor Maté, MD, the root word of "healing" means "returning to wholeness" (Maté 2022). The World Health Organization Constitution (2020) defines health as "a state of complete physical, mental, and social well-being and not merely the absence of disease or infirmity."

> Health and illness are not random states in a particular body or body part. They are, in fact, an expression of an entire life lived, one that cannot, in turn, be understood in isolation: it is influenced by—or better yet, it arises from—a web of circumstances, relationships, events and experiences. (Maté 2022)

The perspective of this book considers health as a healing process, not an achievement of eliminating disease states. Diane Lee, BSR, FCAMPT, states: "Restoring health is about more than removing disease; creating optimal strategies for function and performance is about more than removing pain. What it means to be 'in health' is individually defined. It is linked to individual values and goals" (Lee 2011). As co-editors, we realize we are responsible for creating a book that addresses the complex health conditions facing Pilates teachers today. Many of these conditions were not prevalent when Joseph Pilates developed his system in the years from 1929 to 1967 (NPCE Study Guide 2021).

This book is distinct from all other Pilates resources. We value the uniqueness of the equipment designs and choreography of Joseph H. Pilates. We support a critical examination and application of the Pilates Method. We invited contributors with expertise grounded in years of experience and research studies to design, teach, and document Pilates movement programs. Our intent was to examine gait efficiency and its relationship to specific health conditions. Each contribution demonstrates how a customized Pilates program may fulfill movement potential, supporting the process of healing and living with a health condition.

For 40 years, Joseph Pilates taught his movement system of body conditioning (Contrology) in his New York gym (New York Times 1967).

> The period from the late nineteenth century until the beginning of World War I was characterized by optimism and new technology and medical discoveries. A cultural revolution in health and well-being developed during this period, especially in Germany. Joseph Pilates was one of many Europeans intertwining physical practice and discipline. (Larkam 2017)

He championed that the Pilates Method "corrects and vitalizes the human body" (Larkam 2017). Mr. Pilates' perspective to "correct" the human body was derived from the culture of his time. "The back would be flat if the spine were kept as straight as a plumb line, and its flexibility would be comparable to that of the finest watch spring steel" (Pilates 1945). Mr. Pilates' publications describe movement practices that mold a body into his ideal alignment for the purpose of improved health. The cultural environment and lifestyle practices prevalent today have impacts on human health even Mr. Pilates did not predict. A postural strategy of sustained lumbar flexion contributes to a loss of torso reflexive activity. A study by Maaswinkel *et al.*, published in the *Journal of Biomechanics* in 2015, states that "the muscle pre-activation prior to the onset of perturbation was significantly lower in the flexed posture compared to neutral."

Appreciating and understanding how a person organizes themselves helps the movement teacher design effective movement sequences with a whole-person perspective. Evolving awareness of influences from past and present cultural biases impacts how we move and approach healing.

In contrast to the theory of biomechanics, current paradigms articulate new perspectives on human movement and its relationship to health. Both laboratory and clinical research publications have shown that static alignment and "straight spine" are not required for efficient movement or good health. Efficiency of movement requires an integrated neuromyofascial system to transfer forces through the tissues adapting to stimuli. The Integrated Model of Function developed by Diane Lee explains how form and force closure, together with motor control and emotional states, influence how loads are transferred through the lumbopelvic-hip complex (Lee 2011).

Stephen M. Levin, MD, conceived and defined the algorithm of biotensegrity in 1974 as a force vector model (Scarr 2018).

The language of Biotensegrity is the language of soft matter physics. It is tension and compression with continuity. The premise of Biotensegrity is non-linear continuous matter that is self-generated, self-organising, self-stressing, hierarchical, load distributing and low energy consuming. There are no shear moments, no bending moments, no levers, and no joints. (Sharkey 2015)

The compilation of movement programs in this book addresses the unique expression of gait as a human self-organizing and load distributing movement reflective of the healing process. This book contributes to the process of moving from the past belief systems and embracing new paradigms.

Madeline Black
Elizabeth Larkam

References

Larkam, E. (2017) *Fascia in Motion: Fascia-Focused Movement for Pilates*. Edinburgh: Handspring Publishing, p. 32, Figure 2.1; p. 31.

Lee, D. (2011) *The Pelvic Girdle: An Integration of Clinical Expertise and Research*. 4th Ed. Churchill Livingstone Elsevier, p. 52, Box 22; pp. 49–50, 164.

Maaswinkel, E., van Drunen, P., Veeger, D., van Dieën, J. (2015) "Effects of vision and lumbar posture on trunk neuromuscular control." *Journal of Biomechanics, 48,* 2, 298–303.

Maté, G., with D. Maté (2022) *The Myth of Normal: Trauma, Illness & Healing in a Toxic Culture*. New York City: Avery Publishing, Penguin Random House, pp. 9–11.

New York Times (1967) "Joseph H. Pilates, Body Builder, 86; Developer of 'Contrology' Operated 8th Ave. Gym." *New York Times*, October 10, 1967, p. 47. www.nytimes.com/1967/10/10/archives/joseph-h-pilates-body-builder-86-developer-of-contrology-operated.html. [Accessed August 1, 2023].

NPCE Study Guide (National Pilates Certification Exam Study Guide) (2021) Miami, FL: National Pilates Certification Program, Inc., pp. 94–97.

Pilates, J. H. (1945 [2010]) *Return to Life Through Contrology*. Miami, FL: Pilates Method Alliance, Inc., pp. 1–35.

Scarr, G. (2018) *Biotensegrity: The Structural Basis of Life*. 2nd Ed. Edinburgh: Handspring Publishing, p. xiii.

Sharkey, J. (2015) *Biotensegrity—the fallacy of biomechanics: Part 2*. December 23, 2015. www.johnsharkeyevents.com/research/2015/12/23/biotensegrity-the-fallacy-of-biomechanics-part-2. [Accessed August 1, 2023].

World Health Organization (2020) *WHO Director-General's opening remarks at the Empire Club of Canada*. November 20, 2020. www.who.int/director-general/speeches/detail/who-director-general-s-opening-remarks-at-the-empire-club-of-canada. [Accessed August 1, 2023].

Introduction

Madeline Black and Elizabeth Larkam

I only went out for a walk and...going out, I found, was really going in.

Hippocrates proclaimed that "walking is man's best medicine" (McCarthy 2023). Living day to day involves continuous adaptation and response. Individuals and social systems respond unconsciously and consciously to both internal states and external environments. This book focuses on human movement adaptations and responses influenced by health conditions. Specifically, gait is considered in relationship to health and the process of healing. Numerous studies indicate gait patterns are associated with early detection of health conditions, including Parkinson's disease (Gilat *et al.* 2017), cognitive decline (Bridenbaugh and Kressig 2015), and dementia (Kondragunta and Hirtz 2020). Each of the Pilates movement programs in this book documents the client's movement and gait adaptations. Each program reflects the client's experience of their healing process.

As co-editors we initially designed the methods and materials following the case report format. During the editing process we realized that the program documentation required for a cohesive, practical manuscript had evolved and no longer satisfied case report guidelines.

Each movement contributor followed the format of assessment, program design, teaching, and reassessment. Documents were provided to record the 12-session process (see Chapter 4 in Volume 1). Each client program began with health history and an observational assessment of gait. Each contributor observed and documented their client's movement and gait strategies. Program design and pedagogy were developed based on the findings. During the home program and equipment practice, each client was guided to notice their self-organizing movement strategies. The teacher and client worked together as a team to consciously shift toward more efficient movement patterns. The final assessment documentation indicated a more efficient gait. Clients' self-reports expressed an improved attitude toward their healing process and health. The practice of skills acquisition promoted an uplifted sense of hope and self-efficacy.

We invited additional experts to provide perspectives on Pilates movement programs. Dr. Sherri Betz, DPT, details a history of Pilates research. Graham Scarr, DO, considers human movement within the paradigm of biotensegrity. Ken Endelman explains the variable resistance of springs. Variable spring resistance in the frame of Pilates equipment designs is distinct from other forms of resistance prevalent in exercise environments. The contributed movement programs reference J. H. Pilates' exercises and incorporate the pedagogy developed by Eve Gentry, Kathy Grant, Romana Kryzanowska, and Carola Trier. Sarita Allen wrote about working for Kathy Grant, her teacher and mentor. Alycea Ungaro contributes her perspective on her teacher, Romana Kryzanowska.

In this book you will find:

- Pilates movement programs of home exercise and studio equipment sequences for different health conditions
- An assessment observation guide you can use with your clients

- A glossary of terms and a list of abbreviations
- Photos
- Anatomical illustrations references (see Volume 1)
- A list of equipment and props for each movement program
- A delineation of the J. H. Pilates' movement vocabulary as documented in the *National Pilates Certification Exam Study Guide* (NPCE Study Guide 2021)
- Reference to teachers who studied with J. H. Pilates whose vocabulary is included in the contributed programs (Gentry, Grant, Kryzanowska, Trier)

Timeline of the book

The development of the book spans the years prior to and throughout the global pandemic. The book is shaped by the pandemic timeline and trends in health care. The global pandemic affected each book contributor and the program they designed, taught, and documented for their client. This book reflects how the global pandemic shaped the interactions of Pilates teachers and clients. Contributors started their programs prior to and during the pandemic. Some programs were conducted entirely in person prior to the pandemic. Some programs were hybrid, starting in person and completing on screen. Some programs were conducted entirely on screen.

How to use this book

This book is a thorough resource designed for in-depth study. It is a studio companion providing guidance and inspiration to Pilates teachers as they design, implement, teach, and document client programs. Become acquainted with the book, getting an overview by looking at the photos accompanying each of the programs. Become familiar with the anatomical illustrations in Appendix 1 (see Volume 1).

When you are ready to settle in and study:

- Focus on Chapter 4, assessment, in Volume 1
- Complete the assessment documentation form included in Appendix 2 with yourself as the client (see Volume 1)
- Implement the assessment documentation; make video clips of your own gait
- Read the health condition program that is most interesting to you
- Prior to implementing any movement sequence during a client session, practice on yourself. Become familiar with the kinesthetic logic and cues
- Practice each suggested movement sequence noticing how your gait is influenced.
- With your client's permission, make video documentation of your client's gait. Both you and the client can observe changes in movement efficiency
- Repeat this process for each program included in the book
- Study the references for more detail and understanding
- Continue to study with references noted in this book

Allow for the possibility that interacting with this book may upgrade your own practice and teaching skills and contribute to each client's healing process. As Pema Chodron wrote, "The truth you believe in and cling to makes you unavailable to hear anything new."

With gratitude
Madeline and Elizabeth

References

Bridenbaugh, S. A. and Kressig, R. W. (2015) "Motor cognitive dual tasking: Early detection of gait impairment, fall risk and cognitive decline." *Zeitschrift für Gerontologie und Geriatrie, 48,* 1, 15–21.

Chödrön, P. (1991) *The Wisdom of No Escape: How to Love Yourself and Your World.* Shambhala Publications, USA.

Gilat, M., Bell, P. T., Ehgoetz Martens, K. A., Georgiades, M. J. *et al.* (2017) "Dopamine depletion impairs gait automaticity by altering cortico-striatal and cerebellar processing in Parkinson's disease." *Neuroimage, 152,* 207–220.

Kondragunta, J. and Hirtz, G. (2020) "Gait parameter estimation of elderly people using 3D human pose estimation in early detection of dementia." *Annual International Conference of the IEEE Engineering in Medicine & Biology Society. 2020,* 5798–5801.

McCarthy, A. (2023) "Whatever the problem, it's probably solved by walking." *New York Times*, March 25, 2023. www.nytimes.com/2023/03/25/opinion/walking-hiking-spring.html. [Accessed August 1, 2023].

NPCE Study Guide (National Pilates Certification Exam Study Guide) (2021) Miami, FL: National Pilates Certification Program, Inc.

Contributor Biographies

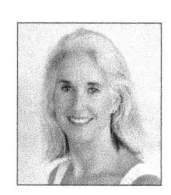

Madeline Black

A Nationally Certified Pilates Teacher, Madeline Black's life pursuit is the discovery of how the human body moves. Over 30 years in the field of movement, her curiosity has explored all aspects of movement in dance, Pilates, yoga, Gyrotonic®, fitness training, and, from studies of human biomechanics, applied biotensegrity, human cadaver dissection labs, and osteopathic and manual therapies. Madeline developed the Madeline Black Method™, a movement method that improves function and strength based on intelligent assessments, manual techniques, and exercise sequences that help people achieve their fullest movement potential. Her extensive study and widely respected accomplishments in the field of movement and fitness have fueled her rise as an international leader in movement and exercise education. She is the author of *Centered* (Handspring Publishing), now in its second edition.

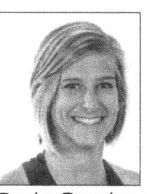

Stephanie Behrendt Comella

Stephanie Behrendt Comella holds a BS in Exercise Biology from UC Davis and is a Nationally Certified Pilates Teacher trained through Balanced Body. Stephanie worked exclusively with spinal cord injury (SCI) and neurological conditions for several years at a specialized rehab facility before switching to a Pilates-based model in 2015. She now teaches from her Pilates studio in the Bay Area. Together with a long-time SCI client, Stephanie co-authored *From the Ground Up: A Human-Powered Framework for Spinal Cord Injury Recovery* (Zebrafish NeuroRecovery), published in 2020. The book aims to educate individuals with SCI and movement professionals on methods for body-reconnection after paralyzing injury (see zebrafishneuro.com).

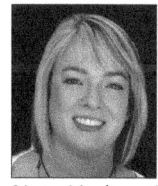

Christine Egan

Christine Egan, MPH, PT, C/NDT, is a pediatric physical therapist with 40 years of experience in the field of pediatric rehabilitation. A native New Yorker, Christine has been in private practice in Marin County, CA for the past 30 years and is highly regarded by both parents and professionals. The cornerstone of her treatment is Neurodevelopmental Treatment (NDT), a technique that requires an intimate knowledge of normal development and uses sensory-motor facilitation to elicit desired motor behaviors. Christine also specializes in posturel and alignment using orthotics, manual therapy, and a host of traditional and complementary approaches. She has been a pioneer in the use of Pilates with children who have neuromuscular and orthopedic disorders. Please visit her website at www.christineegan.com.

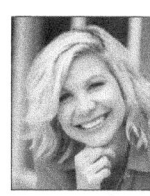

Emilee Garfield

Emilee Garfield, NCPT, is a two-time cancer survivor who teaches movement as medicine to women worldwide through her online courses, teacher training, retreats, and workshops. She is a nationally certified Pilates teacher, author, movement educator, and founder of Cancer Core Recovery® Method, serving women in the cancer community and medical clinics across the globe by offering scholarships to her healing movement

Contributor Biographies

programs and donating copies of her book, *Reclaim Your Strength and Hope: Exercises for Cancer Recovery* (Balboa Press). Emilee's mission is to educate professionals and help other women in cancer recovery have a better quality of life. Contact Emilee at www.emileegarfield.com.

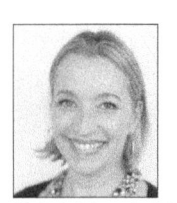

Dawn-Marie Ickes

Dawn-Marie Ickes, MPT, PhD, NCPT, is recognized as an expert in integrative health promotion and wellness. An Assistant Professor at Mount Saint Mary's University, LA, she teaches Advanced Orthopedics, Complementary Medicine, and Integrative Wellness in the PT Environment and directs the MSMU Pilates Pro Bono Clinic. Her integrative method of habitual pattern analysis for the purpose of restoring function and whole-body health utilizes Visceral Manipulation, CranioSacral Therapy, and other integrative therapeutic techniques to support the movement reeducation integral to optimizing the effects of treatment. Years of study in kinesiology, fascial mechanics, dissection, osteopathic manual therapies, and Pilates guided the development of her comprehensive approach.

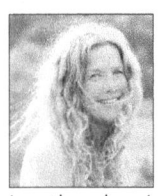

Kelly Kane

Kelly Kane started the Kane School of Core Integration in 1993. The Kane School Pilates certification is a rigorous training program combining the classic principles of Pilates with a modern, clinical perspective on the body. The program crafts advanced teachers with X-ray vision—teachers with solid knowledge of anatomy, biomechanics, and injuries as well as the skills to perceive and improve them. Graduates work in a variety of settings across the fitness, wellness, and medical worlds. The full training includes Foundation Training (Core Muscle Anatomy), Comprehensive Mat, and Basic Training equipment certifications. Kelly has worked with varied populations over the course of her career from athletes to prehab and rehab clients. She is currently obsessed with helping individuals in their "Prime Time" optimize their health. Her primary focus is stewarding women in creating health and happiness after fertility.

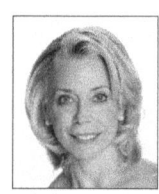

Elizabeth Larkam

Elizabeth Larkam, NCPT, is internationally recognized as an innovator of movement education. Elizabeth began her Pilates studies in 1985 while teaching dance at Stanford University, where she had received her bachelor's and master's education. A Gold Certified Pilates Method Alliance teacher, she was educated by the first-generation Pilates teachers. Elizabeth co-founded and co-owned Polestar Education. When Balanced Body Pilates Education was founded in 2004, she became a Master Teacher and Mentor, conducting courses throughout the world. Elizabeth is a Feldenkrais® practitioner, Franklin Method teacher, and Gyrotonic® and Gyrokinesis® instructor. She is qualified in Gyrotonic® II and Gyrotonic Specialized Equipment. She is the author of *Fascia in Motion: Fascia-Focused Movement for Pilates*, also published by Handspring.

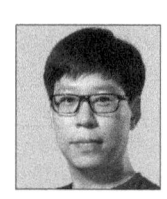

William Li

A sports medicine surgeon and physical therapist for over ten years, Dr. Li, MD, PT, has a wealth of experience in sports medicine, rehabilitation, and functional anatomy. Being a Pilates master instructor, he is devoted to the promotion of Pilates exercise in China as well as the research of applying Pilates exercise in physical rehabilitation. He is now running his own Pilates academy in China and helping the athletes and his patients return to the field.

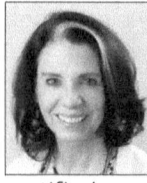

Suzanne Clements Martin

Dr. Suzanne Clements Martin, DPT, NCPT, has a special interest in human movement and potential. As a doctor of physical therapy, certified exercise physiologist, and gold-certified

Pilates expert, she presents internationally, as well as being an award-winning author and video producer. For 40 years, she continues to blend art and science into her works from the fine arts, health, and movement fields. Her specialties include performance arts enhancement, foot issues, spinal asymmetries, and cancer survivorship. She is the author of *Spinal Asymmetry and Scoliosis: Movement and Function Solutions for the Spine, Ribcage and Pelvis* (Handspring). You can find her teaching information at www.pilatestherapeutics.com.

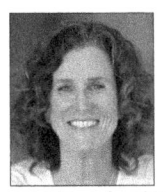

Kathleen McDonough

Kathleen McDonough, PT, MAPT, NCPT, has integrated Pilates and orthopedic physical therapy for 35-plus years. A graduate of UC Davis and Stanford University, the Pilates Center, Boulder, and Polestar Pilates, she serves as secretary on the NPCP Certification Commission and chairs the NPCP Exam Item Writing Committee. Kathleen created and taught spine stabilization programs nationally, and brought Pilates into a major spine specialty practice. She has presented at APTA, World Confederation for Physical Therapy, and PMA conferences, and UCSF's PT and Kaiser Orthopedic Residency Programs. Kathleen is passionate about youth sports, and has brought Pilates into her community schools, running clinics and injury prevention programs.

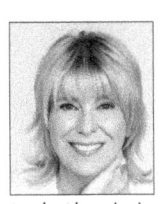

Ann McMillan

Ann McMillan, MSc, NCPT, discovered Pilates while pursuing a dance career in New York City in the 1980s, and went on to complete her master's thesis in Exercise Science at the University of Montreal where she continues to lecture today. Her graduate work was the first to establish a scientific link between Pilates and improved dynamic posture in ballet dancers. Ann is a Pilates coach to Olympic and elite technical artistic sports athletes. "In my professional opinion, Ann McMillan is at the absolute top of the field in integrated Pilates and related fitness training," says three-times Olympic Gold Medalist Ice Dancer Tessa Virtue.

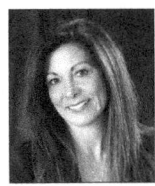

Christine Romani-Ruby

Christine Romani-Ruby, PT, DEd, MPT, ATC, NPCT, is an internationally renowned teacher with 30 years of experience in clinical practice, fitness, and wellness. Dr. Ruby has successfully integrated physical therapy and Pilates to create innovative rehabilitation and wellness programs such as the YUR® Back program for clients recovering from spinal conditions. At her practice, PHI® Pilates Wellness and Rehabilitation in Pittsburgh, PA, Christine has created a cash-based practice and Pilates studio. Among her clients are professional athletes in the NFL and NHL, professional dancers, equestrians, high school athletes, weekend warriors, and those recovering from neurologic and orthopedic conditions. Dr. Ruby is also a professor in the exercise science and sports studies department at Penn West University.

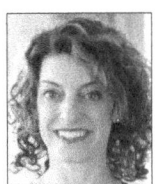

Rebekah Rotstein

Rebekah Rotstein, NCPT, is the creator of the medically endorsed Buff Bones® system, with hundreds of trained instructors around the world. Diagnosed with osteoporosis at age 28, she now presents at hospitals and conferences, advocating for others with low bone mass through innovative education and programming. She has participated in eight cadaver dissections and completed programs and coursework in fascia research, somatic studies, and visceral manipulation. Rebekah was one of the first visiting instructors at Pilates Anytime, is a long-standing ambassador for American Bone Health, and worked as a partner of the U.S. Department of Health and Human Services.

Contributor Biographies

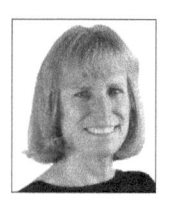

Lise Stolze

Lise Stolze, MPT, DSc, NCPT, is a certified scoliosis therapist through the Barcelona Scoliosis Physical Therapy School (BSPTS) and the Scientific Exercise Approach to Scoliosis (SEAS). Her research on low back pain and Pilates was published in the *Journal of Orthopedic and Sports Physical Therapy*. Lise serves on the Pilates Method Alliance Research Committee and is an educator for Polestar Pilates Education. She is an active member of the International Society on Scoliosis Orthopaedic and Rehabilitation Treatment (SOSORT) and presenter internationally at SOSORT conferences. Lise owns Stolze Therapies in Denver, Colorado.

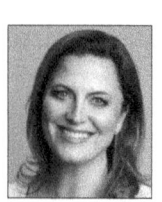

Jo Strutt

Jo Strutt has worked in the field of movement rehabilitation for more than 20 years and is passionate about facilitating the journey from pain and limitation to optimizing physiological health in her Broken to Brilliant™ and Beyond treatment programs. Her own life took her down a path of early success dancing and singing on London's West End stage, and then to tragedy when an accident left her with career and life-changing injuries. This was the beginning of her search for embodied truth in the process of rehabilitation. Jo's experience is authentic and personal in the world of physical rehabilitation, integrating Pilates and osteopathy in the award-winning multi-disciplinary practice Bridgeham Clinic. Jo has worked with elite athletes, professional dancers, and clients healing from injuries and surgery. She hosts educational workshops at Pilates and Osteopathy conferences and mentors practitioners in the holistic health field.

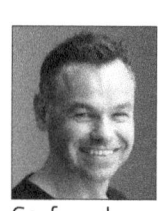

Glenn Withers

Glenn Withers, B Physiotherapy MAPA, MCSP, MHPC, MAPPI, has been leading the world of rehabilitation-based Pilates for over 21 years. Co-founder and creator of the world-renowned APPI Pilates Method, Glenn has been inspiring thousands of clinicians around the world to change their clinical practice to incorporate Pilates into the medical world. Having analyzed all of the traditional Pilates moves, and broken them down based on pain, pathology, and function, Glenn and his wife, Elisa, have created one of the world's most widely used Pilates programs delivered through 23 countries worldwide. Most importantly Glenn is married to his amazing wife Elisa and is the proud father of five beautiful children.

Chapter 1

Pilates and Spinal Asymmetry and Scoliosis: Effect on Gait

Suzanne Clements Martin

Spinal asymmetry and accompanying body-wide neuromyofascial asymmetries are a universal phenomenon. A spiraling curve of the spine from a normal vertical line may be observed from behind. Several factors may contribute to the development of scoliosis. The initial spiral may be attributed to handedness and the innate anatomy of the respiratory diaphragm. Scoliosis is determined when diagnosed with the medical gold standard X-ray Cobb angle measurement of greater than 10 degrees. Roughly 1–2 percent worldwide, largely female, represent the scoliosis condition (Sung *et al.* 2021). It manifests in infancy, childhood, adolescence, and adulthood often after childbirth, cancer treatment, auto-immune activation, joint replacements, menopause, and aging. It can be inherited. Roughly 40 percent of twins develop scoliosis (Greenwood and Bogar 2014). It occurs at times of low bone density and estrogen blood levels, such as in childhood, adolescence, and menopause (Burwell *et al.* 2009). Often triggered by physical accidents, scoliosis can also have onset due to emotional trauma.

The anatomical effects radiate out into many body systems. One side of the vertical spine line develops a relatively stiff convexity causing the shoulder girdle to rotate with respect to the thorax, while the ribs and one humerus grow longer. More progressed spiraling deforms the actual vertebral bony shape and landmarks. On the concave side, the fascia thickens and becomes adherent internally around vital organs. The entire neuromyofascial system is affected including postural musculature. Proximal asymmetries also affect all myofascial continuities. Concavities house disorganized tendon fibers, tissues struggling to make additional vascular pathways to receive oxygen (Martin 2018). The proximal tissue patterns may create a differing gravitational input of each hemipelvis terminating in differing vertical foot loads (Bialek, Pawlak, and Kotwicki 2009). The head also responds to these asymmetrical forces. Nasal cavities, soft palate, eye orbits, and auditory meatuses develop asymmetries, revealing vestibular unsteadiness affecting balance, spatial awareness, and coordination (Pope 2003).

Client description:	18-year-old biological female, identifies as female; pre-professional conservatory cello student
Dates of case report:	March 10, 2020; interruption March 20–May 1, 2020 (COVID SIP); ended June 23, 2020; all in-person sessions

Chapter 1

Studio apparatus and props
Pilates equipment

- Universal Reformer
- Trapeze Table
- Pilates Arc

Props used with equipment

- Mat
- Magic Circle
- Heavy resistance band, 6 ft (1.82 m)
- Foam roller
- Set of wedges
- Wobble board
- 9 in. (23 cm) party balloon
- Raised pad or platform

Home program props

- Mat
- Magic Circle
- Pilates Arc
- Foam roller, 6 ft (1.82 m)
- 2 tennis balls
- Wobble board
- Heavy resistance band, 6 ft (1.82 m)
- 9 in. (23 cm) party balloon

Methods and materials

Session 1/12
1. Health history interview

- 2016: pain in coccyx area prompting medical diagnosis of scoliosis
- Late 2016: medical diagnosis (age 16) of right (dextro) S-curve thoracic scoliosis via radiograph; primary thoracic curve 32-degree Cobb angle; lumbar secondary curve at 15-degree Cobb angle
- Achieved regular periodic menses in late 2015
- Sanders wrist closure complete at time of diagnosis
- 2017: night brace therapy prescribed
  - Dosage: 8–9 hours per night for approximately 6 months
    - Compliancy attained via self-report
  - Symptoms in brace: neck gets sore and is aware of it 1–2 times per night
  - Stopped usage voluntarily due to the right concave waistline seeming to deepen more
- 2017–2019: sought and received intermittent chiropractic, craniosacral therapy, eye/vision and breathing exercise instruction
- Home program: swimming 3 times a week, nightly eye/vision and breathing exercises
- 2017: Vitamin D level low: started calcium, magnesium (1000 mg CA++), Vitamin D 1000IU supplementation
- Hand dominance: right
- Worried about physical repercussions of diagnosis
- Hours playing instrument exposure: 4 hours per day, 5–6 days per week

> **Author note**
> The Sanders wrist closure is a sensitive radiographic skeletal growth measure indicating completion of skeletal growth in order to rule out likelihood for scoliosis progression. End of growth spurt is significant for determining if the scoliosis will worsen. The client reported that the physician determined the adolescent was at the end of her growth spurt using multiple factors such as age, time since onset of menses, apparent physical maturation, plus a radiographic Sanders score.

2. Symptoms

- Worried about scoliosis interfering with profession choice
- No present pain
- Pain in left low back after practice for 2 hours, but does not awaken in the night and less pain upon arising in morning
- Reports no fatigue
- Reports no problem with walking long distances

3. Movement aids

- None

4. Observations

The client is a pre-professional conservatory cello student. The combination of idiopathic scoliosis and her hours of cello practice influences posture and movement patterns.

◆ Cello activity observations

- Seated
    - Right foot forward of left
    - Torso organized in left rotation to stabilize the cello
    - Holds bow with right hand, relative pronation
    - Right upper extremity (UE) abducted/internally rotated
    - Left hand in supination
    - Left humeral head depression

◆ Scoliosis observations (Martin 2018)

- Supine
    - Leg-length difference: right longer than left (0.5 in./1.25 cm)
    - Standing
    - Head position in relation to sternal notch: left
    - Thorax shifted to left of center line
    - Horizontal shoulder tilt: left shoulder higher
    - Anterior lower ribcage protrusion: left
    - Anterior lower ribcage compression: right
    - Lateral waist concavity: right
    - Winging shoulder blade: left
    - Ankle pronation: left
    - Pelvic obliquity: right higher
    - Left hand lower down thigh with neutral palm
    - Right elbow in pronation
    - Eye dominance: right

Final result of case report

The client displayed more ease and appropriate rotation. She increased ankle dorsiflexion and internal femoral rotation on the left leg and the swing of the left humerus. She decreased the left flat foot upon heel strike. She reported less discomfort after cello practice and felt more confident about her health as a professional musician.

Session 2/12: Initial assessment

1. General observations of gait

- Compromised foot load on left side about 40 percent less
- Limited left dorsiflexion with mid-stance
- Decreased ankle extension in mid-swing, minor foot drop
- Decreased left stride compared to right
- Limited torso rotation
- Limited left humeral swing compared to right
- Cervical bracing, chin down
- Right palm and forearm supinated

Author note

Foot loading is an important marker for the impact on scoliosis. Research from physiotherapists Marianna Bialek and Andres M'Hango provides insight into the discrepancies of altered foot loading in those with scoliosis which encourages possible remediation of the limb length functional limitation. Gait kinematics can be affected by addressing the longer leg as the first contact with the ground. In this case, it was the right foot (Azizan, Basaruddin, and Salleh 2018).

2. Standing tests

- Full torso rotation
    - Observations of inefficient side: both
        - Left
            - Shoulder girdle continues in the transverse plane after rotation stops
            - Decreased left pelvifemoral internal rotation
            - Thorax: excessive translation to right
        - Right

Session 12/12: Post-assessment

1. General observations of gait

- Improved foot load on left side about 90 percent
- Increased left dorsiflexion with mid-stance
- Eliminated foot drop
- Equalized stride right to left
- Improved torso rotation
- Still decreased left humeral swing yet improved
- Increased cervical buoyancy
- Supination of right palm and forearm less pronounced

2. Standing tests

- Full torso rotation
    - Observations of inefficient side: left
        - Right preferred
        - No excessive translation of thorax in either direction
        - Left
            - Left rotation range about equal to right
            - Appropriate internal femoral rotation

- Left knee flexion with limited left ankle pronation

- Hemipelvis motion inferior
    - Observations of inefficient side: left
        - Scoliosis pattern, torso asymmetry increases
        - Left innominate remains in place
        - Pelvis shifts to right
        - Thorax translates left relative to pelvic shift

- Hemipelvis motion superior
    - Observations of inefficient side: both
        - Right
            - Scoliosis pattern, torso asymmetry increases
            - Left pelvic rotation in transverse plane
        - Left
            - Difficulty elevating left innominate
            - Restricted left pelvifemoral glide
            - No left ankle supination

- Lateral pelvic shift
    - Observations of inefficient side: both
        - Left
            - No adaptation of the thorax
            - Limited left pelvifemoral lateral and right medial glide
            - Limited right ankle pronation
        - Right
            - Thoracic translation to left
            - Limited right pelvifemoral adduction

3. Seated tests

- Thoracic rotation

- Appropriate shoulder girdle glide with thoracic rotation

- Hemipelvis motion inferior
    - Observations: both sides efficient
        - Right and left improved midline orientation
        - Head and thorax centrally accommodate both sides
        - Left pelvifemoral adduction slightly compromised with right knee bend, yet improved
        - Left thoracic translation less pronounced

- Hemipelvis motion superior
    - Observations: both sides efficient
        - Left side remains higher than right yet less pronounced
        - Pelvifemoral glides appear more equal
        - Right improved with no pelvic rotational compensations
        - Right and left ankle supination improved
        - Left shows appropriate increase in lumbar lateral flexion

- Lateral pelvic shift
    - Observations of inefficient side: left
        - Left
            - Improved left pelvifemoral lateral and right medial glide
            - Improved lumbopelvic translation
            - Increased left pelvifemoral adduction
        - Right ankle adapts in both directions

3. Seated tests

- Thoracic rotation

- Observations of inefficient side: left
  - Seated heavier on left ischial tuberosity
  - Excessive right thoracic translation
  - Right scapula lacks glide
    - Right scapula medial border abducts

- Hip joint and knee flexion
  - Observations of inefficient side: both
    - Left hip flexion
      - Pelvis anteriorly rotates
      - Abdominal bulge may indicate a change in intra-abdominal pressure (see Volume 1, Chapter 10 Editor Note)
      - Increased left dorsiflexion may be compensatory pattern (Martin 2018)
    - Right
      - Left thoracic translation

4. Sit and stand

- Lateral view
  - To standing
    - Anterior thoracic translation
  - To sitting
    - Thoracolumbar junction right rotation with anterior lower ribcage protrusion (Martin 2018)
    - On descent pelvis translates right
    - Shifts weight to the right foot

- Anterior view
  - To standing
    - Transverse plane pelvic rotation left
    - Left hemipelvis anterior
    - Left femur adduction and ankle pronation

- Observations of inefficient side: left
  - Improved weight distribution on ischial tuberosities
  - Thorax organizes toward midline
  - Left displays increased scapula glide with diminished winging
  - Bilateral rotation approximately equal, right slightly less

- Hip joint and knee flexion
  - Observations of inefficient side: left
    - Left
      - Improved pelvifemoral organization
      - Central organization with no abdominal bulging (Martin 2018)
      - Decreased left ankle dorsiflexion
    - Right
      - Central organization thorax over pelvis

4. Sit and stand

- Lateral view
  - Improved appropriate sequential lumbar to thoracic extension
  - Decreased left anterior lower ribcage protrusion
  - Force transfer evenly distributed

- Anterior view
  - Centralized pelvis organization

- Head favors being right of central line

Author note
Cervical rotation to the right and left was added to assess the influence of cervical-thoracic eye dominance.

- Right cervical rotation with upward chin tilt
- Left cervical rotation limited, no chin tilt

5. Standing balance

- Two-leg stance, eyes open
  - 60 seconds

- One-leg stance, eyes open
  - Left leg: 30 seconds
  - Right leg: 30 seconds
    - Left leg more efficient with little wobble
    - Right leg improved with no touch-down of foot
    - Right leg initially displayed wobble, yet able to correct
    - Right leg compensations with several shoulder-level tilts to right

- Improved left pelvifemoral organization and left ankle pronation
- Head over pelvic center of gravity

5. Standing balance

- Two-leg stance, eyes open
  - 60 seconds

- One-leg stance, eyes open
  - 30 seconds
  - Left leg more efficient with little wobble
  - Right leg improved with no touch-down of foot
  - Right leg initially displayed wobble, yet able to correct
  - Right compensations with several shoulder level tilts to right

Chapter 1

Session 3/12: Home program

Fatigue scale	4
Pain scale	1
Client self-report	• "As I continue to do the exercises, I believe that I will continue to feel more strength and movement control"
Key changes observed by author at end of Session 3/12	• No discomfort • Non-dominant right lateral hemipelvis motion superior appeared challenging • Tried new strategies and engaged when given multiple cues or commands • Appeared orientated to midline after one session
Reason behind choice of sequencing	• Break up directional bias • Preparation for new activations • Breathing exercises followed by wedge and balloon prepare internal torso pressures that optimize the excursion of the diaphragm • Supine, seated, side, kneeling, and standing exercises follow a neurodevelopmental sequence to optimize gait • Optimize foot loading accuracy • Writing by the non-dominant left hand reinforces neuroplasticity

Author note

The vertical area of the respiratory diaphragm contains the central tendon located at the anterior lower thorax, which is about one-quarter to one-third of the total surface area of the thorax. In an asymmetrical thorax as with scoliosis, Thomen *et al.* (2020) found the lung surface area is reduced in comparison to those without scoliosis affecting breathing. The organization of the respiratory diaphragm relative to the pelvis facilitates an improved excursion of the breath and internal pressures.

Session movement sequence

1. Lateral rolling with Side Lying Imprinting	(See Chapter 5 in Volume 1, Gentry: Side Lying Imprinting)
Intent	• Safe rotary spinal articulation • Torso-pelvis movement • Cross-brain developmental movement • Coordinated eye tracking related to rotation

Gait reasoning
- Improve counter-rotations of thorax and pelvis
- Vestibular input for vertical stance
- Rotation promoting heat generation and myofascial recoil

Starting position
- Lying on right side on mat
- Head supported
- Hip and knee flexion
- Lumbar region in slight flexion
- Hands cupped onto knees with elbow flexion
- Head and eye gaze to right

Author note
Generalized *organizational cues* are pre-activation for structural integrity during movement. Cues are to: 1. imagine magnets drawing the ischial tuberosities medial; 2. imagine two pelvic parachutes with a gentle superior lift of the anterior and the posterior pelvic diaphragm (Martin 2018).

Movement description
- Prepare with organizational cues (see Author note above)
- Soft breathing throughout
- Imprinting in a sequential movement
  - Weight the lateral-posterior right ilia
  - Pelvis initiates left rotation
- Slowly abduct left femur
- Head and gaze to right
- Weight the posterior pelvis-lumbar region and thorax
- Gently pull right femur to left with right hand to lie on left side
- Head lingers to the right for upper scapular girdle gliding
- Slowly roll head to left with soft gaze
- Arrive in starting position on left side
  - Reverse the motion
- Continuous motion for 6 sets

2. Supine circular foot and hip slides
(See Chapter 5 in Volume 1, Gentry: Knee fold and leg slide)

Intent
- Pelvifemoral articulation
- Improve internal hip rotation
- Facilitate myofascial gliding

Gait reasoning
- Influence pelvic inlet tissues through abduction and adduction
- Improve thoracic to pelvic counter-rotation

Chapter 1

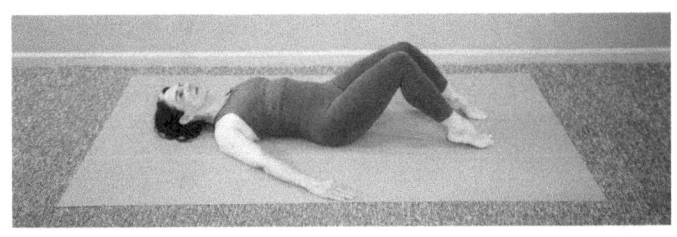

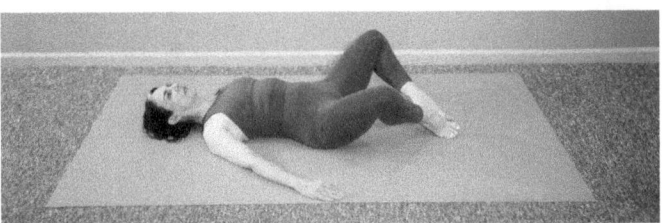

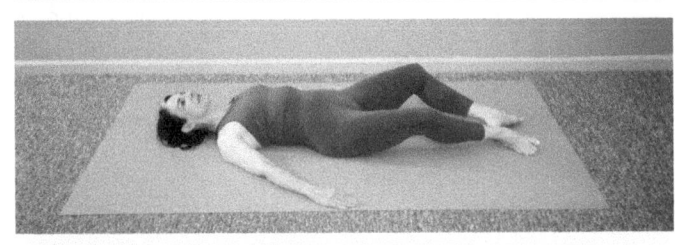

Figure 1.1
Editor note: Refer to text for details of movement sequencing.

Starting position	• Supine on mat
	• Knee flexion, 45 degrees, feet flat
	• Thumbs at lower anterior ribcage
	• Gentle pressure on iliac crests with 3rd fingers
	• Soft breathing with internal eye gaze
Movement description	• Inhale, prepare with organizational cues (see Author note, exercise 1)
Variation 1	• Exhale, let knees fall open
	• Lateral edges of feet slide upon mat
	• Extend lower extremities (LE)
	• Allow feet to widen apart
	• Inhale, adduct and internally rotate femoral joints with knee extension
	• Flex and internally rotate femoral joints with knee flexion
	• Feet remain on mat
	• Repeat circular action 4 times
	• Reverse

Variation 2
- Exhale, consciously abduct/externally rotate femurs
- Extending, adduct and internally rotate LE
- Feet slide toward each other
- Inhale, abduct and externally rotate femurs with knee flexion
- Slide feet along mat
- Adduct femurs to starting position
- Repeat 4 times

3. Supine with wedge placement

Intent
- Improve torso organization
- Articulation of thorax
- Proprioceptive awareness and interoception of individual scoliotic pattern
- Improve breathing into concavities of the torso

Gait reasoning
- Improve counter-rotations
- Facilitate midline orientation

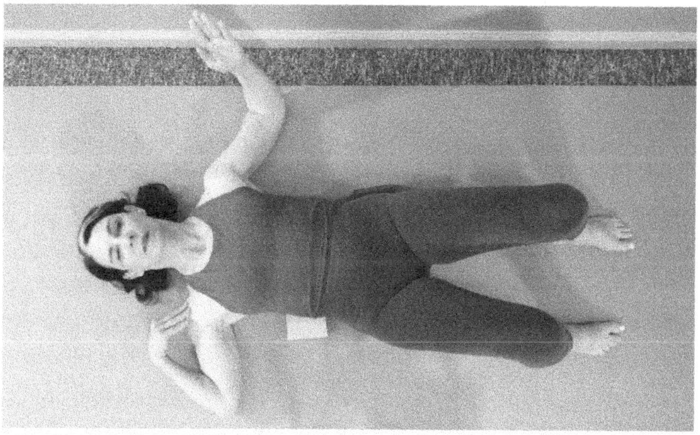

Figure 1.2

Starting position
- Supine on mat
- Feet hip-width apart
- Place a wedge underneath area of perceived lightness (see Chapter 5 in Volume 1, Gentry): propping with soft ball
  - This client placed wedges posterior right at mid- to lower thorax and left ilia

Movement description
- Gentle rocking of anterior and posterior pelvis
- Cease rocking to allow pelvis to settle
- Prepare with organizational cues (see Author note, exercise 1)
- Close right dominant eye
- Place tongue behind right upper teeth
- Gentle posterior increase of weight into wedges
- Place right hand on right shoulder to counteract right scapula protraction
- Leave humerus in 45 degrees abduction and externally rotate flexed elbow
- Facilitate left scapula external rotation with activation of left axilla connective tissue
- Inhale
- Follow a soft exhale from inferior to superior
    - Pubis
    - Umbilicus
    - Sternum
    - Glottis
    - Ears
- Pause for a count of 4
- Repeat 4 times

Author note
The exhale from inferior to superior is following a central line of the torso (Martin 2018). Tissue activation into the wedges facilitates local, subtle isometric contractions.

Author note
Chawla and Deepak (2022) describe a difference in the efficiency of the bilateral organs, where the limbs are effector organs, lateralized, yet the eyes are receptor organs, receiving input bilaterally. In sum, there exists a fundamental difference between the dominance of the limbs and the dominance of the eyes; however, the muscles affecting the eye direction occupy the contralateral motor hemisphere. Therefore, empirical evidence exists, yet this author suggests more research is warranted to better understand the interplay of effect of eye dominance and gaze upon thoracic rotation.

4. Articulating pelvic bridge breathing into a balloon

Author note
Research shows the addition of balloon breathing is effective for alteration of both intra-thoracic and intra-abdominal pressures (Boyle, Olinick, and Lewis 2010).

Intent
- Torso articulation
- Midline orientation of scoliosis curve transition points
- Improve thoracic osteokinematics and arthrokinematics with breathing
- Regulate internal thoracic and abdominal cavity pressures

Gait reasoning
- Thoracic organization relative to the pelvis for improved rotation
- Hip joint congruency for activation of LE with torso
- Improve torso rotation and UE swing
- Improve medial and lateral femoral glide which is compromised in scoliosis
- Improve left arm swing

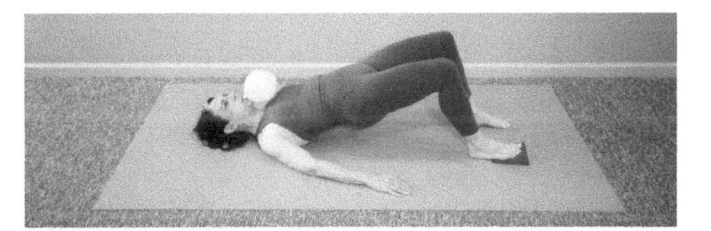

Figure 1.3

Starting position
- Supine on mat
- Feet hip-width apart
- Place wedge underneath left forefoot to enhance dorsiflexion
- Stretch balloon neck several times and place aperture in mouth
- Place arms by sides or rest left arm overhead

Movement description
- Inhale, prepare initiating cues
- Exhale into balloon and begin coccyx flexion
- Continue torso flexion through sacrum and lumbar region
- Extend the hip joints
- Mid- to upper thorax in contact with mat
- Hold bridge position
- Remove balloon from mouth to release air
- Inhale into nose without balloon
- Exhale into balloon and articulate down to starting position
- Remove balloon from mouth to release air
- Finish in starting position, maintaining organizational cues
- Repeat 3 times

5. Seated Spine Stretch

Derivative of J. H. Pilates Spine Stretch (NPCE Study Guide 2021, p. 47)

Intent
- Distribute weight evenly in sitting
- Proprioceptive awareness of laterality and head over center of gravity
- Articulate posterior translation thorax in sagittal plane
- Improve breathing
- Organizing the thoracolumbar junction (TLJ) to midline

Editor note
The term *laterality* refers to the preference for one side of the body over the other. Examples include left- or right-handedness and left- or right-footedness. It is task-specific. It may also refer to the primary use of the left or right hemisphere in the brain.

Author note
Handedness and limb preferential task strategy tend to reinforce a scoliosis pattern. While Johari *et al.* (2016) found that those with scoliosis do not experience significant pathology such as in COPD until a curve is severe, those with curves at 40 degrees exhibit more fatigue with activity, impacting quality of life.

Gait reasoning
- Reorganize scoliosis curve transition points
- Improve torso rotation
- Coordinate head weight over moving center of gravity

Pilates and Spinal Asymmetry and Scoliosis: Effect on Gait

Starting position	• Sitting on mat, shoulders flexed to 75 degrees • Palms face toward each other • Ankles in dorsiflexion with calcaneus on mat
Movement description	• Inhale and prepare with organizational cues (see Author note, exercise 1) • Close dominant eye, tongue touching right upper teeth • Exhale, sternum in direction of the pubis/torso • Slight posterior pelvic rotation with simultaneous neck flexion • Reach forward with 3rd fingers and soles of feet • Stay for 3 breath cycles • Return to starting position initiating with head and pelvis to midline organization • Repeat 4 times

Editor note
The dynamics of the tongue-mandible-hyoid system are managed by a dense and complex neural network which is not often found in other body structures (Pilat 2022). The author incorporates tongue movements to enhance motor control. Tongue articulation can fulfill the demands of phonation, breathing, swallowing, and chewing.

6. Lateral bridge with UE arc

Derivative of J. H. Pilates Side Bend (NPCE Study Guide 2021, p. 50)

Intent	• Teach efficient lateral torso flexion • Improve thorax on scapula glide • Reduce laterality
Gait reasoning	• Improve counter-rotations • Improve left arm swing • Activate the region of serratus posterior • Improve breathing capacity
Starting position	• Sit on right side on mat • Right hand on floor close to pelvis with flexed elbow • Stack legs to side with left foot on right arch • Right scapula in contact with thorax • Left palm supinated with slightly flexed elbow

Author note
Experiment with the client to determine the easier side to push off the mat. It is important to provide a sense of success. Start on the easier side.

Chapter 1

Movement description
- Exhale, prepare to inhale with organizational cues (see Author note, exercise 1)
- Inhale, press into right hand and elevate pelvis
- Simultaneously abduct and flex left UE in an arc superiorly
- Exhale, rotating torso to right and placing left hand on mat
- Press into the right 3rd finger
- Inhale, abduct left UE rotating torso to left into side bridge position
- Lower pelvis to mat flexing right elbow
- Repeat 3 times
- Hold last repetition for 4 breath cycles
- Repeat for the other side

7. Quadruped Knees Off with scoliosis cues

Author note
The scoliosis cue for this client relates to a protrusion of the lower ribs 7–10 due to narrowed ribs lateroposteriorly, thereby pushing the anterior portions ahead of the right anterior sagittal-coronal body surface. The rotation of the thorax is three-dimensional. The vertebrae in the concavity illustrates RASO (right anterior spine overgrowth), widening the distance between the right mid- to lower ribs, the thoracic convexity, while narrowing the left thorax in this region. The left ischial tuberosity relates to the concave side of the body creating a left lumbar lateral flexion, elevating the left lateral pelvis, taking the left ischial tuberosity with it, moving away from the midline. The client places wedges underneath the concave thoracic region and the light pelvic side, then holds the right dominant eye closed while keeping the tongue up behind the top right teeth. The client learned to feel how to self-adjust her left anterior ribcage and left ischial tuberosity to reorganize toward a central orientation.

Editor note
The dynamics of the tongue-mandible-hyoid system are managed by a dense and complex neural network which is not often found in other body structures (Pilat 2022). The author incorporates tongue movements to enhance motor control. Tongue articulation can fulfill the demands of phonation, breathing, swallowing, and chewing.

Intent	• Coordinate limbs to torso activation
	• Lumbar region dynamic stability
	• Activation of thoracic and abdominal pressures in altered gravitation orientation
	• Load non-dominant arm
Gait reasoning	• Create proprioceptive input from limbs to torso
	• Organize feet for even load transfer
Starting position	• Quadruped position on mat
	• Ankles in dorsiflexion
	• Extend phalanges and metatarsals on mat
	• Head in vertical line in front of hands
	• Elbows slightly flexed
Movement description	• Prepare to initiate cues
	• Close the right dominant eye
	• Tongue to top right back teeth
	• Implement scoliosis cues (see Author note above)
	• Inhale
	• Exhale and hover knees about 2 in. (5 cm) above the mat
	• Stay for 3 breath cycles and lower
	• Maintain torso activation
	• Repeat 3 times

8. Tall kneeling with pendulum arms

Intent	• Create proprioceptive input from femurs into pelvis
	• Hip congruency
	• Stimulate hip retinacula and surrounding tissues
	• Head-to-pelvis vertical organization
	• Torso adaptation with arm motion
Gait reasoning	• Torso adaptation with thoracic rotation
	• Equalize foot load distribution
	• Improve humeral counterswing
Starting position	• High kneeling position on mat with one-quarter of wedge underneath shorter leg
	• UE by sides with externally rotated palms anterior
Movement description	• Exhale, prepare with organizational cues (see Author note, exercise 1)
	• Alternate rhythmic short-range 40 degrees UE flexion and extension
	• Inhale 2 quick sniffs, exhale 2 quick "ha's"
	• 10 sets

9. Tall kneeling with pendulum arms reciprocal variation

Intent
- Create proprioceptive input from femurs into pelvis
- Hip congruency
- Stimulate hip retinacula and surrounding tissues
- Head-to-pelvis vertical organization
- Torso adaptation with arm motion

Gait reasoning
- Equalize foot load distribution
- Promote humeral swing and counter-rotation with phonation
- Improve breathing pattern
- Promote balance with perturbation and distraction

Starting position
- High kneeling position on mat with one-quarter of wedge underneath shorter leg
- UE by sides, palms facing lateral femurs

Movement description
- Exhale, prepare with organizational cues (see Author note, exercise 1)
- Initiate quick, small-amplitude reciprocal arm swings
- 32 swings
- Sniff 2 inhales and "ha-ha" exhale through mouth every 4 arm swings

10. Femoral glide with Magic Circle (Black 2022)

Intent
- Promote central vertical line organization
- Break up laterality
- Improve femoral glide

Gait reasoning
- Facilitate lateral pelvic shift to improve lateral translation in stride exchange
- Optimize pelvic transverse rotation
- Facilitate scoliosis cues to organize T12–L1 junction for improved counter-rotation
- Promote head weight over pelvic center of gravity

Starting position
- Stand on mat with left side facing wall
- Place Magic Circle between greater trochanter (GT) and wall
- Bring feet under hip sockets pressing into Magic Circle
- Drape left UE over head to touch right ear
- Place right palm at side of right thorax

Movement description	• Prepare with organizational cues (see Author note, exercise 1) • Close right eye and place tongue at back of right top teeth • Engage gentle pressure with the right hand on thorax toward the left • Rhythmically pulse left GT 20 times in toward the wall • Change to right side • Engage gentle pressure with the right hand on thorax toward the left • Repeat 20 pulses

11. Seated writing with non-dominant hand

Intent	• Break up laterality • Promote neuroplasticity through eyes, proprioception, and integration of fine motor skills • Promote counter-rotation to inefficient side
Gait reasoning	• Balance and coordination for strides • Integration of motor skills promotes gait initiation and progression • Integration spares energy and lessens fatigue
Starting position	• Seated at writing surface with wedge between left GT and lateral femur • Close right dominant eye • Position tongue behind upper right teeth
Movement description	• First exercise: write "My name is _____" 10 times • Spontaneous writing continues for another 2 minutes (set timer)

12. Foot exercises

Intent	• Improve left foot limitation and excessive pronation • Improve dorsiflexion and limitation of right mid-foot • Glide foot joints and lower limb myofascial compartments • Increase awareness of foot position, and in motion

Chapter 1

Gait reasoning
- Prepare foot for optimal foot loading
- Promote talus glide for tibial progression
- Practice left phalangeal extension for minor left foot drop in mid-swing
- Activate foot intrinsically bilaterally
- Pre-activation practice for foot and leg myofascial compartments

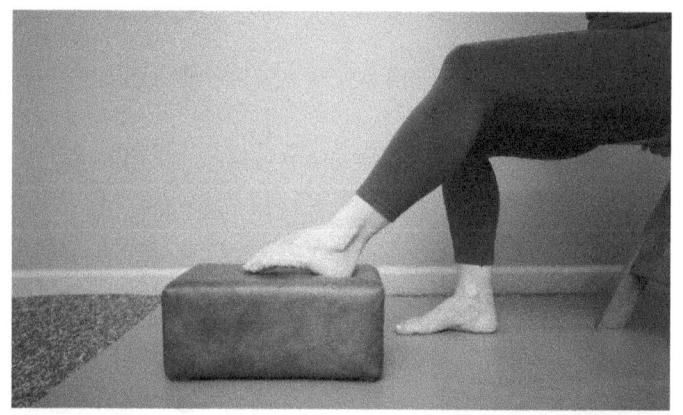

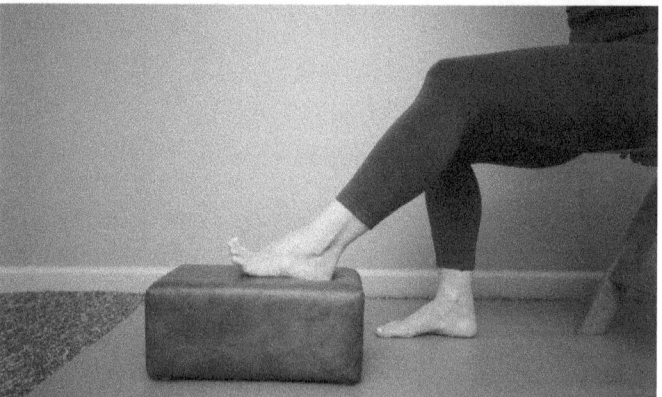

Figure 1.4

Starting position
- Sit toward the edge of a chair
- LE parallel, feet hip-width apart
- Place right foot on a raised pad or platform

Movement description	• Observe and sense the 5 arches of the right foot: 2 longitudinal and 3 transverse
	• Press right rear foot and distal phalanges into pad
	• Cup plantar side of foot activating all 5 arches
	• Hold for 4 breath cycles
	• Anchor the calcaneus
	• Draw forefoot toward heel until 1st distal phalange flexes to touch pad
	• Observe lateral arch for accuracy of rise
	• Maintain the cupped foot
	• Dorsiflex the ankle
	• Maintain dorsiflexion, laterally spread the metatarsals and phalanges
	• Extend proximal interphalangeal (PIP) joints, touching pad with metatarsals
	• Touch phalanges on pad
	• 3 slow repetitions
	• 10 quick repetitions ending in dorsiflexion
	• Reverse
	• From dorsiflexion, flex the phalanges
	• Lower forefoot until 1st distal phalange flexes to touch pad
	• Extend phalanges to touch pad
	• Extend PIP joints with metatarsals on pad
	• Maintain extension and dorsiflex the ankle
	• Hold dorsiflexion, flex the phalanges
	• Repeat the action 3 more times slowly and 10 times briskly

Session 11/12: Studio session

Fatigue scale	3
Pain scale	0
Client self-report	• "The motions are more familiar, easier to do, and I feel more space in my left side and more freedom of motion."
Key changes observed by author at end of Session 11/12	• Decreased flat foot in left stride foot loading
	• Increased and greater ease in thoracopelvic counter-rotation
	• Increased pendulum motion in left humerus

Chapter 1

Reason behind choice of sequencing	• Culmination of previous movement • Breaking up laterality pattern with breathing • All exercises on Universal Reformer to foster reproduction • The new school environment allows her Universal Reformer use

Session movement sequence

1. One Lung Breathing on Pilates Arc (Martin 2018)

Intent	• Improve organization of thoracic curves • Optimize thorax organization relative to pelvis • Pre-activate torso • Coordinate the four diaphragmatic activities (Black 2022)
Gait reasoning	• Encouragement for consistent daily practice • Promote thoracic counter-rotation • Promote optimal breathing for increased energy
Set-up	• Pilates Arc on mat • Towel to support neck and head
Starting position	• Lying on left (concave) side with height of arc at breast level • Left humerus lies over arc • Towel roll underneath cervical region • Right hand holds onto rim of arc • Practitioner kneels behind client with flat palms on lateral thorax T4–T9 • Hips and knees extended • LE adducted
Movement description	• Inhale for 4 counts focusing on right lung • Exhale slowly • Practitioner's hand remains in contact for 4 breath cycles • Perform 4 repetitions on each side CUES ♦ Imagine blowing up a balloon into the left posterior thorax ♦ Imagine squeezing a wet washcloth at the end of exhalation ♦ Breathe into posterior left back thorax and left scapula

Author note
The left thoracic concave side was in contact with the arc first, to affect the convex side, allowing depression of the right thoracic convexity. The use of supported lateral flexion is recognized as a beneficial element in physiotherapy scoliosis specific exercise (Berdishevsky *et al.* 2016). During practice on the second side, the concave side receives stimulation of connective tissue, specifically tendons and vascular (Khosla *et al.* 1980).

2. Footwork on Universal Reformer

Derivative of J. H. Pilates Footwork on Universal Reformer (NPCE Study Guide 2021, p. 52)

Intent
- Promote full dorsiflexion bilaterally
- Promote full plantar flexion bilaterally
- Address leg length discrepancy, which is common in scoliosis

Gait reasoning
- Closed kinematic chain in non-gravitational position for new strategies
- Improve foot loading bilaterally

Set-up
- Supine
- Place wedge perpendicularly under concavity of left thorax and right pelvis
- Pad underneath left metatarsals

Starting position
- Bilateral metatarsals at width of footbar
- Hip flexion/abduction/external rotation
- Knee flexion

Movement description
- Extend knees
- Stay in position
- Dorsiflex the ankles
- Plantar flex the ankles
- Flex the knees to return to starting position
- Repeat 9 times

CUES
- Imagine the medial sides of the LE coming together into the pelvis
- Maintain torso activation as hips flex
- Feel like the heels are coming up behind the knees in plantar flexion
- Whole foot hugging the bar, especially the 4th and 5th metatarsals
- Maintain weighted contact with the thoracic wedge
- In deep hip joint flexion, feel the pelvic wedge into the carriage

Author note
Cue the femoral adduction during external rotation and extension. Adducting during femoral external rotation and knee extension activates the neuromyofascial continuity from the foot to the pelvis. The second position in ballet training (hip abduction/external rotation) translates to standing activities involving balance and transfer of body weight (Watson *et al.* 2017). The combination of the scoliosis cues with ankle dorsiflexion and plantar flexion facilitates fascial gliding throughout the entire system.

3. Mermaid on Universal Reformer
Derivative of J. H. Pilates Mermaid on Universal Reformer (NPCE Study Guide 2021, p. 58)

Intent
- Fascial gliding
- Hemipelvic counter-rotation
- Thoracic rotation and lateral flexion bilaterally

Gait reasoning
- Challenge rotation and balance
- Improve hemipelvic movement for counter-rotation in oppositional strides

Set-up
- 1 medium spring in 1st gear

Starting position
- Sitting with right side facing toward footbar
- Right hip in external rotation, hip and knee flexion
- Left hip in internal rotation, hip and knee flexion
- Right hand on the footbar elbow, slightly flexed
- Left humerus in 90 degrees abduction with elbow extension and supination
- Close right eye, move tongue to right

Author note

Research shows that eye use has an effect on cervical region rotation (Bexander, Mellor, and Hodges 2005).

Movement description

- Right hand on footbar
- Press carriage away
- Inhale into left lateral thorax as torso laterally flexes to right
- Left UE abducts and flexes overhead
- Rotate thorax to right
- Exhale, return to start
- Perform 6 times
- Repeat on the other side

CUES

- Imagine an elastic band attached to each elbow, stretch the band
- Rotate with ease
- Round under, look at the navel, deepen, exhale
- Inhale, lengthen the tongue up into the palate
- Drop the elbow down into the well to return the shoulders against the imaginary wall

Author note

Although it is not recommended to offer Mermaid as a beginning exercise for scoliosis, this client was sufficiently advanced by lesson 11 to allow it. Her 30+ degree curve, age, and flexibility did not contraindicate the exercise. Due to the endurance rotation needed for cello practice, Mermaid is a good exercise to counteract the overuse effect.

Although this exercise is performed on both sides, the right was chosen first due to the client's ease to rotate right. The addition of her scoliosis cues made the exercise specific to her needs. The same scoliosis cues are used for both sides. Mermaid facilitates the counter-rotation of the hemipelvises needed for optimal gait. The hypothesis is that functional leg-length difference is addressed with hemipelvic mobility exercise, since most leg-length discrepancies are functional by nature (Khamis and Carmeli 2017).

4. Articulating bridge with balloon breathing on Universal Reformer

(See Chapter 5 in Volume 1, Gentry: Spinal articulations/hip escalator)

Intent
- Balloon provides resistance to aid expiration
- Torso articulation in sagittal plane
- Activate abdominal region and pelvic diaphragm
- Breathing optimization
- Efficiency of intra-abdominal pressure

Author note
Research shows the addition of balloon breathing is effective for alteration of both intra-thoracic and intra-abdominal pressures (Boyle *et al.* 2010).

Gait reasoning
- Thoracic organization relative to pelvis for improved sagittal plane organization

Set-up
- Springs: 2 medium and 1 light in 1st gear
- Stretch neck of balloon

Starting position
- Supine on carriage
- Feet hip-width apart, 45 degrees external rotation
- Knees flexed with forefeet on footbar
- Left hand holds balloon neck to lips

Movement description
- Inhale, prepare initiating cues
- Exhale into the balloon, begin coccyx flexion
- Continue torso flexion through sacrum and lumbar region
- Extend the hip joints
- Mid- to upper thorax in contact with the mat
- Hold bridge position
- Hold air in balloon
- Press carriage away from footbar 3 times
- Return carriage to stoppers in bridge position
- Remove balloon from mouth to release air
- Inhale into nose without balloon
- Exhale into balloon and articulate down to starting position
- Remove balloon from mouth to release air
- Finish in starting position maintaining organizational cues
- Repeat 3 times

Author note
To hold air in the balloon during carriage movement, use the lips not the teeth. Then press the legs into extension and flexion 3 times.

CUES
- At the height of the bridge encourage continuous organizational cues activation
- Maintain thorax and scapulae in contact with the carriage at the height of the lift and while lowering
- Articulation down sequentially cueing from sternum, umbilicus, pubis, and hip joints
- Relax the forehead and eyes, gaze back into the head

Author note
In scoliosis the continuity of the connective tissues of the torso is organized differently making the transverse movement inefficient. The right hemipelvis is rotated anteriorly causing a decrease in tissue glide, facilitating ineffective torso control (Hides *et al.* 2019).

5. Short Spine Massage on Universal Reformer

J. H. Pilates Short Spine Massage (NPCE Study Guide 2021, p. 56)

Intent
- Facilitate articulation and suspension of torso during flexion
- Increase proprioception through flexion
- Exploring and discovering the transition points of the scoliosis curves is beneficial for self-management
- Inversion for internal organ stimulation

Gait reasoning
- Articulating the thoracic region promotes facet congruency for improved three-dimensional motion
- Promote midline orientation

Set-up
- Springs: 1 medium and 1 light in 1st gear
- Feet in loops
- Headrest down

Starting position
- Supine on carriage with arches of feet in foot loops
- LE adducted in parallel, 45 degrees flexion
- Knees extended
- UE by sides
- Palms pressing into carriage

Chapter 1

Movement description
- Exhale, prepare with organizational cues
- Inhale, begin hip joint flexion to point of pelvis posterior rotation
- Allow pelvis to be lifted off carriage
- Maintain pressing into feet loops
- Stop at mid- to upper thorax
- Flex knees maintaining tension in straps
- Exhale, press head into headrest, and arches of feet into loops
- Slowly articulate down from mid-thorax to pelvis
- Linger and acknowledge transition points
- Continue exhaling softly
- Press feet into straps to extend knees
- Return to starting position
- Repeat 3 times more

CUE
- Back of the head, back of the thorax, back of the pelvis heavy against the mat

Author note
Supported torso flexion with an increase in the weight of the posterior skull against the mat and by pressing the 5th metatarsals of the feet into the loops coordinates full body activation. The goal is to help proprioception and interoception to centralize the torso. The client then "embodies the spine" (Martin 2023). It is critical, and fortunate, to experience this somatic inner awareness to find resolution and a sense of well-being, even in dysfunction or deformity (Hearn and Cross 2020).

6. Short Spine Massage on Universal Reformer variation

Derivative of J. H. Pilates Short Spine Massage on Universal Reformer (NPCE Study Guide 2021, p. 56), J. H. Pilates Long Spine Massage (NPCE Study Guide 2021, p. 60), and Overhead/Jackknife (NPCE Study Guide 2021, p. 53)
(See Chapter 5 in Volume 1, Trier), Short spine massage variations

Intent
- Facilitate articulation and suspension of torso during flexion
- Increase proprioception through flexion
- Exploring and discovering the transition points of the scoliosis curves is beneficial for self-management
- Inversion for internal organ stimulation

Pilates and Spinal Asymmetry and Scoliosis: Effect on Gait

Gait reasoning	• Coordination of flexion and extension • Eccentric loading for extensors • Increase in difficulty for self-organizing • External spatial development to counter laterality • Centralization of gravitational unloading
Set-up	• Springs: 1 medium and 1 light in 1st gear • Headrest down
Starting position	• Supine on carriage with arches of feet in foot loops • LE adducted in parallel, 45 degrees flexion • Knees extended • UE by sides • Palms pressing into carriage
Movement description	• Exhale, prepare with organizational cues • Inhale, begin hip joint flexion to before the point of pelvis posterior rotation • Exhale, use the pressure against the foot loops, ascend upward aiming to line up the feet over the face (Jackknife position) • Maintain Jackknife position • Externally rotate femurs, heels together, plantar flex ankles • Hip joint flexion, abduction, external rotation • Flex knees aiming toward shoulders • Maintain pressing into feet loops • Lower sequentially, press head into headrest, thorax, then pelvis into carriage • Maintain the flexion, rotation, and abduction as the legs extend to 45 degrees • Return to the starting position • Repeat 4 times

CUES
- Sense the scoliosis cues throughout
- Close right eye and place tongue to the right
- Notice the transition points and try to soften them
- Feel the sequential activation of flexion from pubis to sternum
- Find a floating quality

Chapter 1

Author note
Although it is not recommended to perform inversions in a beginning program or with an older adult with bone complications, this client is flexible and young enough to perform the more stringent inversions due to her age and condition. It is beneficial to do so when possible due to the effect of mobility and motility upon the internal organs (Burwell *et al.* 2009).

In addition, the ability to see the body veering off of the central line and auto-correct is invaluable for the client's body and self-awareness. Exercises in auto-correction are a mainstay of the physiotherapy scoliosis-specific exercise catalog (Romano *et al.* 2015).

7. Unilateral straps: feet in loops holding balls on Universal Reformer

Intent
- Balance hemipelvic motion
- Enhance centrality
- Coordinate central orientation of torso with pelvic archway
- Enhance full body even extension

Gait reasoning
- Gait requires hemipelvic motion in opposition to one another
- Scoliosis may amplify while in gravity during verticality; improve organization in verticality
- Improve vestibular disequilibrium that creates compensatory head position and distorted patterns

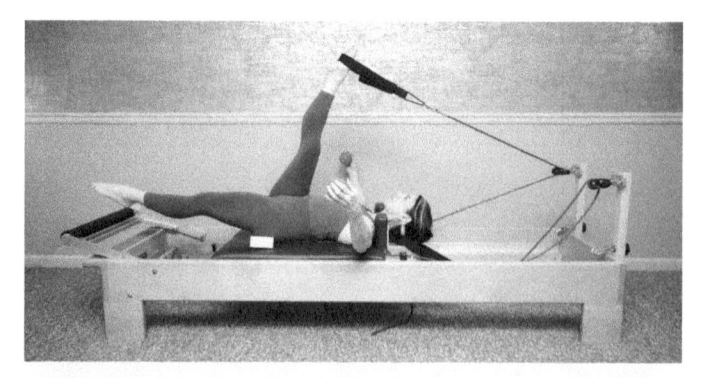

Figure 1.5

Set-up	● 1 medium spring ● Headrest up
Starting position	● Supine on carriage ● Place right foot arch in foot loop on same side pulley ● Femurs 45 degrees externally rotated ● Hip joints at 20–35 degrees flexion ● Knees remain extended throughout exercise ● Adduct both femurs to align feet with midline ● Right femur on top ● Hold tennis balls with UE abducted/externally rotated 30 degrees in coronal plane
Movement description	● Exhale, prepare with organizational cues ● Left hip joint maintains 20–35 degrees flexion ● Right LE is the mover ● Inhale, right hip joint flexes to 45 degrees ● Exhale, right hip joint extends to 20–35 degrees flexion ● Repeat 5 more times ● Change sides ● Repeat 6 times

CUES

- Sense the back of the head, posterior thorax, and pelvis heavy into mat
- Feel like the bottom leg is lifting to meet the top

Author note

Crossing the midline is beneficial for vestibular stimulation and brain neuroplasticity in scoliosis (Carry *et al.* 2020; Hadders-Algra 2018).

Each hemipelvis must be coordinated with the other for balanced gait. Sagittal balance is critical for gait and good stance in verticality (Le Huec *et al.* 2019).

8. Scooter on Universal Reformer variation

(See Chapter 5 in Volume 1, Gentry: Eve's Lunge)

Editor note

Eve's Lunge and Scooter are often referred to as the same exercise. In this case, the author focused on the torso relationship to movement of the UE assisting extension and foot loading to drive the carriage movement.

Chapter 1

Intent
- Mobilization and balance of hemipelvic contralateral motion
- Myofascial gliding

Gait reasoning
- Improve good reciprocal hemipelvic motion
- Improve foot loading addressing leg length differences
- Closed kinematic chain exercise

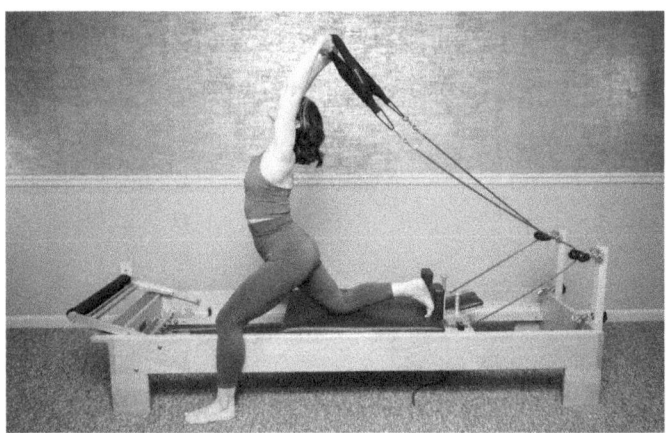

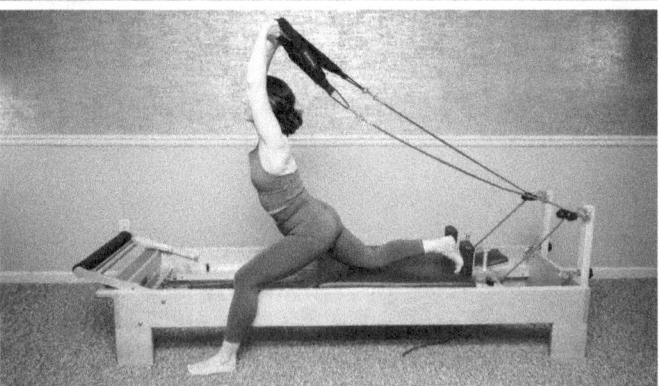

Figure 1.6

Set-up
- Springs: 1 medium and 1 very light

Starting position	• Stand on right side of Universal Reformer
• Left foot on floor in line with bottom of carriage
• Knee is flexed
• Left foot in line with hip joint
• Right foot against shoulder stop on ipsilateral side
• Right knee flexion, knee on carriage
• Rope lengths measured to shoulder stops
• Both hands inside both loops, left palm on right dorsum
• 140–150 degrees shoulder flexion, elbows flexed
• Establish tension in loops by pressing against loops
Movement description	• Prepare with organizational cues
• Inhale, extend torso; following with the gaze allow loops to assist extension
• Exhale, right foot presses into floor to move carriage backward
• Maintain the arcing of the body
• Repeat 3 times more
• Repeat for the other side

CUES

- Maintain pressure against the loops with the hands
- For the left leg forward cues: keep the left femur away from the side of the Universal Reformer
- Keep the weight onto the front of the right thigh
- Imagine a circle around the torso from the crown of the head to the tail
- Allow the foot loops to pull the torso into extension
- Soft breathing: the motion is small, quiet, and sustained

Author note

Dr. Lewton-Brain, DO, showed in a 2008 MRI presentation the difference in torso extension when performing full body extension with and without conscious focus (Martin 2018). Especially in this exercise, the intention is to coordinate the input of the upper and lower limbs into the torso. See Author note in Session 2.

9. Wobble board standing sequence

Intent	• Dynamic vertical foot load
• Challenge balance
Gait reasoning	• Dynamic foot loading training through unlevel surfaces better approximates community ambulation

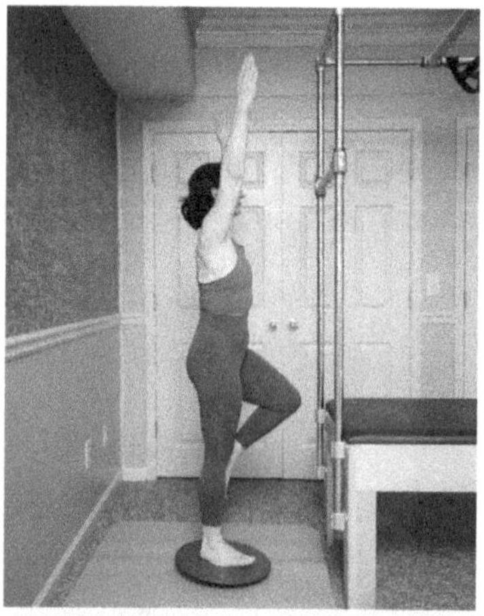

Figure 1.7

Set-up	• Wobble board stationed at narrow end of Trapeze Table
Starting position	• Standing on wobble board
	• Hold on to vertical frame poles
Movement description	• Two legs

- Two legs
  - Rock board side to side allowing knees to bend and be soft 10 times
  - Extend knees and rock board side to side 10 times
  - Extend knees and tip board front to back (dorsiflexion/plantar flexion)
- One leg
  - All performed with extended knee
  - Stand on right foot in center
  - Left hip joint flexed, abducted/externally rotated (FABER) with plantar side of foot on right mid-shin
  - Parallel leg: tip front and back with ankle, not pelvifemoral joint
  - Alternate both legs from external rotation to internal rotation 4 times
  - End in external rotation and remain in external rotation for next set
- Left foot to medial right knee
  - Extend left hip joint posterior to place sole of foot upon floor behind board
  - Rebound quickly to bring left foot to front of right tibia
  - Repeat 4 times
- Reverse the whole series using left leg as stance leg

Author note

Gait is directly influenced by alterations in center of gravity and center of pressure from dynamic vertical body displacements (Winter 1995). Since scoliosis is accompanied by an altered balance system, it benefits to manage these alterations through multi-directional and variable speed shifts of weights. This aspect is important as the client ages. Fall prevention in older adults with scoliosis is of primary importance. This exercise is a good habit to acquire throughout the lifespan.

The journey to Session 11

Session 4/12
Client self-report

- Fatigue scale 0
- Pain scale 2
- "Felt more aware of a lot of different muscles in my foot"
- "Gained more mobility in my ankles"

Key changes observed

- Feet proprioception in non-weight bearing versus weight bearing

Reasoning behind choice of movements

- Increase proprioception of left LE
- Increase mobility of left ankle dorsiflexion
- Improve bilateral hip glide
- Focus on left lumbar area and hemipelvis

Session movement sequence

1. Foot exercise recap and review

2. Foot posture: 5 arches of feet

3. Talar motion in dorsiflexion versus plantar flexion

4. Universal Reformer

- Footwork
- Stomach Massage variations with small box against shoulder stops

5. Trapeze Table

- Bend and stretch in bilateral and unilateral side lying
- Monkey addressing torso concavities and leg lengths through scoliosis cues (NPCE Study Guide 2021, p. 63)

6. Additional movements

- Mat
  - Roll-Up: unable to do on own, assisted with forearm clasp and client's legs braced in adduction
- Gait integration
  - Making music with middle of arch for each step

Session 5/12
Client self-report

- Fatigue scale 4
- Pain scale 2
- "Felt much more movement in my feet"

Chapter 1

- Gained much more physical awareness of exercises from the last session

Key changes observed

- Increased ability for coordination and attention
- Proprioception and body awareness visibly obvious
- Integrating multiple scoliosis cues for eye, tongue, thorax, ankle, and lumbopelvic-femoral region
- Compliance of integration of foot exercise into home program, doing maintenance home program

Reasoning behind choice of movements

- Advancing Pilates vocabulary
- Increase of left pelvifemoral glide
- Increase of left pelvifemoral internal rotation to facilitate pelvic transverse rotation
- Increase left dorsiflexion

Session movement sequence
1. Brief review of foot-ankle exercises with resistance band

2. Bilateral quick rotational circles of foot

3. Universal Reformer

- Footwork

4. Stomach Massage variations with small box

- Feet in parallel, externally rotated heels together with spinal flexion and extension

5. Trapeze Table

- Straps: feet in loops
    - Bilateral hip flexion and extension

6. Mat

- Single Leg Stretch on mat
- Bend and Stretch
- Bilateral or unilateral
- Side lying

7. Universal Reformer

- Supine straps: feet in loops series

8. Additional movement

- Seated breathing with percussive exhalations
- Gait integration with breathing with stepping

Session 6/12
Client self-report

- Fatigue scale 4
- Pain scale 2
- "Felt a new motion through the inversion exercises"
- "New use of my core muscles that I hadn't experienced before"

Key changes observed

- Increased awareness of scoliosis curve transition points
- Increased awareness of inverted pelvic position pressures
- Increased awareness of imbalances

Reasoning behind choice of movements

- Used many options for gravitational and anti-gravitational positions
- Address the numerous imbalances that occur from one gravitational load to another

Session movement sequence

1. Pilates Arc for torso support added

2. Adaptation of Hundred

- Pelvic elevation with shoulders remaining on mat

3. Pilates Arc: Breathing

- Supine
  - Sternal extension breathing, torso and head supported
- Lateral position
  - One Lung Breathing exercises in lateral flexion, torso-supported lateral flexion
  - Mid-pelvis on apex, thoracolumbar breathing
- Supine
  - Posterior pelvis on apex, thorax on mat breathing

4. Universal Reformer

- Pelvic bridging with exhalations into balloon

5. Trapeze Table

- Assisted Rollover holding side upright poles
- Rollover with feet on cross bar, single leg extend and flex (Martin 2023)

6. Universal Reformer

- Assisted Short Spine
- Assisted Jackknife

7. Additional movement
- Mat, teacher-assisted Rollover

Session 7/12
Client self-report

- Fatigue scale 4
- Pain scale 1
- "Felt much more expansion and flexibility in my ribcage"
- Gained more awareness of rotational motions

Key changes observed

- The stiffness of the convex area thorax complied to accept the Mermaid
- Left ischial tuberosity was higher off of the mat as expected
- Right rotation was restricted as expected, but gave insight and meaning to client for need for rotation exercises

Reasoning behind choice of movements
- Increase awareness of rotation limitations
- Improve rotation of both sides
- Safe development of the ability for cognizant and intentional rotational exercise

Session movement sequence
1. Modified Mermaid

2. Universal Reformer

- Footwork
- Stomach Massage
- Bridging: spinal articulation
- Mermaid
- Straps: feet in loops series

3. Additional movements

- Addition of scoliosis cues, closing right dominant eye and right tongue position during Universal Reformer exercises (see Author note, Session 3/12, exercise 1)

Chapter 1

- Addition of torso placement of wedge for Footwork
- Gait integration with breathing: inhale for 4 steps, exhale for 4 steps

Session 8/12
Client self-report

- Fatigue scale 4
- Pain scale 0
- Increased range for rotational motions
- "Felt more strength and agility in the repeated exercises"

Key changes observed

- Left femoral glide in all planes and ilia superior/inferior motion limited, yet responded to standing rotation exercise
- Lack of hip congruency, yet responded to variations in transverse pelvic motion especially in combination with the upper body weighting of the ball and torso rotation

Reasoning behind choice of movements

- Improved femoral congruency
- Activate posterior lateral pelvifemoral tissues
- Reduce left hemipelvis motion superior to improve the lateral pelvic translation
- Optimize ability to progress femur forward for swing
- Increase lumbopelvic transverse rotation to right, allowing more even stride

Session movement sequence
1. Review and reinforce feet slides

2. Functional Footprints

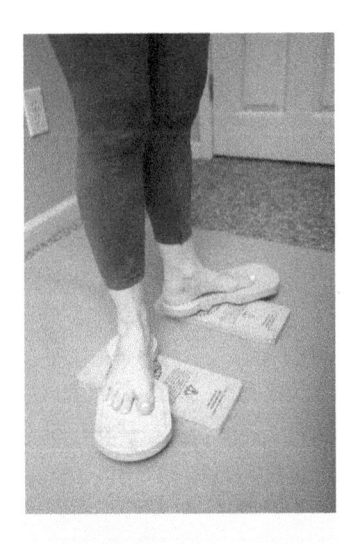

Figure 1.8

- Assessment of femur on pelvis
- Pre-intervention
  - Hip joint rotation: left internal rotation 40 degrees, right internal rotation 30 degrees
  - Assessed ilial rotation and found decreased ilial internal rotation of femur, on left more than right

3. Universal Reformer

- Footwork with ethmoid emphasis

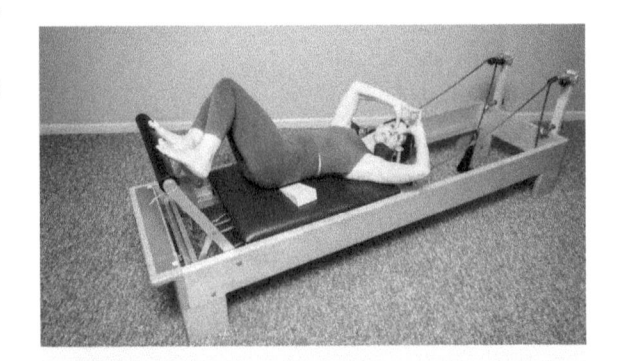

Figure 1.9

Pilates and Spinal Asymmetry and Scoliosis: Effect on Gait

- Use wedges for scoliosis cues
- Hands in ethmoid hold with head 50 degrees rotation right, then left fixed
- Alternating rotation right to left with ethmoid hold
- Fixed cervical thoracic position with eye and tongue/girdle correction

> **Author note**
> Ethmoid hold on the head (Figure 1.9) is a fixed hand position with the thumbs grasping and pulling ventrally the soft tissue of the medial superior orbits and the index fingers exerting firm placement upon the hairline, abducting the digits while approximating the distal phalanges of the 5th digits.

- Footwork with tongue emphasis

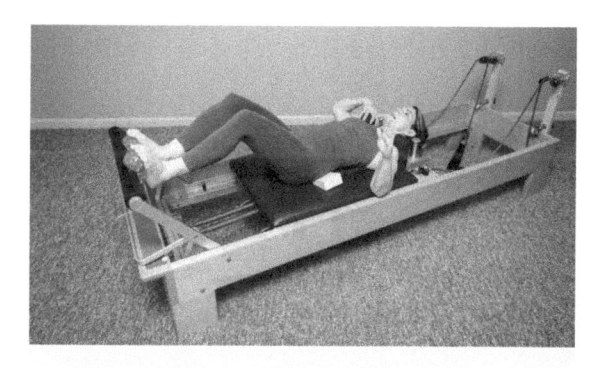

Figure 1.10

- Dominant eye closed
- Tongue position toward mandibular molars
- Right UE abducted, elbow flexion ball on skin directing subtle pressure caudally
- Left UE 45 degrees abducted with elbow flexion

> **Author note**
> Place balls underneath feet on bar to challenge leg length and uneven foot loading. Wedge is underneath left pelvis to challenge right transverse lumbar rotation.

4. Additional movements

- Reassess on Functional Footprints
  - Increased range in both measures of ilial rotation
  - Hip joint rotation: left internal rotation 40 degrees; right internal rotation 35 degrees
  - Left less restricted
- Gait integration
  - Find middle of head between ears over anterior sacrum
  - Initiate motion from T12

Session 9/12
Client self-report

- Fatigue scale 4
- Pain scale 1
- "Felt more comfortable in my repeated movements"
- "Felt a lot of stretch in my legs as well"

Key changes observed

- Improved coordination of scoliosis cues (see Author note, Session 3/12, exercise 1)
- Able to implement the closure of dominant eye and placement of tongue position

Reasoning behind choice of movements

- Preparation for self-practice
- Create a cohesive Pilates experience with individualized scoliosis attention for addressing professional overuse

Chapter 1

- Centralize weight shift and transfer in cadence
- Equal foot loading during stride

Session movement sequence
1. Review program components to prepare for self-practice at conservatory

2. Universal Reformer

- Footwork
- Stomach Massage
- Mermaid
- Pelvic Press
- Short Spine/Long Spine
- Straps: feet in loops series

3. Additional movement

- Stand, balance, and rock on foam roller

Session 10/12
Client self-report

- Fatigue scale 3
- Pain scale 0
- "The usual motions are becoming easier to do"
- "My left side feels more spacious"

Key changes observed

- Small regression
- Increased home practice in anticipation of beginning at conservatory
- Displays right scapula winging and lower right side of torso impacting left foot load in gait

Reasoning behind choice of movements

- Hemipelvic lateral articulation with contralateral ilial motion
- Challenge midline organization
- Addressing effects of consistent practice to cello profession, stance, and general gait
- Emphasize new proprioceptive awareness of scoliosis imbalances relating to both gait and conservatory life

Session movement sequence
1. Vibratory dowel use as suggested by cello coach

2. Track and field stick for fascial glide

3. Visual self-measure of arms overhead for observation of torso lateral flexion

4. Proprioceptive supine measure of right scapula winging into floor

5. Pilates Arc

- Supine chest and anterior pelvic breathing
- Side Lying One Lung Breathing

6. Universal Reformer

- Footwork
    - Pulse tempo variations
- Mermaid
- Pelvic Press with breathing into balloon
- Unilateral straps: feet in loops holding balls
- Eve's Lunge

7. Additional movements

- Gait integration
    - Left ankle extension during swing
    - Left foot push-off
    - Left humeral swing
    - Thoracic counter-rotation

References

Azizan, N. A., Basaruddin, K. S., and Salleh, A. F. (2018) "The effects of leg length discrepancy on stability and kinematics—kinetics deviations: A systematic review." *Applied Bionics and Biomechanics, 2018*. DOI: 10.1155/2018/5156348.

Berdishevsky, H., Lebel, V. A., Bettany-Saltikov, J., Rigo, M. *et al.* (2016) "Physiotherapy scoliosis-specific exercises—a comprehensive review of seven major schools." *Scoliosis, 11*, 20. DOI: 10.1186/s13013-016-0076-9.

Bexander, C. S. M., Mellor, R., and Hodges, P. W. (2005) "Effect of gaze direction on neck muscle activity during cervical rotation." *Experimental Brain Research, 167*, 3, 422–432.

Bialek, M., Pawlak, P., and Kotwicki, T. (2009) "Foot loading asymmetry in patients with scoliosis." *Scoliosis, 4* (Suppl. 1), O19. DOI: 10.1186/1748-7161-4-S1-019.

Black, M. (2022) *Centered: Organizing the Body through Kinesiology, Movement Theory and Pilates Techniques.* 2nd Ed. Edinburgh: Handspring Publishing, pp. 89, 91, 170–173.

Boyle, K. L., Olinick, J., and Lewis, C. (2010) "The value of blowing up a balloon." *North American Journal of Sports and Physical Therapy, 5*, 3, 179–188.

Burwell, R. G., Aujla, R. K., Grevitt, M. P., Dangerfield, P. H. *et al.* (2009) "Pathogenesis of adolescent idiopathic scoliosis in girls—a double neuro-osseous theory involving disharmony between two nervous systems, somatic and autonomic expressed in the spine and trunk: Possible dependency on sympathetic nervous system and hormones with implications for medical therapy." *Scoliosis, 4*, 24. DOI: 10.1186/1748-7161-4-24.

Carry, P. M., Duke, V. R., Brazell, C. J., Stence, N. *et al.* (2020) "Lateral semicircular canal asymmetry in females with idiopathic scoliosis." *PLoS ONE, 15*, 4. DOI: 10.1371/journal.pone.0232417.

Chawla, O. and Deepak, D. (2022) "Ocular dominance: A narrative review." *Himalayan Journal of Ophthalmology, 16*, 1, 16–19.

Greenwood, D. and Bogar, W. (2014) "Congenital scoliosis in non-identical twins: Case reports and literature review." *The Journal of the Canadian Chiropractic Association, 58*, 3, 291–299.

Hadders-Algra, M. (2018) "Early human motor development: From variation to the ability to vary and adapt." *Neuroscience & Biobehavioral Reviews, 90*, 411–427.

Hearn, J. H. and Cross, A. (2020) "Mindfulness for pain, depression, anxiety, and quality of life in people with spinal cord injury: A systematic review." *BMC Neurology, 20*, 1, 32.

Hides, J. A., Donelson, R., Lee, D., Prather, H., Sahrman, S. A., and Hodges, P. W. (2019) "Convergence and divergence of exercise-based approaches that incorporate motor control for the management of low back pain." *Journal of Orthopedic and Sports Physical Therapy, 49*, 6, 437–452.

Johari, J., Sharifudin, M. A., Ab Rahman, A., Omar, A. S. *et al.* (2016) "Relationship between pulmonary function and degree of spinal deformity, location of apical vertebrae and age among adolescent idiopathic scoliosis patients." *Singapore Medical Journal, 57*, 1, 33–38.

Khamis, S. and Carmeli, E. (2017) "A new concept for measuring leg length discrepancy." *Journal of Orthopedic Science, 14*, 2, 276–280.

Khosla, S., Tredwell, S. J., Day, B., Shinn, S. L., and Ovalle, W. K., Jr (1980) "An ultrastructural study of multifidus muscle in progressive idiopathic scoliosis: Changes resulting from a sarcolemmal defect at the myotendinous junction." *Journal of the Neurological Sciences, 46*, 1, 13–31.

Le Huec, J. C., Thompson, W. D., Mohsinaly, Y., Barrey, C. and Faundez, A. A. (2019) "Sagittal balance of the spine." *European Spine Journal, 28*, 9, 1889–1905.

Lewton-Brain, P. (2008) IADMS 18th Annual Meeting, Cleveland, OH, October 23–25, 2008.

Martin, S. C. (2018) *Spinal Asymmetry and Scoliosis: Movement and Function Solutions for the Spine, Ribcage and Pelvis.* Edinburgh: Handspring Publishing, pp.15, 35–36, 53–54, 57, 59, 78–79, 86, 89–108, 126, 137, 140, 142, 154.

Martin, S. C. (2023) Quote from discussions with Handspring Publishing during editing process.

NPCE Study Guide (National Pilates Certification Exam Study Guide) (2021) Miami, FL: National Pilates Certification Program, Inc.

Pilat, A. (2022) *Myofascial Induction: Volume 1—The Upper Body.* Edinburgh: Handspring Publishing, pp.338–341.

Pope, R. (2003) "The common compensatory pattern: Its origin and relation to the postural model." *American Academy of Osteopathy Journal.* Winter, 19–40.

Romano, M., Negrini, A., Parzini, S., Tavernaro, M. *et al.* (2015) "SEAS (Scientific Exercises Approach to Scoliosis): A modern and effective evidence-based approach to physiotherapic specific scoliosis exercises." *Scoliosis, 10*, 3. DOI: 10.1186/s13013-014-0027-2.

Sung, S., Chae, H. W., Lee, H. S., Kim, S. *et al.* (2021) "Incidence and surgery rate of idiopathic scoliosis: A nationwide database study." *International Journal of Environmental Research and Public Health, 10*, 3. DOI: 10.3390/ijerph18158152.

Thomen, R. P., Woods, J. C., Sturm, P. F., Jain, V. *et al.* (2020) "Lung microstructure in adolescent idiopathic scoliosis before and after posterior spinal fusion." *PLoS ONE, 15*, 10. DOI: 10.1371/journal.pone.0240265.

Watson, T., Graning, J., McPherson, S., Carter, E. *et al.* (2017) "Dance, balance and core muscle performance measures are improved following a 9-week core stabilization training program among competitive collegiate dancers." *International Journal of Sports Physical Therapy, 12*, 1, 25–41.

Winter, D. A. (1995) "Human balance and posture control during standing and walking." *Gait and Posture, 3*, 4, 193–214.

Chapter 2
Pilates and Kyphosis: Effect on Gait

Lise Stolze

Scheuermann's disease, like idiopathic scoliosis, has no known cause and is believed to be a developmental disorder of spinal overgrowth (Brink *et al.* 2017). Thoracic kyphosis changes considerably during growth, from its minimum around age 10 to a maximum around age 15. Girls grow fastest when the thoracic kyphosis is at its minimum. If spinal overgrowth occurs at this time, it will present in the anterior vertebral body causing vulnerability to the development of idiopathic scoliosis. Boys complete their growth spurt much later when the thoracic kyphosis is maximizing. This can make them vulnerable to posterior spinal overgrowth or hyperkyphosis (Schlösser *et al.* 2015), and the incidence of Scheuermann's disease is higher in boys than girls (Liu *et al.* 2014). Mild thoracic scoliosis often coexists with hyperkyphosis. Bracing is used in severe cases during the growth phase in adolescents to prevent progression.

Scheuermann's disease is the primary cause of thoracic hyperkyphosis. There are two types of Scheuermann's kyphosis:

Type I: Apex between T7 and T9 (most common)
Type II: Apex between T10 and T12

Radiological criteria for Scheuermann's disease (Liu *et al.* 2014):

1. Thoracic spine kyphosis greater than 40 degrees and...
2. At least 3 adjacent vertebrae demonstrating wedging of greater than 5 degrees

Other signs include:

1. Vertebral endplate irregularity and Schmorl's nodes
2. Intervertebral disk space narrowing anteriorly
3. Association with scoliosis and spondylolisthesis
4. Reduced lateral ribcage expansion (Brink *et al.* 2017)

Clinical measures of hyperkyphosis include:

1. C7 to wall distance (Suwannarat *et al.* 2018)
2. Rib to pelvis distance (Siminoski *et al.* 2003)
3. Debrunner kyphometer (Tran *et al.* 2016)
4. Kyphotic index (Tran *et al.* 2016)

Sagittal plane spinal curves influence the distribution of force through the spine. The thoracic spine has a natural flexion curve—or kyphosis of about 26–46 degrees (Bernhardt and Bridwell 1989)—caused by mild anterior wedging of the vertebral bodies. The lumbar spine has a natural lordosis (relative extension) of about 32–56 degrees (Bernhardt and Bridwell 1989). Excessive thoracic kyphosis may be the result of poor postural positioning, but if it cannot be passively reduced, it is considered a structural "hyperkyphosis." This can be caused by stress fractures, osteoporosis, or Scheuermann's disease.

Vertebral wedging in Scheuermann's kyphosis reduces thoracic mobility and restricts the distribution of force through the spine. The cervical and lumbar spine segments can become hyperlordotic or hypermobile. Consequently, Scheuermann's kyphosis is associated with low back pain and forward head posture (Liu *et al.* 2014). Thoracic anterior chest muscles are short and over-active while posterior torso extensor muscles are long and inhibited. Conversely, posterior lumbar and cervical muscles are short and over-active while anterior muscles become long and inhibited. Intervention consists of lengthening shortened muscles, reducing inhibition, and stabilizing hypermobile segments (Katzman *et al.* 2016). For adolescents with a 55-degree Cobb angle and adults with pain and disability, hyperkyphosis bracing may be indicated (Bettany-Saltikov *et al.* 2017).

Thoracic expansion in Scheuermann's kyphosis can be facilitated with specific exercises focused on shoulder girdle and respiration (Bezalel *et al.* 2019). Limited shoulder flexion is often a consequence of thoracic hyperkyphosis (Otoshi *et al.* 2014). Improving shoulder flexion can facilitate upper thoracic extension and help reduce lower cervical hypermobility and forward head posture. Gravity produces an axial load that can influence the progression of hyperkyphosis. Ultimately, the ability to self-regulate body organization and breathing are priorities for the client with Scheuermann's kyphosis (Bezalel *et al.* 2019).

Client description: 62-year-old female psychologist, identifies as a female

Dates of case report: Session 1: March 5, 2021; Session 12: April 10, 2021

Studio apparatus and props
Pilates equipment

- Universal Reformer
- Trapeze Table

Props used with equipment

- Mat
- Pillows
- Dowel
- Mirror
- 6 in. (15 cm) ball

Home program props

- Mat
- Pillows

- Heavy resistance band, 4 ft (122 cm)
- Mirror
- Dowel
- Wall bar

Methods and materials

Session 1/12
1. Health history interview

- August 2008: client reports first feeling back pain "at bottom of bra line" and neck pain at base of neck when singing in choir, which she had done much of her adult life
- She remembers "always having bad posture"
- She mostly sits during her job as a psychologist and experiences little pain with this

- X-rays, March 2014: Scheuermann's kyphosis (thoracic spine Cobb angle = 66 degrees); mild primary thoracic scoliosis (Cobb angle = 12 degrees) with apex at T8 and left pelvic prominence
- DEXA scan 2014: osteoporosis at left femoral neck (T score = −2.8) and total left hip joint (T score = −2.6); osteopenia in the lumbar spine (T score = −2.2)
- Prescribed a hyperkyphosis brace, which provided some initial temporary pain relief
- She refused bisphosphonate treatment for her osteoporosis and chose treatment of supplements and weight-bearing exercises, especially walking
- Jan 2020: reported pain and "tingling" in right arm
- MRI, January 2020: degenerative disc disease at C5–C6
- February 2020: physical therapy including cervical traction, manual therapy, and posture exercises provided some relief
- She has stopped singing in the choir
- Goals: walk daily for more than 20 minutes without pain, return to singing in the choir

2. Symptoms

- Pain at base of bra line and base of neck
- Pain worse with standing and walking for more than 20 minutes
- Pain worse with overhead activities: putting dishes away, cleaning ceiling fan
- Pain better with sitting
- Occasional tingling in right arm "off and on" throughout the day

3. Movement aids

- None

Final result of case report

Client stands and walks up to 40 minutes with minimal pain daily. She has returned to singing in the choir, taking sitting breaks as needed. She is now able to control pain with overhead activities by dynamic stabilization of the transitional areas of the torso regions. Reporting minimal right arm tingling. Pre-height measured was 5 ft 4.1 in. (1.62 m). Post-height measured is 5 ft 4.7 in. (1.64 m).

Chapter 2

Session 2/12: Initial assessment

1. General observations of gait

- Hyperextension at occipitoatlantal (OA) junction and hyperflexion at cervicothoracic (CT) junction (forward head posture)
- Hyperkyphosis of the thoracic spine
- Scapular protraction with anterior humoral head, right more than left
- Limited hip joint extension bilaterally
- Pelvis shifts left with left lower extremity (LE) weight bearing
- Right foot pronates

2. Standing tests

- Full torso rotation
- Observations of inefficient side: both
  - Right thoracic rotation greater than on left due to mild right thoracic scoliosis
  - No sequential rotation in thorax
  - Excessive rotation occurs at thoracolumbar junction (TLJ)
- Hemipelvis inferior motion
- Observations of inefficient side: right
  - Excessive translation of ribs to the right during right hemipelvis inferior motion amplifying scoliosis pattern
- Hemipelvis superior motion
- Observations of inefficient side: both
  - Right: more difficult to hike due to scoliosis right thoracic

Session 12/12: Post-assessment

1. General observations of gait

- Able to better control sagittal plane alignment at OA and CT junctions
- Hyperkyphosis of thoracic spine
- Maintains more neutral shoulder and scapular alignment
- Improved hip joint extension bilaterally
- Able to maintain frontal plane pelvic organization with LE weight bearing
- Increased control of right foot pronation

2. Standing tests

- Full torso rotation
- Observations of inefficient side: both
  - Right thoracic rotation greater than left
  - No sequential rotation in thoracic region
  - Client can control excessive movement at TLJ during rotation
- Hemipelvis inferior motion
- Observations of inefficient side: right
  - Able to control translation of ribs to the right during right hemipelvis inferior motion
- Hemipelvis superior motion
- Observations of inefficient side: both

- Left: increased right thoracic translation during hike

◆ Lateral pelvic shift

● Observations of inefficient side: left
  - Pelvis in lateral shift left as part of scoliosis pattern
  - Shifting pelvis left accentuates right thoracic translation

3. Seated tests

◆ Thoracic rotation

● Observations of inefficient side: both
  - Range of motion (ROM): right greater than left due to scoliosis pattern
  - No sequential articulation through thorax
  - Rotation occurred at transition of cervical and lumbar regions
  - Excessive TLJ right rotation
  - Weight bears on right ischial tuberosity

◆ Hip joint and knee flexion

● Observations of inefficient side: both
  - Right hip flexion amplifies scoliosis pattern
  - Left hip flexion reduces scoliosis pattern
  - Left ROM flexion: right greater than left

4. Sit and stand

◆ Lateral view

● Hyperextension of CT junction with forward head posture

- Right: more difficult to hike
- Left: able to control translation of ribs to the right

◆ Lateral pelvic shift

● Observations of inefficient side: right
  - Pelvis laterally shifts: left more than right

3. Seated tests

◆ Thoracic rotation

● Observations of inefficient side: both
  - ROM: right greater than left due to scoliosis pattern
  - Controls excessive motion at TLJ
  - Weight bears on right ischial tuberosity

◆ Hip joint and knee flexion

● Observations of inefficient side: both
  - Can consciously reduce scoliosis pattern when lifting right leg
  - Demonstrates more midline organization

4. Sit and stand

◆ Lateral view

● Reduced forward head posture

- Hyperkyphosis of thoracic spine

◆ Anterior view

- Pelvis shift left
- Adducts left femur
- Right ankle pronates

5. Standing balance

◆ Two-leg stance, eyes open

- 60 seconds

◆ One-leg stance, eyes open

- Right leg: more than 30 seconds
- Left leg: 3 seconds

- Able to control thoracic flexion, but kyphosis remains

◆ Anterior view

- Reduced pelvis shift
- Centration of femoral joint
- Reduced right ankle pronation

5. Standing balance

◆ Two-leg stance, eyes open

- 60 seconds

◆ One-leg stance, eyes open

- Right leg: more than 30 seconds
- Left leg: more than 30 seconds

Session 3/12: Home program

Fatigue scale	5
Pain scale	6 (when standing or walking for more than 20 minutes)
Client self-report	• Client states she is concerned about her inability to walk due to pain because weight-bearing exercises are part of her treatment plan for osteoporosis. Yesterday, she stood in the kitchen cooking for about 90 minutes which exacerbated her neck pain
Key changes observed by author at end of Session 3/12	• Demonstrates ability to control hypermobile areas of compensation • Reduction of lateral pelvic shift during standing
Reason behind choice of sequencing	• Exercise in gravity-eliminated position to reduce compensatory habitual patterns while standing and sitting • Improve proprioception of torso organization • Increase awareness of breath • Integrate the changes into upright position

Session movement sequence

1. Hundred (modified)	Derivative of J. H. Pilates Hundred (NPCE Study Guide 2021, p. 46) (See Chapter 5 in Volume 1, Gentry: Bellows breathing)
Intent	• Supine position reduces sagittal plane curves • Facilitate dynamic stabilization of transition areas of the cervical and lumbar regions • Increase awareness of breath
Gait reasoning	• Reduce sagittal and frontal plane postural compensations out of gravity • Transference of new strategies to standing and walking
Starting position	• Supine on mat with head pillow to reduce suboccipital hyperextension • Feet on floor, hip joints and knees flexed • Resistance band tied around ribcage • Upper extremities (UE) by sides with palms up

Chapter 2

Movement description	• Inhale, sensing the expansion of the thorax into the band • Exhale, maintaining the expansion • Imagine the ribs are an umbrella • Imagine holding an orange between chin and sternum without squeezing the orange • Lift hands with elbows extended slightly off the mat • Maintain scapulae on thorax and humeral head congruency • Pulse arms anterior and posterior a few degrees in both directions • Traditional Hundred breath pattern, 5 counts inhale, 5 counts exhale • 10 repetitions

2. Resistance band arm arcs (See Chapter 5 in Volume 1, Grant: Ribcage Arms)

Intent	• Challenge the thoracolumbar transition area with overhead movement • Improve sagittal control of hypermobile cervical and thoracolumbar transition areas

Author note
Shoulder flexion facilitates upper thoracic extension (Edmondston *et al.* 2012), reducing lower cervical flexion (part of forward head posture).

Gait reasoning	• Improve thorax rotation with arm swing • Increase proprioception of midline

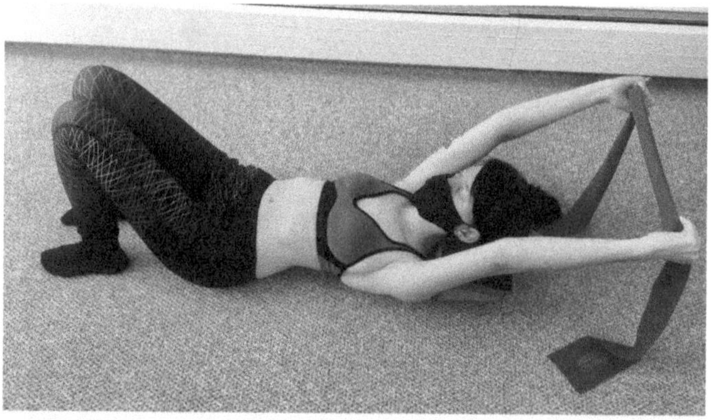

Figure 2.1

Pilates and Kyphosis: Effect on Gait

Starting position
- Supine on mat with head pillow
- Feet on floor, hip joints and knees flexed
- Hold resistance band with thumbs up grip, hands slightly wider than shoulder width
- Flex UE to 90 degrees placing slight tension on the band
- Feel scapulae equally weighted on mat

Movement description
- Exhale, flex UE to a range maintaining control of TLJ
- Inhale to return to starting position
- 6–8 repetitions

3. Supine shoulder articulations

Intent
- Reduce anterior humeral head and head forward orientation
- Control thoracolumbar hyperextension

Gait reasoning
- Improve anterior thoracic articulation
- Facilitate clavipectoral myofascial glide
- Improve glenohumeral joint external rotation
- Encourage lateral ribcage expansion
- Challenge to control thoracolumbar hyperextension

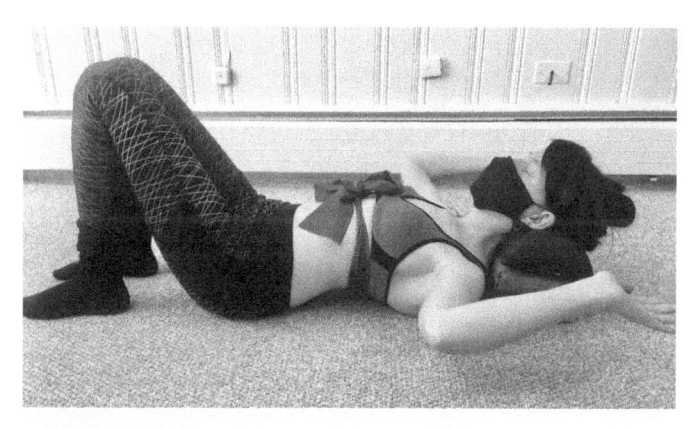

Figure 2.2

Starting position
- Supine on mat
- Humerus abducted to 90 degrees with elbows flexed to 90 degrees
- Humeral joint congruent to maintain humeral external rotation
- Feet on floor, hip joints and knees flexed

Movement description
- Horizontally adduct UE and exhale
- Horizontally abduct UE and inhale
- Focus on organization of thorax, shoulder girdle, and arms

4. Quadruped with dowel

Intent
- Challenge sagittal plane organization in gravity
- Improve scapular awareness with weight bearing through the UE
- Use of dowel for proprioception

Gait reasoning
- Improve sagittal plane organization

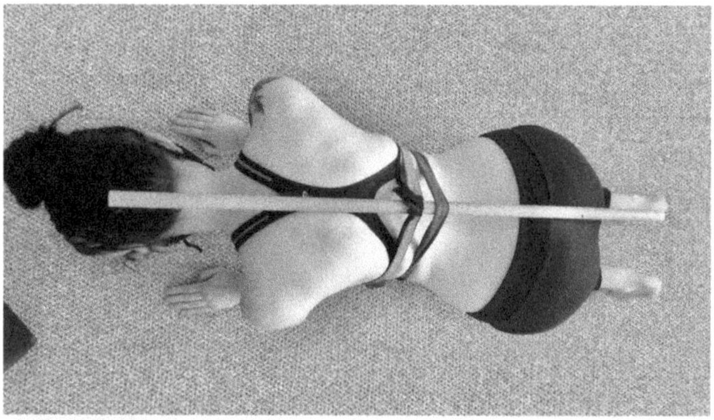

Figure 2.3

Starting position
- Quadruped on mat
- Dowel placed in midline at sacrum, at mid-thorax
- Head will not touch, so imagine head against stick
- Imagine holding an orange between chin and sternum
- Resistance band around ribcage to hold stick and provide proprioception for breathing

Movement description
- Remain in position
- Breathe slowly
- Maintain contact with dowel
- 6–8 breaths

5. Semi-hanging (Lehnert-Schroth 2007)

Editor note
Katharina Schroth, born February 22, 1894, in Dresden, Germany, was suffering from a moderate scoliosis herself and developed a more functional approach of treatment for herself. She recognized that postural control can only be achieved by changing postural perception and breathing. Katharina and her daughter, Christa Lehnert-Schroth, developed the Schroth Method (Weiss 2011).

Intent
- Facilitate reorganization of the torso toward midline
- Challenge control of thoracolumbar hyperextension
- Translate sensory input from hanging into standing between sets

Gait reasoning
- Reduce sagittal plane distortion
- Improve midline orientation

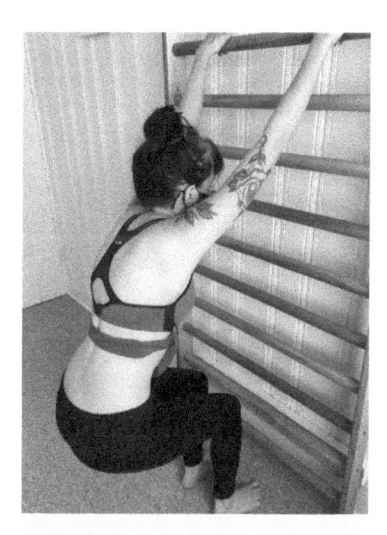

Figure 2.4

Starting position
- Hold wall bar and hang in squat position
- Elbows extended
- Hip and knee joints at 90 degrees flexion
- Hands shoulder-width apart or wider
- Knees positioned under hands
- Equal weight on each foot

Movement description
- Focus on thoracic expansion with breath
- Exhale, depress scapulae
- Inhale, relax
- 6–8 breaths, 3 sets
- Minimize hyperextension at TLJ
- Avoid flexion and posterior pelvic tilt
- Stand between sets to integrate orientation

6. Standing against wall (See Chapter 5 in Volume 1, Kryzanowska: Wall Series)

Intent
- Find sagittal plane organization against gravity using wall for proprioception

Gait reasoning
- Improve sagittal plane orientation for midline organization

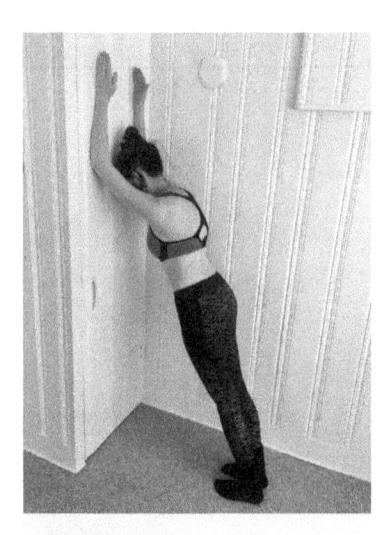

Figure 2.5

Starting position
- Stand with heels close to wall, aligned under hip joints, with pelvis and thorax against wall
- Imagine holding an orange gently between chin and sternum to reduce cervical hyperextension
- Imagine head reaches toward wall only as far as upper cervical region maintains integrity
- Weight evenly distributed on feet
- UE by sides, palms face inward

Pilates and Kyphosis: Effect on Gait

|Movement description|• Focus on expansion of breath
• Maintain wall contact and awareness of foot position
• Flex arms toward wall without losing control of TLJ
• Palms remain facing each other, keeping elbows extended
• Exhale to flex, inhale to extend
• 8 times|

7. Single leg stance in mirror

Editor note
Mirror monitoring plays an important role in the original Schroth program to allow synchronizing the corrective movement and perception with the visual input (Weiss 2011).

|Intent|• Improve sagittal plane orientation
• Use of mirror stimulates the tectospinal motor pathway, which mediates reflex responses to visual stimuli
• Single leg stance challenges postural alignment|

Author note
The tectospinal tract is one of several extrapyramidal tracts—pathways by which motor signals are sent from the brain to lower neurons. These tracts originate in the brainstem, carrying motor fibers to the spinal cord, and are responsible for the involuntary and automatic control of all musculature, such as muscle tone, balance, posture, and locomotion. The tectospinal tract mediates reflex movements in response to visual stimuli. It helps orientate the head and torso toward visual or auditory stimuli and is responsible for coordinating head and eye movements (Fitzgerald, Gruener, and Mtui 2007).

|Gait reasoning|• Improving sagittal and frontal postural alignment in single leg stance will help with stance phase of gait
• Aligning foot in single leg stance will help reduce pronation tendency|
|Starting position|• Stand in sagittal plane alignment
• Find frontal plane alignment using mirror
• Equal weight on tripod of feet: heel, 1st metatarsal and 5th metatarsal
• Feet aligned with knees and hip joints|
|Movement description|• Unweight one foot
• Find balance while maintaining sagittal and frontal plane alignment
• Repeat 3 times each side|

Chapter 2

Session 11/12: Studio session

Fatigue scale	2
Pain scale	0
Client self-report	• Walking for up to 40 minutes before feeling pain at base of neck and across mid-thorax. Discomfort while standing to cook is lessened. She feels less frequent tingling in right arm. Focusing on reorganizing her body reduces any discomforts. She would like to try returning to choir
Key changes observed by author at end of Session 11/12	• Forward head adjusted toward central axis by control of placement • Less left lateral pelvic shift • Reduced right anterior humeral head • Less right foot pronation • Improved hip joint extension during push-off • Able to stand on one LE for up to 30 seconds each, maintaining sagittal and frontal planes
Reason behind choice of sequencing	• Exercise in gravity-eliminated position to reduce compensatory habitual patterns while standing and sitting • Feeling feet contact on Universal Reformer footbar for load transference through LE and torso • Prepare for load transference in upright • Progression from supine to quadruped, sitting and standing to gradually challenge organization • Balance

Session movement sequence

1. Footwork on Universal Reformer	J. H. Pilates Footwork on Universal Reformer (NPCE Study Guide 2021, p. 52)
Intent	• Supine position reduces sagittal plane curves • Prepare thorax for breathing expansion • Use of the footbar to improve foot proprioception
Gait reasoning	• Re-educate the tendency for lumbar region hyperextension during hip joint extension • Footwork improves foot and ankle proprioception/organization to prepare for ground reaction forces • Supine position prepares the body for ease in organization of head, neck, and shoulders against gravity • Focusing on reduction of left lateral pelvic shift during alternating ankle dorsiflexion and plantar flexion

Pilates and Kyphosis: Effect on Gait

Set-up	• 3 medium springs
	• Headrest up, with 2 pillows to reduce upper cervical hyperextension
Starting position	• Supine with feet on footbar
	• Heels elevated, with 6 in. (15 cm) ball between malleoli
	• Hip and knee joints in flexion
	• UE by sides
Movement description	• Press into the feet and move the carriage back
	• Extend LE
	• Dorsiflex ankles with extended knees
	• Plantar flex with extended knees
	• Flex hip and knee joints
	• Return to starting position
	• Repeat 10 times
	• Add flexion of hip and knee joints
	• Add single LE variations

CUES

- Imagine gently holding an orange between chin and sternum for optimal head position
- Expand and widen the thorax while breathing

Author note
The ball between the malleoli ensures there is no pronation during dorsiflexion and plantar flexion. The ball is removed for alternating dorsiflexion/plantar flexion with hip and knee joints flexion. Cue to remain toward midline to reduce left lateral pelvic shift.

2. Bridge on Universal Reformer

(See Chapter 5 in Volume 1, Gentry: Spinal articulations/hip escalator)

Intent	• Improve active hip extension while controlling lumbar extension
	• Pelvic rotational control during single LE variation
Gait reasoning	• Improve hip extension during push-off
	• Reduction of excessive left lateral pelvic shift
Set-up	• Springs: 2 medium and 1 light
	• Headrest up with 1 pillow (1 less than with Footwork) to reduce upper cervical hyperextension caused by hyperkyphosis

CUES

- Exhale, pressing carriage away and maintaining the reduced sagittal curves
- Inhale on the return and control the springs on the return
- Single LE variation: pelvis remains in frontal orientation

Starting position	• Supine with heels on footbar hip-width apart • UE by sides
Movement description	• Extend hip joints to lift pelvis off carriage • Carriage remains at stoppers • Press the carriage back and forth by extending hip joints and flexing knees • Variation: single leg, with opposite leg in hip and knee flexion to 90 degrees

Author note

Bridge requires hip joint extension to elevate the pelvis. Bridge can improve extension during gait without accessing excessive motion at the TLJ. Since a structural hyperkyphosis cannot be sufficiently reduced, a single pillow may still be required to reduce upper cervical hyperextension.

3. Hundred preparation: Arm arcs on Universal Reformer	Derivative of J. H. Pilates Hundred (NPCE Study Guide 2021, p. 46)
Intent	• Challenge lumbar dynamic stability under an extension load • Gliding of shoulder girdle and UE
Gait reasoning	• Control of lumbar hyperextension • Shoulder flexion ROM increases thoracic extension
Set-up	• Headrest up • 2 pillows to reduce upper cervical hyperextension due to hyperkyphosis • Medium spring • Straps
Starting position	• Supine in hip and knee flexion to 90 degrees • Shoulders flexed to 90 degrees • Elbows extended • Holding straps
Movement description	• Inhale, shoulder extension • Exhale, shoulder flexion

Pilates and Kyphosis: Effect on Gait

Author note
The 90 degrees hip and knee flexion position challenges the thorax and pelvis relationship. This exercise is preparation for Chest Expansion in tall kneeling.

CUE
- Posterior surface of both scapulae and both innominates are equally weighted on the carriage

4. Mermaid on Universal Reformer

Derivative of J. H. Pilates Seated Mermaid/Side Arm Sit on Wunda Chair (NPCE Study Guide 2021, p. 73)

Intent
- Improve lateral thoracic expansion
- Improve cervical and thoracic integration in lateral flexion
- Challenge head, neck, and shoulder organization in the frontal plane
- Challenge control of convexity expansion

Gait reasoning
- Lateral thoracic expansion to reduce thoracic kyphosis

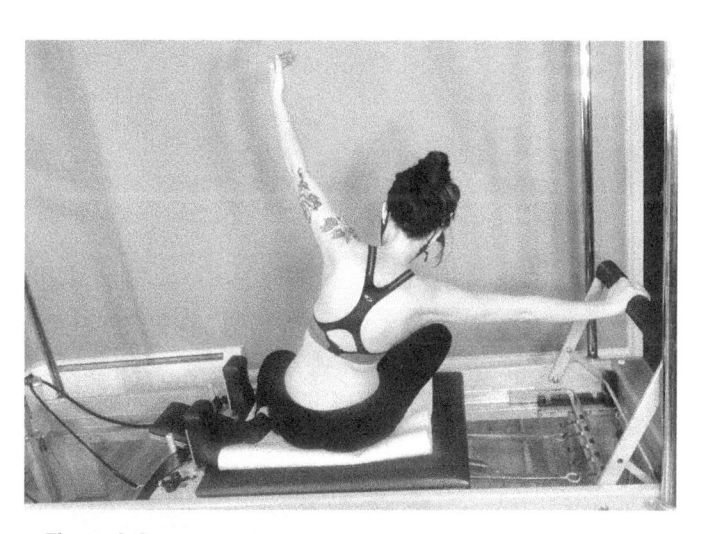

Figure 2.6

Set-up
- Medium spring
- Footbar up

Chapter 2

Starting position
- Sitting facing right side toward footbar
- Right hip joint in external rotation, flexion, and knee flexion
- Left hip joint in internal rotation, flexion, and knee flexion
- Right hand on the footbar
- Left humerus in abduction to 90 degrees with elbow extended
- Head and torso organized in sagittal plane

Movement description
- Right hand on footbar presses the carriage away
- Inhale into left lateral thorax as torso laterally flexes to right
- Left UE abducts and flexes overhead
- Exhale, return to start
- 5 times
- Repeat on the other side

CUES
- Aim ischial tuberosities down as UE abducts and flexes overhead
- Imagine you are against a wall, maintaining alignment of head and torso
- Left lateral flexion: refrain from expanding right convexity and compressing left concavity
- Right lateral flexion: expand and breathe laterally into the left concavity

Author note
The tendency for the client with hyperkyphosis is to move excessively at the TLJ and cervical region. Mermaid challenges both sagittal and frontal plane control at these junctions while moving into lateral flexion. Due to this client's mild right thoracic scoliosis, the right posterior lateral ribcage is already expanded and the left side approximated. An increase of right thorax/ribs expansion during left lateral flexion needs to be minimized. The left posterior lateral thorax and ribs (concave side) are approximated. Encourage expansion with breath into left side during right lateral flexion.

5. Knee Stretch on Universal Reformer Derivative of J. H. Pilates Knee Stretch Series Kneeling/Forward/Round Back (NPCE Study Guide 2021, p. 60)
(See Chapter 5 in Volume 1, Trier), Knee stretch variations
(See Figure 2.3)

Intent	• Cervical sagittal plane control against gravity
	• Activate spine extensors
	• Shoulder flexion facilitates upper thoracic extension, reducing kyphosis
	• Hip joint extension requires control of hypermobile thoracolumbar transition area
Gait reasoning	• Reduce sagittal plane excessive curve
	• Improve extension
Set-up	• Springs: 1 medium and 1 light
	• Footbar down
Starting position	• Quadruped on carriage with hands on footbar
	• Calcaneus against shoulder stops
	• Metatarsals extended
	• Dowel placed from head along thorax and sacrum in midline (see chapter 10 vol 1 page 321 Editor note)
Movement description	• Exhale, pressing carriage back, extending hip joints, and flexing shoulders
	• Inhale, flexing hip joints, and bringing carriage inward
	• Return to starting position

CUES

- As the carriage moves back, maintain contact of head, thorax, and sacrum against the stick
- Maintain client's optimal position of the lumbar region

Author note

The combination of shoulder flexion and hip joints extension in this exercise challenges the sagittal plane torso organization. Flexion of the shoulders facilitates the upper thoracic region movement into relative extension. Reducing upper thoracic flexion can aid in reducing forward head posture.

6. Prone shoulder extension with elbow flexion holding risers on Universal Reformer

Intent	• Improve shoulder flexion
	• Facilitate shoulder girdle activation to facilitate thoracic expansion
Gait reasoning	• Increase extensor activation
	• Cervical and shoulder girdle organization

Chapter 2

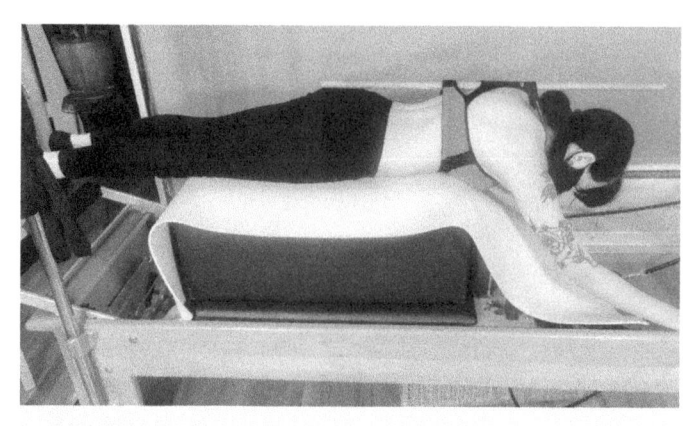

Figure 2.7

Set-up	• Light spring
	• Long box
	• Footbar down
	• Risers up
Starting position	• Prone on long box facing risers
	• Mid-sternum placed at edge of box
	• Hold risers, shoulders fully flexed, elbows fully extended
	• Hip joints and knees extended
Movement description	• Exhale, pull carriage toward risers, flexing elbows
	• Hold to inhale, expanding thorax
	• Extend elbows and shoulders
	• Return to starting position

CUES
- Imagine the dowel on the torso from previous exercises
- Maintain organization of head on cervical region during exhale with elbow flexion

Author note
This exercise requires dynamic stability. In prone position, the head and neck are challenged to maintain orientation against the sagittal force of gravity. Activation of extensors will change the balance of tension and compression of anterior/posterior organization, reducing hyperkyphosis.

Pilates and Kyphosis: Effect on Gait

7. Chest Expansion on Universal Reformer		J. H. Pilates Chest Expansion on Universal Reformer (NPCE Study Guide 2021, p. 67)
Intent	•	Head, neck, and shoulder organization
	•	Increase thoracic and rib motions
	•	Maintaining balance in the tall kneeling position on a moving carriage requires a higher level of coordination against gravity
Gait reasoning	•	Sagittal organization in kneeling to improve stance
	•	Improve UE flexion and extension for arm swing

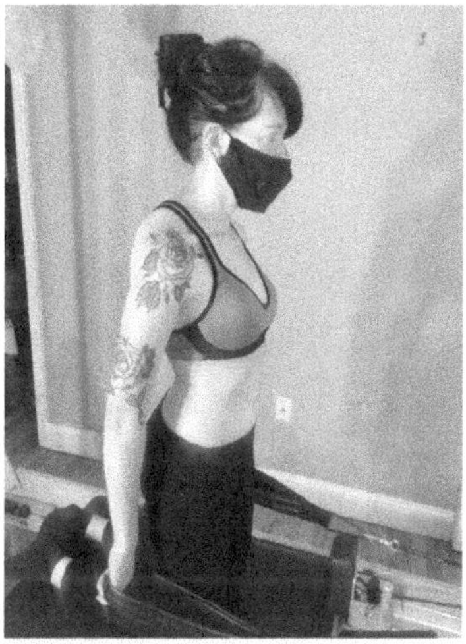

Figure 2.8

Set-up	•	Footbar down
	•	Medium spring
Starting position	•	Tall kneeling facing straps
	•	Feet extend over edge of Universal Reformer
	•	Hold short straps in hands
	•	Shoulder flexion, enough to tension the springs
	•	Elbows extended
Movement description	•	Inhale to extend shoulders and move carriage
	•	Hold position and breath
	•	Turn head right, then left, then return to front
	•	Exhale, flex shoulder moving carriage to stops
	•	Return to start

Chapter 2

CUES
- Inhaling expands the thorax and facilitates upper thoracic extension
- The clavicles are rotating posterior creating a feeling of width
- Imagine you are holding a ball between your knees
- Maintain midline orientation
- Control the recoil of the springs on the return

Author note
This exercise requires spotting for safety. The unstable nature of this exercise is both challenging and informative about the client's habitual compensations due to hyperkyphosis.

8. Splits: Front with and without assistance on Universal Reformer/Trapeze Table	Derivative of J. H. Pilates Splits: Front on Universal Reformer (NPCE Study Guide 2021, p. 62)
Intent	• Standing balance with UE movement challenges • Thoracic expansion
Gait reasoning	• Improve extension in relationship to gravity • Organize foot position in standing to reduce pronation • Challenge sagittal orientation in standing

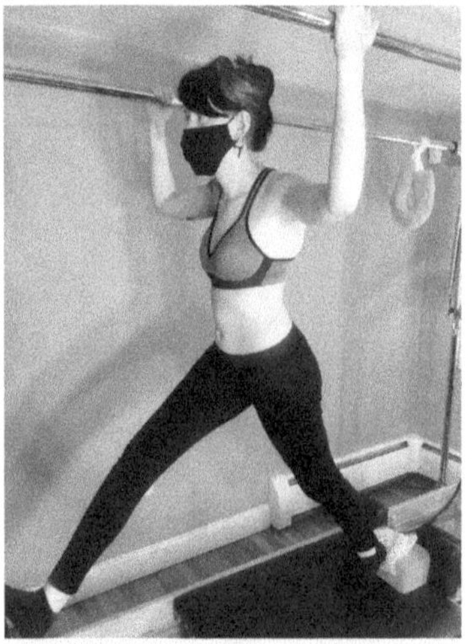

Figure 2.9

Pilates and Kyphosis: Effect on Gait

Set-up	• Universal Reformer/Trapeze Table combination • Footbar up • Springs: 1 medium and 1 light
Starting position	• Standing on Universal Reformer facing footbar • Metatarsals of right foot on footbar • Left calcaneus halfway up shoulder stops • Ankle plantar flexed with metatarsals extended • Hold on to Trapeze Table horizontal bars • Elbow flexion • Right knee and hip joint flexion • Left hip joint and knee extended • Torso organized in sagittal plane midline
Movement description	• Exhale, extend right knee, pressing carriage back • Humerus abducts with elbow flexion to facilitate increased expansion of thorax • Inhale, flex right knee • Return carriage to starting position

CUES
- Imagine a set of headlights on the anterior superior iliac spine (ASIS)
- Shine the light forward to balance the pelvis
- When possible do not hold onto bars to challenge balance and maintain torso orientation to midline

Author note
Holding on to overhead horizontal Trapeze Table bars helps promote thoracic expansion by UE flexion and abduction.

9. Splits: Side on Universal Reformer
J.H. Pilates Splits: Side (NPCE Study Guide 2021, p. 61)

Intent	• Facilitate hip glide • Improve LE closed kinematic chain in standing • Challenge sagittal plane organization in standing
Gait reasoning	• Reduce excessive left lateral pelvic shift • Standing resisted LE abduction/adduction challenges ankle adaption
Set-up	• Springs: 1 medium and 1 light • Standing platform • Footbar down

Starting position
- Stand facing side of carriage with right foot on platform and left foot on carriage
- UE by sides

Movement description
- Press into both feet
- Inhale, abduct LE, moving carriage away from standing platform
- UE abduct to 90 degrees
- Exhale, adduct LE, returning carriage
- UE adduct to sides
- Repeat 10 times
- Repeat on the other side

CUES
- Focus on self-regulation of organization
- Gaze straight ahead
- Place equal weight on both feet

Author note
Splits: Side activate the lumbopelvic-femoral complex prior to following with a practice of single leg standing and general walking for gait integration. This complex activation informs the single leg stance aspect of gait, controlling pelvis shift or pelvic hike on the weight-bearing side.

The journey to Session 11

Session 4/12
Client self-report

- Fatigue scale 5
- Pain scale 1 currently; 4–5 with standing and walking for more than 20 minutes
- Reports she can obtain optimal organization when supine, but having difficulty transferring it to standing and walking

Key changes observed

- Improved thoracic expansion during breathing
- Demonstrates home program with good sagittal plane awareness of midline

Reasoning behind choice of movements

- Eliminate gravity in warm-up exercises to allow for easier sagittal organization
- Transition to sitting and standing to apply learned sagittal organization from gravity-eliminated positions

Session movement sequence

1. Supine breathing

2. Resistance band arm arcs

3. Supine shoulder articulations

4. Quadruped with dowel

5. Semi-hanging

6. Universal Reformer

- Footwork
- Hundred preparation: arm arcs
- Splits: Side

7. Additional movements

- Single leg stance
- Integration with gait

Session 5/12
Client self-report

- Fatigue scale 3
- Pain scale 2 currently; 3–4 when standing and walking for more than 20 minutes
- Has had a difficult and stressful week
- Has been doing home program consistently and feels better afterwards

Key changes observed

- Able to control hyperextension of TLJ with overhead movement
- Able to reduce anterior humeral position during exercises

Reasoning behind choice of movements

- Begin to challenge client's ability to maintain new orientation and awareness of breath

Session movement sequence
1. Supine shoulder articulations

2. Quadruped with dowel

3. Wall plank

4. Semi-hanging

5. Universal Reformer

- Footwork
- Bridging
- Knee Stretch
- Splits: Side

6. Additional movements

- Standing against wall
- Single leg stance
- Integration with gait

Session 6/12
Client self-report

- Fatigue scale 4
- Pain scale 3
- Increased pain due to standing for over 2 hours cooking for family gathering
- Continued home program with relatives in town and sees the benefit of the practice

Key changes observed

- No significant changes today, client appears tired

Reasoning behind choice of movements

- Focus on breath and ribcage expansion
- Supine and prone movements due to fatigue

Session movement sequence
1. Hundred preparation

2. Supine shoulder 90 degrees abduction/external rotation with elbow flexion

Chapter 2

3. Prone shoulder 90 degrees abduction/external rotation with elbow flexion (Figure 2.10)

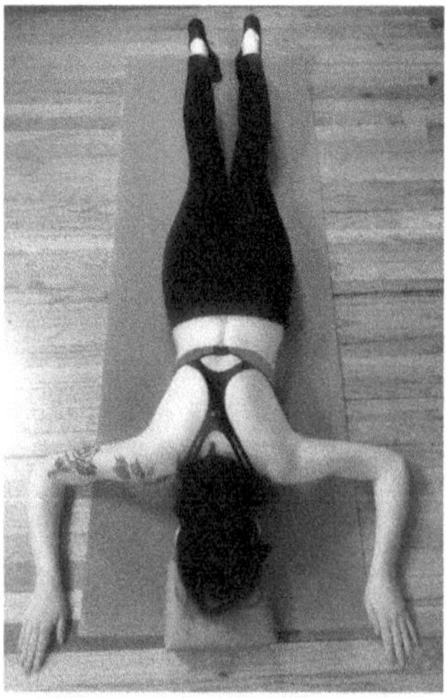

Figure 2.10

4. Universal Reformer

- Footwork
- Hundred preparation: arm arcs
- Splits: Side

5. Additional movement

- Gait integration

Session 7/12
Client self-report

- Fatigue scale 0
- Pain scale 1
- Compliant with home program
- Feels progress with ability to self-regulate organization to lessen pain while standing

Key changes observed

- Able to demonstrate better pelvic frontal plane orientation
- Improved pronation

Reasoning behind choice of movements

- Challenge head, neck, and shoulder awareness in prone
- Challenge extension and foot awareness

Session movement sequence

1. Resistance band arm arcs

2. Supine shoulder articulations

3. Bridge: add single LE variation

4. Prone shoulder extension with elbow flexion holding risers

5. Universal Reformer

- Footwork, added unilateral
- Bridging
- Knee Stretch
- Splits: Side
- Prone shoulder extension with elbow flexion holding risers
- Splits: Front with assist

6. Additional movements

- Standing against wall
- Single leg stance in mirror
- Integration with gait

Session 8/12
Client self-report

- Fatigue scale 1

- Pain scale 0–1
- Walking daily for 15 minutes incorporating new organization
- Feels less tingling in right UE; notices this has improved with her UE exercises

Key changes observed

- Client can demonstrate better organization during gait
- Demonstrates improved extension without hypermobility at the TLJ

Reasoning behind choice of movements

- Continue challenging extensors in prone
- Focus on Chest Expansion with thoracic expansion
- Begin to build endurance

Session movement sequence
1. Semi-hanging

2. Universal Reformer

- Footwork, added unilateral
- Hundred preparation: arm arcs
- Bridging
- Mermaid
- Knee Stretch
- Prone shoulder extension with elbow flexion holding risers
- Splits: Front with assist
- Chest Expansion
- Splits: Side

3. Additional movements

- Wall plank
- Standing against wall
- Single leg stance in mirror
- Gait integration

Session 9/12
Client self-report

- Fatigue scale 1
- Pain scale 0–1
- Walked for 20 minutes and was able to mitigate pain
- Cooking for more than 30 minutes, feels neck pain, takes breaks in sitting but can continue without pain
- Has been practicing single leg stance with home program

Key changes observed

- Less left lateral pelvic shift
- Improved thoracic expansion with breath and during movements

Reasoning behind choice of movements

- Continue to increase endurance
- Challenge foot-ankle to torso organization

Session movement sequence
1. Supine shoulder articulations

2. Prone shoulder extension with elbow flexion holding risers

3. Quadruped: added oppositional UE flexion and LE extension

4. Universal Reformer

- Footwork, added unilateral
- Hundred preparation: arm arcs
- Bridging
- Mermaid
- Knee Stretch
- Prone shoulder extension with elbow flexion holding risers
- Splits: Front with assist

Chapter 2

- Chest Expansion
- Splits: Side

5. Additional movements

- Stand against wall
- Wall plank
- Single leg stance with plantar flexion in mirror
- Integration with gait

Session 10/12
Client self-report

- Reports less arm tingling
- Walking for more than 20 minutes without pain 3 times a week
- Stood for 30 minutes at a church function and was able to control her pain by self-regulating

Key changes observed

- Client demonstrates ability to maintain improved oragnization throughout all exercises
- C7 to wall distance = 7.5 cm, improvement of 1.5 cm since initial visit

Reasoning behind choice of movements

- Maintain focus on thoracic expansion
- Whole-body organization

Session movement sequence
1. Semi-hanging

2. Universal Reformer

- Footwork, added unilateral
- Hundred preparation: arm arcs
- Bridging
- Mermaid
- Knee Stretch

- Prone shoulder extension with elbow flexion holding risers
- Splits: Front with assist
- Chest Expansion
- Splits: Side

3. Additional movements

- Wall plank
- Stand against wall
- Single leg stance in mirror
- Integration with gait

References

Bernhardt, M. and Bridwell, K. H. (1989) "Segmental analysis of the sagittal plane alignment of the normal thoracic and lumbar spines and thoracolumbar junction." *Spine, 14,* 7, 717–721.

Bettany-Saltikov, J., Turnbull, D., Ng, S. Y., and Webb, R. (2017) "Management of spinal deformities and evidence of treatment effectiveness." *The Open Orthopaedics Journal, 11,* 1521–1547.

Bezalel, T., Carmeli, E., Levi, D., and Kalichman, L. (2019) "The effect of Schroth therapy on thoracic kyphotic curve and quality of life in Scheuermann's patients: A randomized controlled trial." *Asian Spine Journal, 13,* 3, 490–499.

Brink, R. C., Schlösser, T. P. C., Colo, D., Vavruch, L. *et al.* (2017) "Anterior spinal overgrowth is the result of the scoliotic mechanism and is located in the disc." *Spine, 42,* 11, 818–822.

Edmondston, S. J., Ferguson, A., Ippersiel, P., Ronningen, L., Sodeland, S., and Barclay, L. (2012) "Clinical and radiological investigation of thoracic spine extension motion during bilateral arm elevation." *JOSPT, 42,* 10, 861–869.

Fitzgerald, M. J. T., Gruener, G., and Mtui, E. (2007) *Clinical Neuroanatomy and Neuroscience.* 5th Ed. Philadelphia, PA: Elsevier Saunders.

Katzman, W. B., Vittinghoff, E., Kado, D. M., Schafer, A. L. *et al.* (2016) "Study of hyperkyphosis, exercise and function (SHEAF) protocol of a randomized controlled trial of multimodal spine-strengthening exercise in older adults with hyperkyphosis." *Physical Therapy, 96,* 3, 71–381.

Lehnert-Schroth, C. (2007) *Three-Dimensional Treatment for Scoliosis: A Physiotherapeutic Method for Deformities of the Spine.* Trans. C. Mohr and A. Reeves. The Martindale Press, p. 167, Figure 477 e 2.

Liu, N., Guo, X., Chen, Z., Qi, Q. *et al.* (2014) "Radiological signs of Scheuermann disease and low back pain: Retrospective categorization of 188 hospital staff members with 6-year follow-up." *Spine, 39,* 20, 1666–1675.

NPCE Study Guide (National Pilates Certification Exam Study Guide) (2021) Miami, FL: National Pilates Certification Program, Inc.

Otoshi, K., Takegami, M., Sekiguchi, M., Onishi, Y. *et al.* (2014) "Association between kyphosis and subacromial impingement syndrome: LOHAS study." *Journal of Shoulder and Elbow Surgery, 23,* 12, 300–307.

Schlösser, T. P., Vincken, K. L., Rogers, K., Castelein, R. M., and Shah, S. A. (2015) "Natural sagittal spino-pelvic alignment in boys and girls before, at and after the adolescent growth spurt." *European Spine Journal, 24,* 6, 1158–1167.

Siminoski, K., Warshawski, R. S., Jen, H., and Lee, K. C. (2003) "Accuracy of physical examination using the rib-pelvis distance for detection of lumbar vertebral fractures." *The American Journal of Medicine, 15,* 115, 233–236.

Suwannarat, P., Amatachaya, P., Sooknuan, T. *et al.* (2018) "Hyperkyphotic measures using distance from the wall: Validity, reliability, and distance from the wall to indicate the risk for thoracic hyperkyphosis and vertebral fracture." *Archives of Osteoporosis, 13,* 1, 25.

Tran, T. H., Wing, D., Davis, A., Bergstrom, J. *et al.* (2016) "Correlations among four measures of thoracic kyphosis in older adults." *Osteoporosis International, 7,* 3, 1255–1259.

Weiss, H. R. (2011) "The method of Katharina Schroth—history, principles and current development." *Scoliosis, 6,* 17. DOI: 10.1186/1748-7161-6-17.

Chapter 3

Pilates for Management of Central Lumbar Spinal Stenosis: Effect on Gait

Christine Romani-Ruby

It has been over 50 years since lumbar spinal stenosis (LSS) was first described. LSS is defined as a narrowing of the space within the spinal canal, intervertebral foramina, or nerve root canal and can occur in any portion of the spine. This narrowing can occur at one or multiple levels and symptoms will worsen as the condition progresses (Chatha *et al.* 2011). Spinal stenosis is the cause of 5 percent of all back disease. LSS is the most common type with an onset age of 50–60 years and a higher prevalence in men. Studies have shown that approximately 20 percent of individuals older than 60 years of age and up to 80 percent of those older than 70 years of age have MRI evidence of LSS. As the population ages and individuals continue their active lifestyles, the incidence of symptomatic spinal stenosis is expected to rise. It is estimated that 103 million people world-wide are diagnosed with spinal stenosis annually (Ravindra *et al.* 2018).

Two types of spinal stenosis are defined in the literature. The first is central spinal stenosis where there is compression of the spinal cord or cauda equina within the spinal canal caused by facet joint arthrosis, the ligamentum flavum buckling, degenerative disc disease, or spondylolisthesis. The second type is lateral spinal stenosis where there is compression of a spinal nerve root within the intervertebral foramen. Spinal stenosis can be either congenital or acquired (Chatha *et al.* 2011). If congenital it can be caused by a malformation of the vertebral arch, a developmental error, or it may be idiopathic. If acquired, it is generally caused by degenerative changes, spondylolisthesis, disc protrusion, post-operative fibrosis, systemic bone disease, tumors, or a iatrogenic problem. There is no specific surgery for spinal stenosis, but surgeries that can repair or slow these acquired or congenital conditions can significantly decrease the symptoms of spinal stenosis (Costandi *et al.* 2015).

The symptoms of central LSS are usually insidious, and they vary greatly with the area that is involved. In the lumbar spine clients generally complain of stiffness or backache that is aggravated by weather change or activity. Many complain of morning stiffness that is relieved by increased activity while other symptoms are aggravated by activity, especially walking (Costandi *et al.* 2015). Central LSS symptoms are associated with midline back pain and radiculopathy. In cases of severe LSS, innervation of the urinary bladder and the rectum may be affected, but lumbar stenosis most often results in back pain with lower extremity weakness and numbness along the distribution of nerve roots of the lumbar plexus. Clients report pain, weakness, and numbness in the legs while walking. The onset of symptoms during gait is believed to be caused by increased metabolic demands of compressed nerve roots that have become ischemic due to stenosis (Costandi *et al.* 2015).

Chapter 3

> Clients often report relief of symptoms with heat or rest and will compensate for symptoms by flexing forward, slowing their gait, leaning onto objects (e.g., over a shopping cart), and limiting distance of ambulation. Generally, lumbar flexion relieves the pressure on exiting nerve roots and centralizes pain for these clients while extension peripheralizes pain (Costandi et al. 2015; Munakomi et al. 2022).

Client description: 54-year-old biological female, identifies as female; therapist working with deaf children in their home

Dates of case report: Session 1: January 19, 2020; Session 12: February 20, 2020; all in-person sessions

Studio apparatus and props
Pilates equipment

- Universal Reformer
- Trapeze Table
- Wunda Chair
- High and low barrel

Props used with equipment

- 1 in. (2.5 cm) head pillow
- Home program props
- Folded towel for head

Methods and materials

Session 1/12
1. Health history interview

- 2006: diagnosed with L5–S1 central spinal stenosis due to mild anterolisthesis and a synovial cyst
- 2009: L5–S1 fusion
- Endometriosis
- 2019: hysterectomy
- 2020: has an exacerbation of low back and left leg symptoms
- MRI shows no problems with the prior fusion
- Edema and narrowing in the L5–S1 foramen bilaterally and degeneration of the sacroiliac joints (SIJs)
- 2019: MRI reveals narrowing L5–S1 bilateral foramen and screws from fusion intact
- Significant degeneration of L5–S1 and SIJs
- Client is normal weight and active: walking, biking, and kayaking
- 1998: gave birth to twins by vaginal delivery

2. Symptoms

- Low back pain greater in left side than right
- Left leg numbness and paresthesia laterally to above the knee
- Most painful moving sit to stand and rolling over in bed
- Standing increases leg paresthesia
- Driving increases pain and paresthesia in left leg
- Night pain when rolling over but can return to sleep

3. Movement aids

- None

> **Author note**
> On observation the client stands in sway-back posture with a right lateral shift. On forward bending the client does not reverse the lumbar curve.

Lateral shift

Clients with acute back pain may present with antalgic posturing (Magee 2008). A loss of the lumbar lordosis, a lateral shift of the torso, or a scoliosis pattern are common presentations. In non-weight-bearing positions, the lateral shift resolves. To reduce the lateral shift physical therapy techniques may be required.

Editor note

Antalgic posturing is a position to avoid pain commonly by shifting laterally. Antalgic gait is a characteristic gait resulting from pain on weight bearing in which the stance phase is shortened on the affected side (Chaitow 2011).

Sway-back posture

Sway-back posture is a common inefficient stance that was originally described by Vladimir Janda (Page *et al.* 2010) and further detailed by Florence Kendall (Kendall *et al.* 2005). Today, it is prevalent due to sedentary lifestyles and sitting occupations. The name *"sway-back"* comes from the appearance of the thorax "swayed back" from the pelvis. The orientation of the pelvis may be either a posterior rotation or organized well in the sagittal plane but displaced anteriorly relative to the thorax. Observing from a side view, the relationship of the lateral malleolus to the greater trochanter in a vertical alignment identifies the sway-back. This reveals the hyperextension of the hip joints and a resultant resting hyperextension in the lumbar region (Kendall 2005).

Sway-back may be contributing to sit-to-stand pain experienced by clients with a diagnosis of LSS. An extension force is placed on the lumbar region which increases the pressure on the spinal nerve roots. From sitting to standing, the client will pull one knee posterior prior to standing and press the pelvis forward on the ascent (Sahrmann 2002). Teaching clients with LSS to reorganize their stance alignment and to move between sitting and standing in an efficient way may lessen or eliminate pain.

Final result of case report

An important component for a client with spinal stenosis is education. This client can explain the cause of her pain as related to movement and knows movements that will relieve and prevent her discomfort. The client demonstrates a reversal of the lumbar curve in forward bending and demonstrates dynamic stability of the torso during slow walking. Her lower extremity range of motion (ROM) has improved significantly, especially in her hip joints and ankles, increasing her ability to ambulate. Thoracic rotation has also improved, allowing a more even and normal arm swing during gait. Her standing posture and sit-to-stand test improved, minimizing excessive extension.

Lumbar reversal

Forward bending from a standing position occurs daily. In an efficient forward bend the pelvis shifts posteriorly as the hip joints flex. In the sagittal plane, the lumbar region reverses its anterior curve to approximately 20–25 degrees posteriorly. The continuation of forward bending occurs primarily at the hip joints (Sahrmann 2002). When a stiffness of the lumbar region and thoracolumbar fascia is present the reversal of the lumbar region is limited. The lumbar region appears flattened or may increase flexion beyond 20–25 degrees. A flexion range beyond 25 degrees may increase the risk of injury.

Session 2/12: Initial assessment

1. General observations of gait

- No right arm swing and minimal left arm swing
- Left lower extremity in external rotation
- Left foot pronated and abducted with reduced toe flexion during push-off
- Left hemipelvis superior motion with right thoracic translation to advance left lower extremity
- No thoracic rotation
- Lumbar instability with left leg swing greater than right
- Left pelvic shift on left heel strike

2. Standing tests

- Full torso rotation
- Observations of inefficient side: left
  - Decreased left torso rotation
  - Elevated left iliac crest
  - Limited left pelvic rotation
  - Excessive motion of ankles
- Hemipelvis inferior motion
- Observations of inefficient side: left
  - Difficulty lowering left hemipelvis
  - Compensates with thoracic rotation to left
- Hemipelvis superior motion

Session 12/12: Post-assessment

1. General observations of gait

- Normal arm swing
- No hemipelvis superior motion or thoracic translation as left lower extremity advances
- Improved thoracic rotation
- Equal leg swing
- Less pelvic shift on left heel strike

2. Standing tests

- Full torso rotation
- Observations of inefficient side: left
  - Increased ROM bilaterally
  - Left iliac crest no longer elevated
  - Ankles improve adaptation
- Hemipelvis inferior motion
- Observations of inefficient side: left
  - Slight improvement in lowering left hemipelvis
  - No compensation with thoracic rotation to left
- Hemipelvis superior motion

- Observations of inefficient side: left
  - Left hemipelvis superior motion elicits pain
  - Left iliac crest already elevated
  - Compensates with right thoracic shift
  - Left ankle stiffness

◆ Lateral pelvic shift

- Observations of inefficient side: left
  - Left foot inverts and supinates
  - Client reports stiffness and lack of balance
  - Compensation of torso rotation and lateral flexion

3. Seated tests

◆ Thoracic rotation

- Observations of inefficient side: left
  - Left limited
  - Pain with left rotation
  - Lumbar and pelvic compensation with both rotations

◆ Hip joint and knee flexion

- Observations of inefficient side: left
  - Left lumbar flexion
  - Right thoracic translation

4. Sit and stand

◆ Lateral view

- Limited hip joint flexion
- Forward translation of the pelvis with hyperextension
- Knee pulling back
- Pain in low back and left hip joint on standing

- Observations of inefficient side: left
  - No pain with left hemipelvis superior motion
  - No longer laterally shifts

◆ Lateral pelvic shift

- Observations of inefficient side: left
  - Shift to left less stiff with greater ROM
  - No compensation of torso rotation and lateral flexion

3. Seated tests

◆ Thoracic rotation

- Observations of inefficient side: left
  - Rotation shows improved ROM
  - No pain with left rotation

◆ Hip joint and knee flexion

- Observations of inefficient side: left
  - No change to left lumbar flexion
  - Less right thoracic translation

4. Sit and stand

◆ Lateral view

- Improved hip joint flexion
- Forward translation of the pelvis: no hyperextension
- Knees remain level
- Reports no pain in low back and left hip joint on standing

Chapter 3

Editor note
See Author note on sway-back posture above for a description of "knee pulling back."

◆ Anterior view

● Right hip joint medial rotation
● Right foot pronation
● Pain in lumbar and left pelvifemoral regions on standing

5. Standing balance

◆ One-leg stance, eyes open

◆ Left leg: 60 seconds

● Right leg: 60 seconds

◆ Anterior view

● No report of pain in lumbar and left pelvi-femoral regions on standing

5. Standing balance

◆ One-leg stance, eyes open
● Left leg: 60 seconds
● Right leg: 60 seconds

Session 3/12: Home program

Pain scale: 3, constant

Client self-report
- Continues to have low back pain in the morning
- Moving sit to stand most of the time with no pain
- Legs sore from last session

Key changes observed by author at end of Session 3/12
- Client able to move sit to stand slowly without excessive extension
- Able to self-organize standing posture

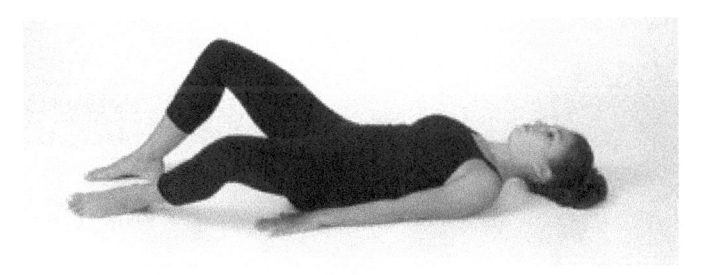

Figure 3.1

Reason behind choice of sequencing
- Improve hip flexion
- Practice hip movement during activities of daily living (ADL)
- Disassociate lumbar and thoracic motion
- Foster independence in exercise that can be performed frequently at home

Session movement sequence

1. Bent Knee Fall-Out

Intent
- Disassociate hip joint and torso motion
- Improve hip ROM
- Increase torso motor control

Gait reasoning
- Improve midline orientation during leg swing
- Minimize excessive transverse plane motion of the lumbar region

Starting position
- Supine
- Hip and knee flexion with feet on mat
- 1 in. (2.5 cm) pillow under head

Movement description	• Externally rotate and abduct right femur without pelvic movement in any plane • Repeat 8–10 times • Repeat on other side • Progress to alternating sides

2. Pelvic tilt

Intent	• Improve torso flexion • Improve torso motor control • Disassociate lumbar and thoracic movement • Promote optimal organization of the thorax in the sagittal plane • Decrease the incidence of sway-back posture
Gait reasoning	• Restore lumbar region curvature to improve lumbopelvic gait motion
Starting position	• Supine • Hip and knee flexion with feet on mat
Movement description	• Posteriorly rotate pelvis initiating from the ischial tuberosities • Maintain the thoracic and cervical position • Encourage abdominal activation using the breath

3. Cat

Intent	• Improve flexion of lumbar region • Disassociate thoracic and lumbar motion • Improve activation of abdominals • Improve ankle dorsiflexion and 1st metatarsophalangeal (MTP) extension
Gait reasoning	• Improve ability for torso to be in midline during leg swing • Improve heel strike and push-off • Reorganize sway-back posture for more optimal stance
Starting position	• Quadruped • Ankles dorsiflexed and phalanges in extension

Pilates for Management of Central Lumbar Spinal Stenosis: Effect on Gait

Movement description	• Exhale, posteriorly rotate the pelvis initiating from the ischial tuberosities • Articulate from the pelvis through the thoracolumbar junction (TLJ) avoiding movement above the TLJ • Return to the starting position avoiding hyperextension of the lumbar region • Avoid hip external rotation by observing the feet moving inward and outward • Repeat 8–10 times

4. Cat rock back

Intent	• Improve pelvifemoral flexion on a dynamic stable torso • Improve arm swing • Disassociate arm and thoracic motion • Improve ankle dorsiflexion and 1st MTP extension
Gait reasoning	• Improve arm swing • Increase hip flexion with torso control • Improve heel strike and toe-off

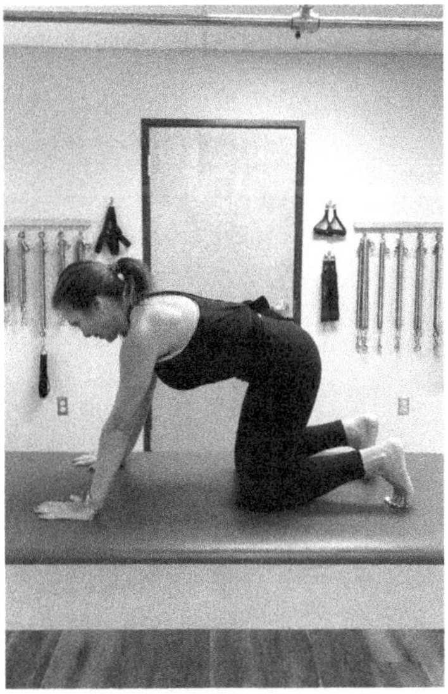

Figure 3.2

Chapter 3

Starting position	• Quadruped • Ankles in dorsiflexion with MTP extension
Movement description	• Posteriorly rotate pelvis initiating with ischial tuberosities • Maintain posterior rotation while rocking back into hip flexion • Return to starting position when posterior rotation can no longer be maintained • Avoid movement of thoracic and cervical regions • Repeat 8–10 times

5. Seated external rotation/abduction/flexion of hip joint

Intent	• Improve external rotation/abduction/flexion of the hip joints • Improve lumbar flexion
Gait reasoning	• Reduce extension of the lumbar region during hip extension
Starting position	• Sit on a hard chair • Place right ankle on left femur • Right hip joint in right external rotation/abduction/flexion • Avoid rotation or abduction of left lower extremity (LE) • Maintain upright torso
Movement description	• Maintain torso position while raising and lowering left heel • Repeat 8 times • Flex torso, hold, and repeat heel raise 8 times • Repeat on other side

6. Standing extension

Intent	• Improve extension
Gait reasoning	• Improve torso control on push-off
Starting position	• Stand facing a counter or railing • Flex right knee and place right ankle on top of a chair
Movement description	• Posteriorly rotate pelvis • Flex right shoulder with elbow extended • Hold for 1 minute • Repeat on other side

7. Bridge	(Romani-Ruby 2008)
Intent	● Improve hip extension with torso control ● Activate extensors
Gait reasoning	● Improve push-off ● Improve torso control with hip extension
Starting position	● Supine ● Hip and knee flexion, feet on mat ● Upper extremities (UE) at sides ● No head support
Movement description	● Inhale, press feet into mat and extend hip joints into bridge ● Press UE into mat ● Keep weight to inside of feet ● Avoid LE adduction/internal rotation ● Exhale, lower whole torso through hip joint flexion ● Repeat up to 30 times

Session 11/12: Studio session

Pain scale	1–2, intermittent
Client self-report	● Mild stiffness in the morning ● No pain when rolling in the afternoon or evening ● No pain moving sit to stand ● Intermittent low back pain ● No paresthesia or numbness in left leg ● Driving can still cause some discomfort but only in the low back; she is able to resolve the low back pain by changing position
Key changes observed by author at end of Session 11/12	● Client moves sit to stand with no pain or paresthesia ● Client demonstrates arm swing with gait ● Client ambulates with good torso control at slow speed
Reason behind choice of sequencing	● Promote effective lumbar flexion ● Decrease lateral shift ● Disassociate lumbar and thoracic motion for improved torso motion

Chapter 3

Session movement sequence

1. Seated push-through and push-up with footboard on Trapeze Table

Derivative of J. H. Pilates Push-Through Seated Front on Trapeze Table (NPCE Study Guide 2021, p. 63) (Romani-Ruby and Ruby 2018)

Intent
- Promote effective lumbar flexion
- Decrease lateral shift
- Disassociate lumbar and thoracic motion
- Promote shoulder and thoracic ROM
- Improve ankle ROM

Gait reasoning
- Flexion is the client's direction of preference that will reduce the lateral shift and centralize symptoms
- Increase ankle motion for improved gait
- Push-up will improve arm swing and thoracic motion for ambulation
- Activation of flexors

Editor note
Peripheralization refers to symptoms of pain or numbness/tingling traveling away from the origin of pain. Centralization essentially refers to symptoms returning toward the origin of pain or resolving completely.

Set-up
- Light spring, top-loaded
- Footboard placed across table against upright side posts

Starting position
- Sitting upright, LE abducted and externally rotated
- Feet against the footboard
- Hold push-through bar with UE abducted

Movement description
- Posteriorly rotate pelvis for lumbar flexion
- Inhale, pressing bar upward
- Anteriorly rotating pelvis increases hip joint flexion without hyperextending lumbar region
- Exhale posteriorly, rotating pelvis into starting position
- Inhale hold
- Exhale, maintaining posteriorly rotated pelvis
- Flex hip joints to push bar down and forward
- Return to the starting position
- Repeat 8 times

Pilates for Management of Central Lumbar Spinal Stenosis: Effect on Gait

CUES
- Avoid hyperextending the torso or dropping the head through the arms on push-up
- In lumbar flexion position maintain the position without increasing thoracic flexion
- Initiate each motion with the ischial tuberosities
- Avoid flexing or hyperextending the knees
- Avoid extending the wrists

Author note
The emphasis of this exercise is on the quality of the lumbar flexion and not on the range of motion. Encourage optimal torso placement and avoid peripheralization of symptoms into the extremities. Watch the neck, shoulders, and wrists on the push-up to avoid flexion of thorax. Keeping the wrists in a neutral position will stimulate external rotation at the shoulder joints with thoracic extension.

2. Push-through with thoracic rotation on Trapeze Table

Derivative of J. H. Pilates Push-Through Seated Front on Trapeze Table (NPCE Study Guide 2021, p. 63) and mat exercise Saw (NPCE Study Guide 2021, p. 48)

Intent
- Improve thoracic articulation
- Improve shoulder ROM
- Reciprocal torso rotation of thorax and pelvis

Gait reasoning
- Increase thoracic rotation
- Improving arm swing

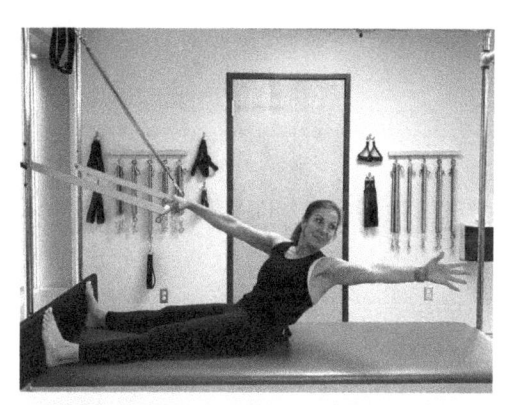

Figure 3.3

Set-up
- Light spring, top-loaded
- Footboard placed across table against upright side posts

Chapter 3

Starting position	• Sitting upright, with LE abducted and externally rotated • Feet against footboard • Hold push-through bar with hands near center of bar
Movement description	• Posteriorly rotate pelvis for lumbar flexion • Maintaining position of ischial tuberosities on the table, let go of right hand and rotate torso to right • Look in direction of rotation • Allow left shoulder to externally rotate • Return to starting position • Perform on other side • Repeat 8 times alternating breath with movement

CUES
- Articulate the rotation from the head to the thoracolumbar junction
- Reach forward into the footboard through the same-side leg

Author note
Encourage outward rotation of the shoulder of the arm holding onto the push-through bar

3. Push-Through Seated Front with legs crossed on Trapeze Table	Derivative of J. H. Pilates Push-Through Seated Front on Trapeze Table (NPCE Study Guide 2021, p. 63) and mat exercise Saw (NPCE Study Guide 2021, p. 48, pp. 20–21) (Romani-Ruby and Ruby 2018)
Intent	• Encourage torso rotation • Activate reciprocal patterns for gait
Gait reasoning	• Reciprocal torso rotation of thorax and pelvis

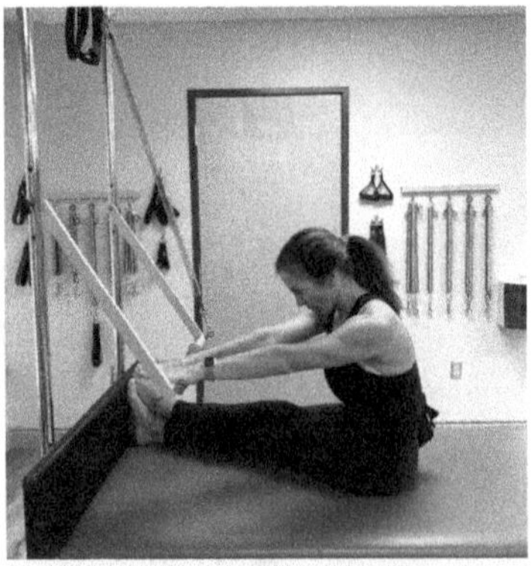

Figure 3.4

Set-up
- Light spring, top-loaded
- Footboard placed across table against upright side posts

Starting position
- Sitting upright, LE abducted and externally rotated
- Feet against foot board
- Left ankle crossed over right ankle
- Hold push-through bar with hands to left side

Movement description
- Posteriorly rotate pelvis for lumbar flexion
- Articulate, flexing torso, lowering toward the table
- Return to starting position
- Repeat 8 times
- Change to right ankle crossed over left ankle
- Repeat 8 times

CUES
- Keep the pelvis orientation toward the footboard
- Reach crossed-over leg in opposition to the torso flexion

4. Standing hip extension on Ladder Barrel

Intent
- Reduce flexor dominance, thus allowing lumbar area to move posteriorly
- Extension of lumbar region narrows foramen where nerve roots are stenosed
- To relieve pressure on stenosed areas

Gait reasoning
- Improve ability to extend during push-off

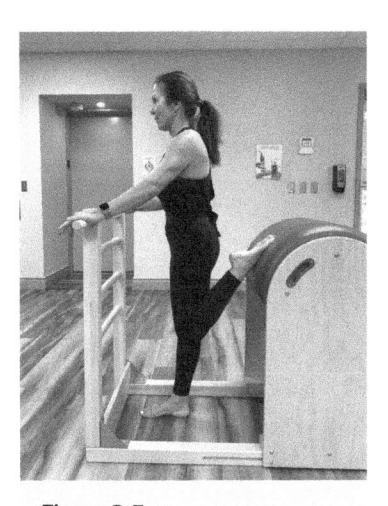

Figure 3.5

Set-up	• Stand in Ladder Barrel facing ladder
Starting position	• Flex left knee and place left foot on top of barrel • Extend right standing leg • Posteriorly rotate pelvis • Raise left arm
Movement description	• Hold position for 1 minute on each side

CUES
- Be sure standing LE is extended and activated
- Level the pelvis to eliminate a hemipelvis hike

5. LE external rotation/abduction/flexion on Wunda Chair	Derivative of J. H. Pilates Washer Woman Over the Chair: Hamstring 2 (NPCE Study Guide 2021, p. 77) (Romani-Ruby 2011)
Intent	• Improve articulation and glide of hip joint • Increase lumbar flexion mobility • Client needs to improve mobility toward lumbar flexion to take stress off lumbar nerve roots
Gait reasoning	• Hip joint glide for improved LE swing
Set-up	• Heavy spring, position 2
Starting position	• Standing at the back of the chair facing the foot pedal • Place left leg on top of the chair in external rotation/abduction/flexion • Right leg is posterior and extended with foot on floor
Movement description	• Flex torso toward chair pedal and touch pedal • Press foot pedal downward • Complete 8 slow repetitions • Return to starting position • Change to other side

CUES
- Watch for excessive head-on-neck extension
- Encourage upward rotation of scapula

6. Knee Stretch on Universal Reformer: variation 1

Derivative of J. H. Pilates Knee Stretch Series: Kneeling/Round Back on Universal Reformer Knee stretch variations (NPCE Study Guide 2021, p. 60) (See Chapter 5 in Volume 1, Trier) (Romani-Ruby 2015)

Intent
- Closed kinematic chain exercise challenges the UE and LE activation during active flexion and extension
- To improve sagittal plane movement
- UE sagittal plane motion

Gait reasoning
- Torso organization with UE and LE sagittal plane motion

Set-up
- Lower the footbar
- Springs: 1 very light and 1 medium

Starting position
- Kneeling in quadruped on carriage with hands on standing platform
- Position body so that knees are directly under hip joints and hands under shoulders
- 1 very light spring

Movement description
- Inhale, move the carriage back as far as you can, activating extensors without changing torso position
- Hold position
- UE flexion moves carriage further back
- Hold the UE position
- Exhale, bring carriage back to where knees are under hip joints
- Pull, closing carriage with UE extension
- Repeat 8 times

CUES
- Maintain the torso orientation to the floor, not allowing it to angle downward when the UE move the carriage
- Limit the movement to a range where the torso position can be maintained

Author note
As the client progresses, this exercise can be done without springs. If there is leg or back pain, increase the tension of the spring.

Editor note
Here increasing the springs supports the body during the movement rather than increasing the challenge. Using no springs increases the load of the torso. See variable spring resistance in Pilates in Chapter 6.

Chapter 3

7. Knee Stretch on Universal Reformer: variation 2

Derivative of J. H. Pilates Knee Stretch Series: Kneeling/Round Back on Universal Reformer (NPCE Study Guide 2021, p. 60) (Romani-Ruby 2015)

Intent
- Reduce extension dominance to decrease stress on lumbar nerve roots

Gait reasoning
- Improved torso extension for midline orientation and improved rotation
- Improved lumbopelvic control in sagittal plane

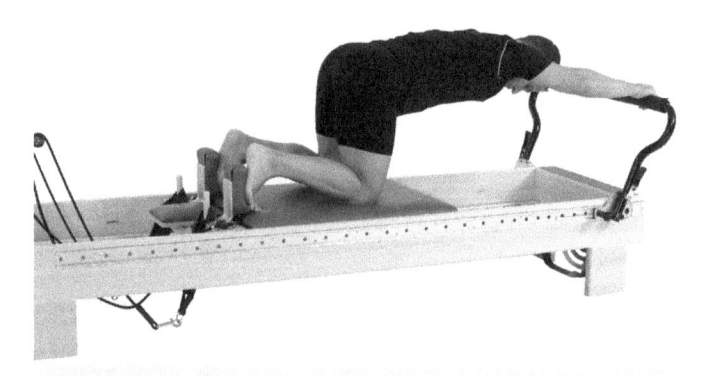

Figure 3.6

Set-up
- Springs: 1 medium and 1 light

Starting position
- Kneeling on carriage in quadruped
- Place feet against shoulder stops and hands wide on footbar
- UE shoulder flexion and elbow extension
- Push carriage open until knees are directly under hip joints

Movement description
- Maintain starting position
- Small-range hip extension and flexion moving carriage in and out
- Repeat 8 times
- Hold 90 degrees of hip flexion
- Pull and push carriage with UE
- Repeat 8 times

CUES
- The carriage will not fully close
- Focus on the femoral glide during extension and flexion
- Inhale with extension
- Exhale with flexion

Author note
If there is back or leg pain, increase the tension of the spring to support the torso.

8. Elephant on Universal Reformer

Derivative of J. H. Pilates Long Stretch Series: Elephant on Universal Reformer (NPCE Study Guide 2021, p. 55) (Romani-Ruby 2015, pp. 33–34)

Intent
- Improve coordination of hip joint movement
- Encourage moving toward torso flexion with hip extension
- Promote minimizing stress to adherent nerve roots

Gait reasoning
- Hip joint articulation and coordination for leg swing
- Increase ankle dorsiflexion for stance phase

Set-up
- Springs: 1 medium and 1 light

Starting position
- Stand on mid-carriage with feet aligned with hip joints
- Hip joint flexion and knee extension
- Place hands on footbar with shoulders over wrists, elbows extended
- Posteriorly rotate pelvis

Movement description
- Maintain shoulders over wrists
- Move carriage outward slightly extending the hip joints
- Return carriage to starting position
- Repeat 8 times
- Maintain feet aligned with hip joints
- Flex and extend shoulders to move the carriage
- Repeat 8 times
- Maintain posteriorly rotated pelvis throughout movement

CUES
- Reach the inferior ischium toward the calcaneus
- Draw in the abdomen
- Head and cervical region follows contour of torso

Author note
Springs can be lightened if the client is unable to move the carriage.

Chapter 3

9. Arabesque on Universal Reformer — Derivative of J. H. Pilates Long Stretch Series: Arabesque on Universal Reformer (NPCE Study Guide 2021, p. 55) (Romani-Ruby 2015)

Intent
- Encourage abdominal activation with hip extension
- Promote minimizing stress to the adherent nerve roots

Gait reasoning
- Improve ankle mobility for transfer of weight from one foot to the other

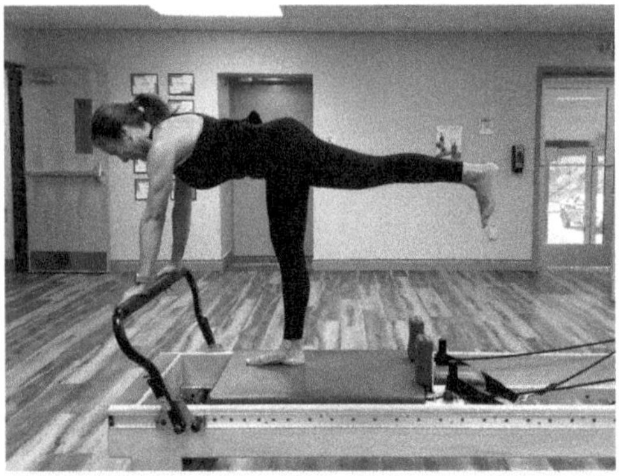

Figure 3.7

Author note
Improving ankle joint articulation will effectively improve the transfer of weight from one foot to the other during gait. This will decrease the stress of the stenotic areas during gait.

Set-up
- Medium spring

Starting position
- Standing on mid-carriage with feet aligned with hip joints
- Hip joint flexion and knee extension
- Place hands on footbar with shoulders over wrists, elbows extended
- Posteriorly rotate pelvis
- Extend left hip joint, leg parallel to carriage

Movement description
- Extend right leg 10 degrees
- Flex right hip joint to return to starting position
- Shoulders remain over wrists
- Repeat 8 times
- Maintain posteriorly rotated pelvis throughout movement

CUES
- Reach the inferior ischium toward the calcaneus
- Draw in the abdomen
- Head and cervical region follows contour of torso

Author note
Springs can be adjusted to meet the ability to perform the task.

10. Eve's Lunge and variations on Universal Reformer
(See Chapter 5 in Volume 1, Gentry, Eve's Lunge) (Romani-Ruby 2015)

Intent
- Increase awareness of flexion and extension
- Improve posterior pelvifemoral strategy

Gait reasoning
- Improve extension for push-off

Set-up
- Medium spring

Starting position
- Stand on left side of Universal Reformer with left foot on floor near footbar
- Left knee centered over left ankle
- Right knee in flexion resting on carriage with foot against the shoulder stop
- Hold on to footbar with both hands

Movement description
- Press into left foot
- Extend right hip joint and knee moving carriage backward
- Return to starting position
- Repeat 8 times
- Repeat on other side

CUES
- Maintain the knee centered over ankle of standing leg throughout movement
- Focus on extending the hip joint rather than extending the knee

Author note
Avoid hyperextension of the leg resting on the carriage. This exercise can be performed both dynamically and statically for challenge variations. Removing the hands from the footbar will increase the difficulty of the exercise. Decreasing the spring tension will also create challenge.

11. Splits: Side on Universal Reformer variation 1

J. H. Pilates Splits: Side on Universal Reformer (NPCE Study Guide 2021, p. 61)
(Romani-Ruby 2015)

Intent	• Increase activation of the hip joint to improve stance, sit-to-stand activity, and gait
	• Activate LE in abduction and adduction
	• Improve medial and lateral glide of hip joints
Gait reasoning	• Improve ability and balance for one-leg stance phase
	• Increase load in standing

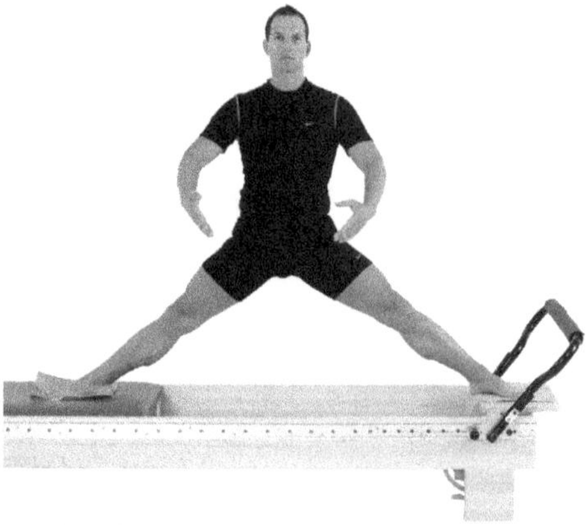

Figure 3.8

Set-up	• Medium spring
	• Lower footbar and attach standing platform
Starting position	• Stand sideways on Universal Reformer with one foot on standing platform and one foot on carriage
	• Externally rotate LE 45 degrees
	• Knees extended
Movement description	• Inhale, pressing carriage out
	• Exhale, resisting carriage closing
	• Repeat 8 times
	• Repeat on other side

CUES
- As the foot presses out the carriage, feel the torso moving with the carriage
- Avoid habitual sway-back position

Author notes
Check that the pelvic crests remain level as the client opens and closes the carriage. The torso maintains its midline orientation. Progress to a heavier spring.

12. Splits: Side on Universal Reformer variation 2

Derivative of J. H. Pilates Splits: Side on Universal Reformer (NPCE Study Guide 2021, p. 61) (Romani-Ruby 2015)

Intent
- Increase activation of hip joint to improve stance, sit-to-stand activity, and gait
- Activate hip joint in various angles and ROM

Gait reasoning
- Improve stance leg balance for leg swing
- Challenge adaptation through various force vectors

Set-up
- Medium spring
- Standing platform

Starting position
- Standing sideways on Universal Reformer with one foot on standing platform and one foot on carriage
- Externally rotate LE 45 degrees
- Knees flexed

Movement description
- Press carriage out while simultaneously extending both knees
- Resist carriage closing with extended knees
- Repeat 8 times
- Repeat on other side

CUES
- When pressing the carriage open, attempt to keep the torso from rising to fully glide in the hip joints
- Observe if the pelvis remains level. If not, the action of the LE is uneven

Author note
- Observe if the pelvic crests remain level as the client opens and closes the carriage
- The torso maintains its midline orientation
- Progress to a heavier spring

13. Splits: Side on Universal Reformer variation 3 (Romani-Ruby 2015)

Intent
- Improve ability to orientate to midline while changing levels
- Challenge pelvic diaphragm through activation of LE

Gait reasoning
- Stimulate ground force reaction from the feet
- Improve plantar flexion, knee and hip extension for push-off

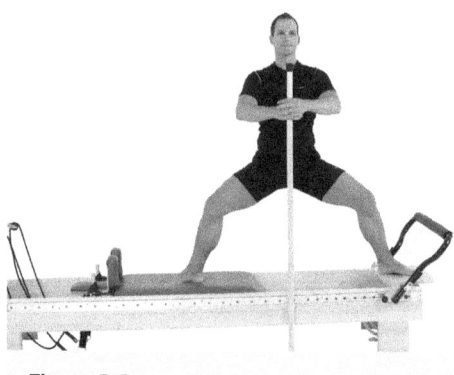

Figure 3.9

Set-up
- Very light spring
- Standing platform

Starting position
- Standing sideways on Universal Reformer with one foot on standing platform and one foot on carriage
- Externally rotate LE 45 degrees
- Knees extended

Movement description
- Carriage remains closed throughout
- Exhale, flex, abduct hip joints, and flex knees
- Inhale, extend, adduct hip joints and knees
- Repeat 8 times
- During knee extension raise the heels in plantar flexion
- Repeat 8 times

Author note
Use a pole for balance if necessary.

CUES
- When pressing the carriage open, attempt to keep the torso from rising to fully glide in the hip joints
- Observe if the pelvis remains level. If not, the action of the LE is uneven

14. Splits: Side on Universal Reformer variation 4

(Romani-Ruby 2015)

Intent
- Improve ability to orientate to midline while changing levels
- Challenge pelvic diaphragm through LE activation

Gait reasoning
- Stimulate ground force reaction from feet
- Improve plantar flexion, knee, and hip extension for push-off

Set-up
- Very light spring
- Standing platform

Starting position
- Standing sideways on Universal Reformer with one foot on standing platform and one foot on carriage
- Externally rotate LE 45 degrees
- Knees extended

Movement description
- Carriage remains closed
- Exhale, flexing hip and knee joints
- Inhale, extending hip and knee joints
- Repeat 8 times
- With extended knees plantar flex the feet by raising heels
- Repeat 8 times

Author note
Use a pole for balance if necessary.

15. Long Stretch on Universal Reformer

J. H. Pilates Long Stretch on Universal Reformer (NPCE Study Guide 2021, p. 55)
(Romani-Ruby 2015)

Intent
- Disassociate shoulder and torso
- Improve torso dynamic stability
- Load adaptation in extension

Gait reasoning
- To improve arm and thoracic awareness in gait
- Create a strategy to eliminate irritation of nerve roots during standing and gait
- To decrease the excessive motion in the lumbar region by improving endurance

Chapter 3

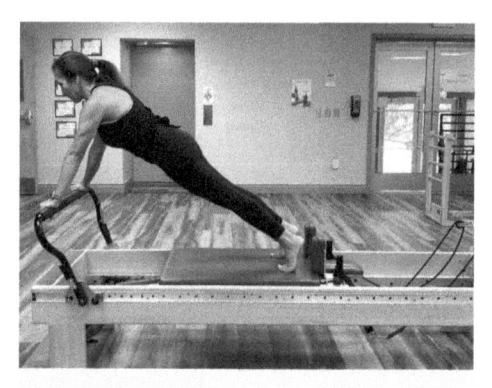

Figure 3.10

Set-up
- Medium spring

Starting position
- Kneel on carriage with knees aligned center of hip joints
- Feet slightly away from shoulder stops with phalangeal extension
- Place hands on footbar shoulder-width apart

Movement description
- Inhale, extend, pressing carriage away into a plank position
- Shoulders directly over the wrists
- Maintain plank position
- Exhale, return carriage inward maintaining plank position
- Repeat 8 times
- Last repetition inward to kneel on carriage

CUES
- The carriage will not fully close during the exercise
- Place thumbs with fingers on the footbar and avoid deep wrist extension

The journey to Session 11

Session 4/12
Client self-report

- Pain scale 2
- Low back pain this morning that eased as she moved
- Headache and fatigue after driving for work today
- Legs feeling sore
- No pain with the home exercises
- Client had no questions on home exercises
- Demonstrated confidence and independence on home exercises so far

Key changes observed

- Client independent with home exercise program
- Sit to stand improved, performed with no pain

Reasoning behind choice of movements

- Improving balance with torso control through LE

Session movement sequence
1. Mat bridge added

- 30 repetitions

2. Trapeze Table

- Bend and Stretch/Footwork with spring from below
- Roll-Down with light leg springs

3. Ladder Barrel

- Standing extension

4. Wunda Chair

- LE external rotation/abduction/flexion

5. Universal Reformer

- Ankle ROM on the jump board

6. Additional movement

- Demonstrated self-correction of sway-back posture (see box Sway-back posture above)

Session 5/12
Client self-report

- Continues to report leg soreness from session
- Pain scale 2
- Pain mostly in the morning
- Fatigue in low back after a long day driving for work
- Home exercises going well

Key changes observed

- Nothing significant

Reasoning behind choice of movements

- Continued reeducation of LE movement
- Adding reeducation of UE movement
- Challenging torso control with UE and LE movement

Session movement sequence
1. Performed mat bridge for home program independently

2. Trapeze Table

- Push-up and push-through, 1 light spring

3. Wunda Chair

- LE external rotation/abduction/flexion

4. Ladder Barrel

- Standing extension

5. Universal Reformer

- Eve's Lunge
- Knee Stretch
- Elephant
- Arabesque
- Splits: Side variation 1
- Splits: Side variation 4

6. Additional movements

- Discussed seated posture at work and in the car: sit on the back of the sitting bones in a slight posterior tilt with the chest open
- Avoid turning out the right LE on the gas pedal
- Match the legs when driving and use cruise control when possible

Session 6/12
Client self-report

- Client can self-manage pain during walking with posterior pelvic rotation and lumbar flexion
- Increased walking time and distance
- Pain scale 2–3
- Pain intermittent at lumbar area only

Key changes observed

- Client reversing the lumbar curve effectively (see box Lateral shift above)
- Standing posture improved

Reasoning behind choice of movements

- Continue lumbar flexion focus as it is proving to be direction of preference
- Progress to more strenuous exercise

Session movement sequence
1. Progressed to single leg bridge

2. Trapeze Table

- Seated push-through and push-up
- Seated push-through with thoracic rotation

3. Universal Reformer

- Knee Stretch variation 2
- Knee Stretch variation 1
- Elephant
- Arabesque
- Splits: Side variation 1
- Splits: Side variation 2
- Splits: Side variation 3
- Splits: Side variation 4

4. Wunda Chair

- Seated Footwork

- LE external rotation/abduction/flexion

5. Ladder Barrel

- Standing extension

6. Additional movement

- Review and recheck sit to stand

Session 7/12
Client self-report

- Pain scale 2–3
- Pain intermittent and only in low back
- Reports decreased stiffness in the morning after performing posterior pelvic rotation in bed before rising
- Client had no questions on home program

Key changes observed

- Client is learning to incorporate exercises into her daily routine

Reasoning behind choice of movements

- Continue lumbar flexion focus as it is proving to be direction of preference
- Progress into more strenuous exercise

Session movement sequence
1. Trapeze Table

- Seated push-through and push-up
- Seated push-through with thoracic rotation

2. Universal Reformer

- Knee Stretch variation 2
- Knee Stretch variation 1
- Elephant

- Arabesque
- Splits: Side variation 1
- Splits: Side variation 2
- Splits: Side variation 3
- Splits: Side variation 4

3. Wunda Chair

- LE external rotation/abduction/flexion

4. Ladder Barrel

- Standing extension

Session 8/12
Key changes observed

- Demonstrates less sway-back posture when standing between exercises

Reasoning behind choice of movements

- Continue lumbar flexion focus as it is proving to be direction of preference
- Progress into more strenuous exercise

Session movement sequence
1. Trapeze Table

- Seated push-through and push-up
- Seated push-through with thoracic rotation

2. Universal Reformer

- Knee Stretch variation 2
- Knee Stretch variation 1
- Elephant
- Arabesque
- Splits: Side variation 1
- Splits: Side variation 2
- Splits: Side variation 3
- Splits: Side variation 4

3. Wunda Chair

- LE external rotation/abduction/flexion

4. Ladder Barrel

- Standing extension

Session 9/12
Client self-report

- Client reports a really good day yesterday
- Walked 4 miles
- Pain scale 1
- Pain intermittent in lumbar area only when standing for longer periods
- States she relieves pain by bending forward or sitting down

Key changes observed

- Client self-organizes during exercises
- She is aware of inefficient movement patterns

Reasoning behind choice of movements

- Check client efficiency of movement for future progressions

Session movement sequence
1. Single leg bridge

2. Universal Reformer

- Knee Stretch variation 2
- Knee Stretch variation 1
- Elephant
- Arabesque
- Splits: Side variation 1
- Splits: Side variation 2
- Splits: Side variation 3
- Splits: Side variation 4

3. Wunda Chair

- LE external rotation/abduction/flexion

4. Ladder Barrel

- Standing extension

5. Additional movement

- Observed client's position seated in her car as this is the place that increases pain. Adjusted the seat to a higher position for knees to be below the pelvis, moved the steering wheel closer, and moved the seat back providing for appropriate leg length, avoiding extension. Practiced posterior pelvic rotation while driving for pain relief

Session 10/12
Client self-report

- Client pleased to be able to walk for exercise without causing back pain
- Driving can still cause back pain, but no leg symptoms
- Pain scale 1–2
- Pain intermittent in lumbar area
- Discussed the importance of keeping the home program up for maintenance

Key changes observed

- Hip flexion ROM is within normal limits

Reasoning behind choice of movements

- Continue lumbar flexion focus as it is proving to be direction of preference
- Progress into more strenuous exercise

Session movement sequence
1. Trapeze Table

- Seated push-through and push-up
- Seated push-through with thoracic rotation

2. Universal Reformer

- Knee Stretch variation 2
- Knee Stretch variation 1
- Elephant
- Arabesque
- Splits: Side variation 1
- Splits: Side variation 2
- Splits: Side variation 3
- Splits: Side variation 4

3. Wunda Chair

- LE external rotation/abduction/flexion

4. Ladder Barrel

- Standing extension

References

Chaitow, L. (2007) "Chronic pelvic pain: Pelvic floor problems, sacro-iliac dysfunction and the trigger point connection." *Journal of Bodywork and Movement Therapies, 11,* 4, 327–339.

Kendall, F. P., McCreary, E. K., Provance, P. G., Rodgers, M. M., and Romani, W. A. (2005) *Muscle: Testing and Function with Posture and Pain.* 5th Ed. Philadelphia: PA: Lippincott Williams & Wilkins.

Magee, D. J. (2008) *Orthopedic Physical Assessment.* 5th Ed. St. Louis, MO: Saunders Elsevier.

NPCE Study Guide (National Pilates Certification Exam Study Guide) (2021) Miami, FL: National Pilates Certification Program, Inc.

Chatha, D. et. al. 2011

Costandi, et al. 2015

Munakomi, et. al. 2022

Page et al. (2010)

Ravindra, et. al. 2018

Romani-Ruby, C. (2008)

Romani-Ruby, C. (2011)

Romani-Ruby, C. (2015)

Romani-Ruby, C. and Ruby (2018)

Sahrmann (2002)

Chapter 4
Pilates and Sacroiliac Joint Dysfunction: Effect on Gait

Kathleen McDonough

Non-specific, chronic low back pain (LBP) is one of the most prevalent orthopedic complaints and a leading cause of absence from work, disability, and decreased quality of life worldwide. The sacroiliac joint (SIJ) is a cause in up to 40 percent of all cases of LBP, yet it is often underdiagnosed and undertreated (Enix and Mayer 2019; Falowski *et al.* 2020; Jonely, Avery, and Desai 2020; Schneider *et al.* 2019). Often, there is poor efficacy in medical treatment of SIJ pain. Symptoms may include LBP, pain in the buttock or whole leg, and pain with standing on or moving something with one leg. Groin and symphysis pubis pain may also be present.

Diagnosis is problematic due to difficulty identifying the source(s) of the pain, consistency in pain referral patterns, and complexity of anatomy, innervation, and functional relationships of the SIJ (Chuang *et al.* 2019; Schneider *et al.* 2019). Chronic LBP, SIJ, and pelvic girdle pain are more prevalent in women worldwide. Causes and risk factors for SIJ pain include leg-length discrepancy, pregnancy, gait abnormalities, obesity, repetitive low-grade trauma (jogging), other trauma including falls, lifting, motor vehicle accidents, previous lumbar surgeries (especially fusion), arthritis, scoliosis, and inflammatory conditions (Enix and Mayer 2019; Gutke *et al.* 2018). Recently, systemic hypermobility, such as in Ehlers–Danlos syndrome, has been identified as a source of SIJ and pelvic girdle pain, and overwhelmingly affects more women than men (Ali *et al.* 2020; Demmler *et al.* 2019).

The pelvic girdle is made up of two ilia, joined anteriorly at the symphysis pubis, and the sacrum at the SIJ posteriorly.

The principles of form and force closure were introduced to describe the complex mechanism of sacroiliac joint (SIJ) stability. Form closure refers to a theoretical stable state of a joint with close fitting articular surfaces, where no extra forces are needed to maintain the stable state of the system during loading and unloading situations. (Vleeming and Schuenke 2019)

Sacral nutation and lumbar lordosis are necessary for effective force closure (sensorimotor control) that allows the pelvis to absorb and transfer loads. "A considerable amount of load transfer between the upper and lower body occurs through the sacroiliac (SI) joint" (Decker and Davidson 2017).

Increased or decreased force closure due to the body's adaptive responses tend to produce positional and movement abnormalities leading to painful stimuli from the articular surface and adjacent soft tissue (Rupert *et al.* 2009). The body's adaptive responses contribute to asymmetric forces that can produce strain on the SIJ. Bilateral exercises that facilitate force closure are indicated.

Visceral impairments, motor control, and emotional states, such as beliefs and fears, particularly about movement, also contribute to optimal or non-optimal load transfer between

Chapter 4

ground and torso, which can manifest as pain or dysfunction in many areas of the body (Hides *et al.* 2019).

Care should be taken to ensure quality of movement without pain, with enough resistance to load without loss of force closure. Bilateral movements, and exercises that focus on whole-body response to loads, are most beneficial. Given the incidence of hypermobility in those with SIJ pain (Enix and Mayer 2020; Falowski *et al.* 2020), contraindicated exercises would be those emphasizing end-range movements (with excessive resistance) and those in less stable positions (without sufficient spring resistance).

Client description: 46-year-old biological female, identifies as female; Pilates teacher with longstanding SIJ and leg pain

Dates of case report: Session 1: January 29, 2021; Session 12: February 22, 2021. All sessions were virtual, due to thoracolumbar junction (TLJ) restrictions.

Studio apparatus and props
Pilates equipment

- Universal Reformer
- Trapeze Table
- Wunda Chair
- Spine Corrector
- Ladder Barrel

Props used with equipment

- Mat
- 9 in. (23 cm) ball, partially inflated
- Magic Circle
- Strap
- 4 in. (10 cm) diameter soft balls
- 22 in. (55 cm) ball
- Non-skid rubberized mat (7.5 x 14 x 0.5 in. (19.05 x 35.56 x 1.27 cm))

Home program props

- Mat
- Wall space
- 9 in. (23 cm) ball, partially inflated
- 22 in. (55 cm) ball
- Magic Circle

- Strap
- Roller, 36 in. (92 cm) long, 6 in. (15 cm) in diameter

Methods and materials

Session 1/12
1. Health history

- Frequent flare-ups with pain
- No numbness, tingling, or difficulty sleeping due to pain
- Pain began with pregnancies, especially her third child, 18 years ago. Three uncomplicated vaginal deliveries with minimum pelvic diaphragm trauma, no stitches, and some problems with urinary urgency
- Previous treatment included physical therapy and massage, but no lasting relief
- Generalized hypermobility
- Aggravating factors: lunge stretches, lower extremity (LE) abduction, side kicks, longer hikes
- Good general health: Graves' disease, pre-menopausal, some nagging right knee pain and pain from bunions (in left foot more than right). No history of trauma.

- Activity: runs on a treadmill for 2 miles 3–4 times a week; stationary cycling or boot camp classes twice a week; weight work or TRX 3 times a week
- Almost zero Pilates recently, mostly due to pain and instability of her pelvis
- Previous yoga, but felt that she could hurt herself doing so
- Work: teaches 25 hours a week and does about 10 hours a week managing two studios
- Goals: longer hikes without leg pain, return to Pilates on equipment, especially Universal Reformer, without pain

2. Symptoms

- Low back pain, left buttock pain, anterior left pelvifemoral pain
- When pain flares up she has whole left leg pain, which can be severe
- Previous tailbone pain, no sensitivity currently

3. Movement aids

- None

Final result of case report
The client's gait was much improved: Increasing hip joint strategy compared to knee strategy improved load transfer from legs to torso and shoulders without hyperextension or excessive rotation at the TLJ. The client successfully returned to Pilates exercises on the apparatus without pain, was able to hike longer distances, and completed intensive yoga training without pain.

Session 2/12: Initial assessment

1. General observations of gait

- Decreased or asymmetric arm swing: right shoulder girdle posteriorly, left anteriorly
- Decreased thoracic rotation, especially the right
- Excessive rotation at the TLJ
- Decreased LE extension in both right and left at push-off
- Decreased left hip joint extension at push-off, with quad dominant
- Knee strategy employed more than hip joint strategy

Editor note
This specific client employs a standing movement strategy of excessive extension at the TLJ and end-range nutation with increased hip joint flexion. Round-back position is appropriate to restore the integrity of the TLJ with respect to the sacrum and force and form closure.

2. Standing tests

- Full torso rotation

- Observations of inefficient side: left
  - Limited pelvis rotation on left femur
  - Lacks internal rotation of left femur
  - Early and increased thoracolumbar extension
  - Feet do not adapt

- Hemipelvis inferior motion

Session 12/12: Post-assessment

1. General observations of gait

- Improved and symmetrical arm swing
- Improved thoracic rotation, right is equal to left
- Excessive TLJ rotation decreased
- Increased right and left push-off
- Increased LE extension both right and left in push-off
- Gait rhythm demonstrates even weight transfer

2. Standing tests

- Full torso rotation

- Observations of inefficient side: both
  - Slightly improved pelvic rotation on left femur
  - Less thoracolumbar extension
  - Better load transfers

- Hemipelvis inferior motion

- Observations of inefficient side: right

- Efficient side: left
- Non-efficient side: right
- Observations of inefficient side: right
  - Left hip joint unable to internally rotate or adduct
  - Right hemipelvis unable to drop, lumbar region restricted in left lateral flexion
  - Thorax translates to right

◆ Hemipelvis superior motion

- Observations of inefficient side: left
  - Left hemipelvis unable to rise
  - Left femur unable to adduct
  - Thorax translates to right, weight shifts to right

◆ Lateral pelvic shift

- Observations of inefficient side: left
  - Avoids internal rotation and adduction of left LE
  - Raises left upper extremity (UE) and laterally flexes right thorax
  - Poor pelvic stability, right hemipelvis drops

3. Seated tests

◆ Hip joint and knee flexion

- Observations of inefficient side: both
  - Weight shifts and rotates thorax right, elevates left UE

Author note
Included dorsiflexion and knee flexion test. Neither were efficient. Knee flexion and dorsiflexion: tibia externally rotates bilaterally. Included hip abduction with external rotation. Right was inefficient: weight shifts left and rotates thorax right.

- Slight improvement of left hip joint adduction and internal rotation
- Right hemipelvis able to lower
- Improved left lateral flexion
- No thoracic translation to right

◆ Hemipelvis superior motion

- Observations of inefficient side: both
  - Hemipelvis rises, equally on right and left
  - Femur adducts, equally on right and left
  - Thorax and weight do not translate to right

◆ Lateral pelvic shift

- Observations of inefficient side: left
  - Left LE able to internally rotate and adduct
  - No raising of left UE
  - Thorax does not right laterally flex but there is slight right thoracic rotation

3. Seated tests

◆ Hip joint and knee flexion

- Observations of inefficient side: both
  - Slight weight shift, no thoracic rotation or elevation of UE

Author note
Included dorsiflexion and knee flexion test. Neither were efficient. Knee flexion and dorsiflexion: tibia externally rotates bilaterally. Included hip abduction with external rotation. Right was inefficient, slight thoracic lateral flexion to right.

Chapter 4

4. Sit and stand

- ◆ Lateral view
  - Knee extension strategy more than hip joint extension strategy on left side
- ◆ Posterior view
  - Rotates pelvis to right and increased weight bearing through right LE to stand
- ◆ Anterior view
  - Less overall use of left LE
  - Knee extension strategy more than hip joint extension strategy on left side

5. Standing balance

- ◆ Two-leg stance, eyes open
  - 60 seconds
- ◆ One-leg stance, eyes open
  - Left leg: 60 seconds
  - Right leg: 60 seconds
- ◆ One-leg stance, eyes closed
  - Left leg: 8 seconds
  - Right leg: 11 seconds

4. Sit and stand

- ◆ Lateral view
  - Improved balance of hip joint extension and knee extension strategy bilaterally
- ◆ Posterior view
  - No pelvic rotation, equal weight bearing in LE to stand
- ◆ Anterior view
  - Equal use of LE from sit to stand
  - Improved balance of hip joint extension and knee extension strategy bilaterally

5. Standing balance

- ◆ Two-leg stance, eyes open
  - 60 seconds
- ◆ One-leg stance, eyes open
  - Left leg: 60 seconds
  - Right leg: 60 seconds
- ◆ One-leg stance, eyes closed
  - Left leg: 20 seconds
  - Right leg: 60 seconds

Session 3/12: Home program

Fatigue scale	1
Pain scale	1
Client self-report	• Ready to work
Key changes observed by author at end of Session 3/12	• Client able to understand instructions • Client able to modify or change previous movement habits, such as posterior pelvic tilt to initiate LE extension • No pain with activity
Reason behind choice of sequencing	• Fundamental movement skills for vocabulary and exercise understanding • Emphasis on symmetrical/bilateral exercises to decrease strain on SIJ • Using props for proprioception of pelvifemoral movement • Challenge with variety of positions from supine, prone, quadruped, full kneeling, and standing

Session movement sequence

1. Breathing	• Knee folds: alternating LE, abduction • Ribcage Arms • Puppet Arms • Upper abdominal curl (See Chapter 5 in Volume 1, Gentry and Grant)
Intent	• Find pain-free mid-range position • Three-dimensional breathing • Challenge torso adaptability with UE and LE movement • Maintain force closure with upper torso flexion
Gait reasoning	• Proprioception of client's pelvifemoral relative positioning in preparation for load transfer during standing • Control of TLJ supine with LE movement
Starting position	• Supine, hook lying, with the feet on mat about 6 in. (15 cm) apart • Explore lumbar-pelvic-femoral anteroposterior movement to determine any pain limits and feel pain-free mid-range position

Chapter 4

Movement description	• Three-dimensional breathing, emphasis on thoracic expansion
• Knee folds marching: single LE
• Abduct one LE, return to midline
• Puppet Arms: UE to ceiling, protract and retract to find mid-range scapular position, humerus congruent, elbows straight, palms facing one another
• Move one UE overhead with inhale, expanding ribs without anterior movement of TLJ; exhale and return to start
• Upper torso flexion: hands behind occiput, nod head on neck, eyes toward knees, articulate in flexion from C1–T3
• Stay in position for 10 breaths (breathing in for a count of 5 and out for a count of 5)
2. Bridge	(See Chapter 5 in Volume 1, Gentry: Spinal articulations/hip escalator)
Intent	• Activate pelvifemoral extension movement without pain
• Facilitate force and form closure
• Torso control without thoracolumbar hyperextension
Gait reasoning	• Hip joint extension for push-off
• Dynamic balance of flexors and extensors
• Balance for stance phase
Starting position	• Supine, hook lying, with the feet on the mat about 6 in. (15 cm) apart
• Equal pressure through medial and lateral longitudinal arches of feet
• Both UE pressing down into mat, elbows extended, posterior axilla pressing into floor
Movement description	• Articulate through torso until hip joints are extended
• No thoracolumbar hyperextension, keep pubis up, ribs low
• Hold for 1 minute, continue pressing into feet and UE/shoulder girdle
• Repeat with Magic Circle on outside of knees, pressing out into circle
• Repeat with 9 in. (23 cm) inflatable ball between knees, inflated enough to align center of distal femurs to femoral joints

Pilates and Sacroiliac Joint Dysfunction: Effect on Gait

3. Pistons (See Chapter 5 in Volume 1, Grant, Pistons)

Intent
- Activate the flexors to normalize the infrasternal angle (ISA)
- Challenge sustaining torso activation with TLJ in contact with mat to reverse thoracolumbar extension

Gait reasoning
- To be more efficient in thoracic rotation by reorientating the TLJ from overextension to central axis
- Practice the motion of alternating LE movement with activation of torso flexors to bring the torso to midline in standing

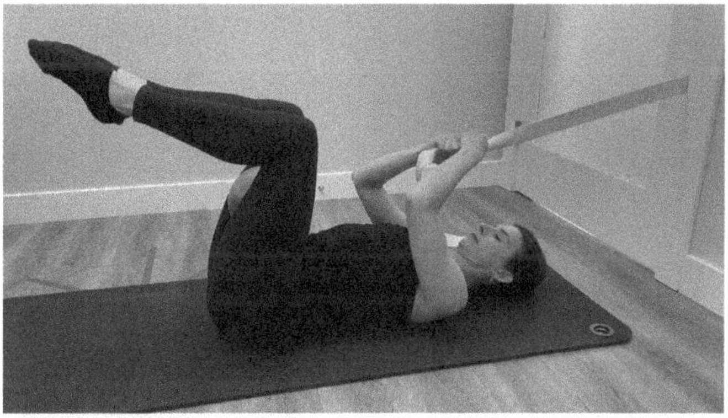

Figure 4.1

Set-up
- Fix a strap approximately 1 ft (30 cm) above level of mat, above the head
- Place a small pillow under head to activate flexion

Starting position
- Supine
- Supine hands hold the strap near the chest with elbows flexed
- Hip and knee joints in 90 degrees flexion
- 9 in. (23 cm) ball placed between the thighs at mid-thigh

Movement description
- Pull down firmly on the strap bringing elbows to sides
- Actively hold the ball at 90 degrees of hip and knee joints flexion
- Emphasize exhalation for facilitating ISA
- Hold for 1–3 minutes, building awareness and endurance
- Add flexion and extension, alternating LE in a piston action

Chapter 4

4. Swan — Derivative of J. H. Pilates Swan Dive (NPCE Study Guide 2021, p. 48)

Intent
- Activate torso extensors through torso articulation
- Facilitating the SIJ force closure through extensor activation from LE and UE

Gait reasoning
- Improve thoracic orientation to pelvis and feet for improved rotation
- Challenging the torso against gravity
- Balanced organization

Starting position
- Lie prone with head turned to the right
- Hip joints externally rotated, adducted
- Knee joints extended
- Ankles plantar flexed
- Palms on mat near shoulders
- Elbows flexed

Movement description
- Inhale, feeling whole body pre-activation
- Exhale, anterior abdominal wall moves away from the mat
- Inhale, press palms into the mat, gaze eyes forward
- Extend torso without hyperextension
- Elbows extend
- Exhale, lower torso to starting position turning head to the left
- Repeat 2 times for each side

5. Quadruped kneeling on roller

Intent
- Bilateral movement
- Improve proprioception of torso adapting to LE movement
- Challenge flexion and extension with control

Gait reasoning
- Challenging midline orientation with active hip joint flexion and extension
- Closed kinematic chain of UE to torso to feel connections of UE to LE through the torso

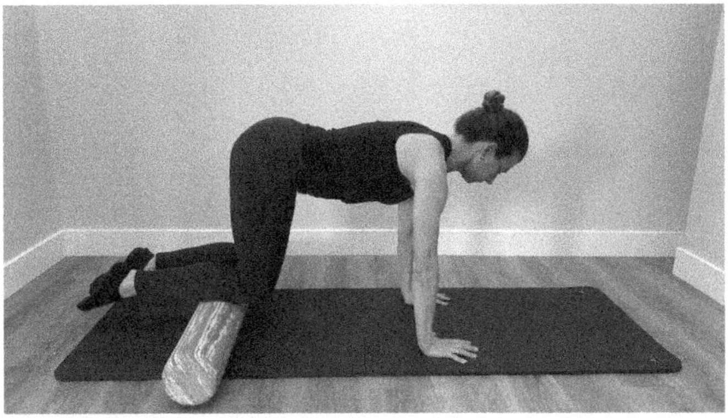

Figure 4.2

|Starting position | • Quadruped on mat with client's optimal organization for the movement task
• Shins on roller crosswise, hip and knee joints flexed at 90 degrees
• Hands on mat under shoulders
• Torso organized with attention to excessive lumbar lordosis and TLJ excessive movement |

|Movement description | • Exhale, feeling torso activation from UE and mid-shins on roller
• Maintain axial elongation of torso
• Inhale, rolling roller slightly back to extend femoral joints
• Exhale, returning to starting position
• Repeat 8 times |

6. Thigh stretch Derivative of J. H. Pilates Thigh Stretch on Universal Reformer (NPCE Study Guide 2021, p. 57)

| Intent | • Bilateral exercise with emphasis on continuity of LE into torso
• Eccentric activation of anterior torso in lean-back
• Posterior challenge to maintain central axis
• Dynamic activation of flexors and extensors |

| Gait reasoning | • Balance for stance phase
• Training to maintain central axis for improved midline orientation |

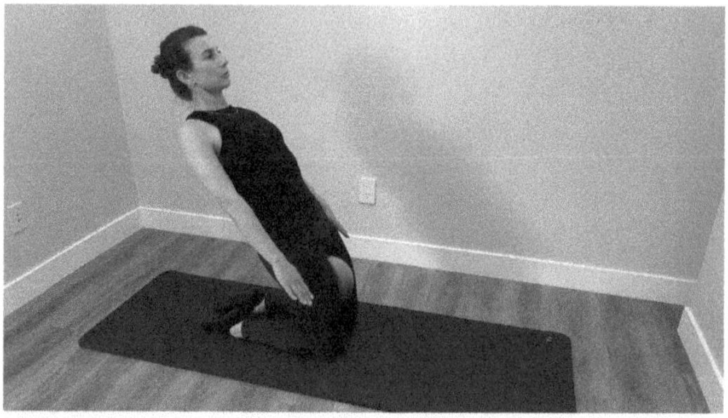

Chapter 4

Figure 4.3

Starting position	- Kneeling with hip joints extended
- Partially deflated 9 in. (23 cm) ball placed between the thighs at mid-femur
- Pad under shins to support the knees
- Reach UE forward with shoulders flexed at approximately 45 degrees
Movement description	- Inhale, extend shoulders, opening the chest and leaning back, keeping hip joints extended and torso in client's optimal organization for the movement task
- Exhale, press shins to mat and return to upright
- Arms return to starting position

7. Standing Footwork

Derivative of J. H. Pilates Footwork on Universal Reformer (NPCE Study Guide 2021, p. 52)

Intent
- Start with small squats
- Increase hip joint strategy versus knee extension strategy
- Bilateral exercise in weight bearing
- Activate from feet to torso

Gait reasoning
- Increasing hip joint extension strategy versus knee extension strategy for more efficient distribution of ground forces
- Pre-load LE articulating from feet
- Proprioception of joint patterning and timing in the sagittal plane

Pilates and Sacroiliac Joint Dysfunction: Effect on Gait

Starting position	• Standing on mat with heels together, balls of feet 2–3 in. (5–7 cm) apart
	• Weight evenly distributed through the feet
	• Torso aligned through central axis
	• Heels press together throughout exercise
Movement description	• Rise onto balls of feet, plantar flex
	• Slight flexion of hip and knee joints with ankle plantar flexion
	• Maintain hip and knee joint flexion, then dorsiflex ankles
	• Extend hip and knee joints initiating return with extension

8. Hundred	J. H. Pilates "Hundred" (NPCE Study Guide 2021, p. 46)
Intent	• Balanced use of flexors
	• Proximal activation of flexion
Gait reasoning	• Diminish hyperextension tendencies during gait

Editor note

In order to safely sustain the Hundred position this client has two options: 1. to initiate the Hundred with a posterior pelvic rotation or 2. to move the TLJ in the direction of flexion. To stimulate force closure in this position, the strategy of moving the TLJ is preferred.

Starting position	• Inhale to prepare
	• Exhale, extend upper extremities to mat and flex torso
	• Hold position
	• Move UE in small range alternating shoulder flexion and extension
	• Inhale 5 counts, exhale 5 counts
	• Repeat 10 cycles of breathing pattern
	• Return to starting position
Movement description	• Rise onto balls of feet, plantar flex
	• Slight flexion of hip and knee joints with ankle plantar flexion
	• Maintain hip and knee joint flexion, then dorsiflex ankles
	• Extend hip and knee joints initiating return with extension

9. Footwork on mat	Derivative of J. H. Pilates Footwork on Universal Reformer (NPCE Study Guide 2021, p. 52)
Intent	• Practice coordinated movement from feet to torso without hyperextension
	• Control and activation throughout the series

Gait reasoning	• Diminish hyperextension tendencies during gait
Starting position	• Supine on mat, hip and knee joints flexion toward chest
	• Heels together
	• Hands behind occiput, nod and curl up head
Movement description	• Inhale, extend LE
	• Exhale, flex LE
	• Perform 4–8 repetitions in three foot positions
	■ Pilates V
	■ Plantar flexion, hip joints adducted, inner edges of feet together
	■ Dorsiflexion, hip joints adducted, inner edges of feet together
	• Maintain torso position throughout series

Editor note
Pilates V is a position of the hip joint in external rotation, abduction. The calcanei are together with the forefeet about 2–3 in. (5–7 cm) apart. The feet appear to be in the shape of a V.

10. Roll-Up J. H. Pilates "Roll-Up" (NPCE Study Guide 2021, p. 46)

Intent	• Torso articulation in the sagittal plane
	• UE and LE continuity with torso
	• Twist variation for eccentric control in flexion or rotation
Gait reasoning	• Coordinated activation of flexion and extension for phases from leg swing to push-off
Starting position	• Supine with hip and knee joints extended
	• Ankles dorsiflexed
	• Shoulders flexed, elbows extended with hands on mat overhead
Movement description	• Inhale to feel whole-body pre-activation
	• Exhale, shoulder flexion with elbows extended to 90 degrees
	• Continue exhale as torso flexes from head to pelvis
	• Hands reach toward feet
	• Inhale
	• Exhale, reverse sequential movement, return to start position
	• Repeat 5 times

Pilates and Sacroiliac Joint Dysfunction: Effect on Gait

11. Spine Stretch	J. H. Pilates Spine Stretch (NPCE Study Guide 2021, p. 47)
Intent	• Improve torso articulation through the midline in the sagittal plane • Maintain SIJ force closure throughout movement by maintaining weight on ischial tuberosities without allowing the weight to shift posteriorly
Gait reasoning	• Find placement of center of mass (COM) over base of pelvic support prior to standing • Proprioception of SIJ force closure throughout torso flexion and extension
Starting position	• Seated upright on mat • Hip joints in flexion, abduction • Knee joints extended • Ankles in dorsiflexion • Shoulders 90 degrees flexion • Elbows extended
Movement description	• Inhale, feeling whole-body pre-activation • Exhale, flex the torso simultaneously from the head and lumbar region • Hands reach for the feet maintaining 90 degree shoulder flexion • Inhale in flexed position • Exhale, articulate the torso from flexion toward extension • Return to starting position • Repeat 5 times
12. Standing Roll-Down against wall	Derivative of J. H. Pilates Roll-Up (NPCE Study Guide 2021, p. 46) (See Chapter 5 in Volume 1, Kryzanowska, Wall series)
Intent	• Torso activation in flexion and extension in standing • Proprioception using the wall for feedback for organizing torso in standing • UE activation in the sagittal plane
Gait reasoning	• Orientating the torso in the sagittal plane, reducing hyperextension • UE mobility and activation in the sagittal plane for arm swing

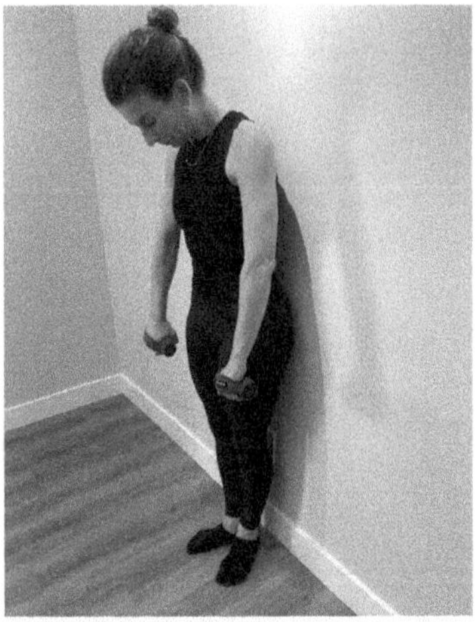

Chapter 4

Figure 4.4

Starting position	- Standing, with feet 10–12 in. (25–30 cm) from wall
- Torso against wall
- LE adducted, slight external rotation
- UE at sides holding 1-pound hand weights
Movement description	- Inhale, lifting hand weights in UE flexion
- Exhale, articulating in flexion from the head through the torso off the wall, down to the lowest ribs, with UE framing the head
- Inhale, articulating in extension from the pelvis to the head and return to wall
- Lower weights, shoulder flexion
- Repeat 5 times

Session 11/12: Studio session

Fatigue scale	4
Pain scale	0
Client self-report	- Home exercise program alternating mat with Universal Reformer without problems

| Key changes observed by author at end of Session 11/12 | • Improved whole-body movement and control on Universal Reformer
• Able to maintain appropriate tension, against resistance, through limbs and torso control
• Consistent load transfer from UE or LE to torso, and control for hypomobility |
|---|---|
| Reason behind choice of sequencing | • Universal Reformer workout without pain was primary goal of client
• Progression from beginner to intermediate Universal Reformer sequence without pain increased client confidence
• Client recognized and felt SIJ support through bilateral movements
• Developed the coordination patterning in bilateral movement and ready to challenge with unilateral movements
• Client recognized and corrected non-optimal movements such as initiating leg movements with posterior pelvic tilt
• Client able to maintain control throughout and into end of range movements while working with spring resistance |

Session movement sequence

1. Footwork on Universal Reformer	J. H. Pilates Footwork on Universal Reformer (NPCE Study Guide 2021, p. 52)
Intent	• Activating hip joint extension without excessive knee extension
• Pre-loading and movement reeducation from feet to torso in supine
• Practice coordinating breath with movement focusing on maintaining torso support
• Bilateral movement
Gait reasoning	• Articulate from feet to torso for improved transfer of weight
• Encourage hip joint strategy more than knee strategy for push-off
• Mobilize and dynamically engage feet for improved adaption to ground surfaces
Set-up	• 4 springs
• Headrest up
• Footbar up

Chapter 4

Starting position	• Supine on carriage • Pilates V • Arches • Heels • Tendon stretch/prehensile • UE press down on carriage
Movement description	• Inhale, extend hip joints and knees moving carriage away from footbar • Exhale and flex, externally rotate hip joints, flex knees returning carriage

Editor note
Pilates V is a position of the hip joint in external rotation, abduction. The calcanei are together with the forefeet about 2–3 in. (5–7 cm) apart. The feet appear to be in the shape of a V.

Arches foot position is the midfoot placed on the footbar with "Janda short foot formation" (Page, Frank, and Lardner 2010).

Heels is the placement of the plantar surface of the midpoint of the calcanei.

Tendon Stretch/Prehensile is the placement of the forefoot on footbar with the distal end of the metatarsals in contact with the bar. The ankle is in dorsiflexion.

CUES
- Pressing femurs toward the floor assists in hip joint extension
- Press arms and lean thorax into the carriage to prevent sliding into shoulder stops

Author note
Client initially had a very strong knee extension movement pattern during gait, in squats, and rising from a chair. She tended to initiate leg movement with posteriorly rotating the pelvis. The posteriorly rotated pelvis resulted in non-optimal position of the sacrum relative to the pelvis (optimum position is necessary for form closure of the SIJ).

2. Hundred on Universal Reformer

J. H. Pilates Hundred on Universal Reformer (NPCE Study Guide 2021, p. 52)

Intent
- Sagittal plane movement
- Activation of flexors with torso control
- LE adduction, external rotation, extension
- Increase depth of breathing
- Axial elongation of torso

Gait reasoning Information not provided

Editor note
In order to safely sustain the Hundred position, this client has two options: 1. to initiate the Hundred with a posterior pelvic rotation or 2. to move the TLJ in the direction of flexion. To stimulate force closure in this position, the strategy of moving the TLJ is preferred.

Set-up
- 3–4 springs
- Footbar down
- Headrest up

Starting position
- Supine
- Hold handles at 90 degrees shoulder flexion
- Elbows extended
- Hips flexed 90 degrees
- Knees extended
- Feet plantar flexed

Movement description
- Inhale to prepare
- Exhale, pull straps extending upper extremities and flex torso
- Hold position
- Move UE in small range alternating shoulder flexion and extension
- Inhale 5 counts, exhale 5 counts
- Repeat 10 cycles of breathing pattern
- Return to starting position

CUES
- Articulate into flexion from head to torso
- Activate legs from inner heels stimulating LE to torso
- On exhale draw anterior abdominal wall posteriorly
- Small range of motion (ROM) of rhythmic shoulder flexion and extension without moving the carriage

3. Short Spine Massage on Universal Reformer

J. H. Pilates Short Spine Massage on Universal Reformer (NPCE Study Guide 2021, p. 56)

Intent
- Facilitates articulation and suspension of torso
- Reduces excessive anterior activation

Gait reasoning
- Torso control through the sagittal plane, especially at TLJ
- Use of hip joint extensors more than knee extensors
- Activation of feet stimulating torso articulation

Set-up
- 2 springs
- Headrest down
- Footbar down
- Straps on feet

Starting position
- Supine on carriage
- Hip joint flexed and externally rotated
- Knees flexed toward chest
- Feet in straps, ankle plantar flexion with calcanei together
- UE presses down into carriage

Movement description
- Inhale, begin hip joints flexion to point of pelvis posterior rotation
- Allow pelvis to be lifted off carriage
- Maintain pressing into feet loops
- Stop at mid- to upper thorax
- Flex knees maintaining tension in straps
- Exhale, press head into headrest and arches of feet into loops
- Slowly articulate down from mid-thorax to pelvis
- Return to starting position
- Repeat 3 times

CUES
- Maintain continuous tension of straps throughout movement
- As knees flex, ischial tuberosities remain high
- Axillas and palms of hands press on to carriage during descent of torso

Editor note
The distribution of peripheral ground forces, with the feet in loops (straps) and the arms on the carriage, informs proximal integrity. The goal is to move with control through an active ROM reducing hypermobility.

4. Stomach Massage: Round Back and Flat Back on Universal Reformer

J. H. Pilates Stomach Massage (NPCE Study Guide 2021, p. 56)

Editor note
According to the NPCE Study Guide, Round Back is torso flexion. In Flat Back the hands press into the shoulder stops to facilitate thoracic extension. The feet on the elevated footbar facilitates hip joint flexion and posterior pelvis action. To maintain force closure in this seated position, place a small box under the pelvis to reduce flexion or place the box between the sacrum and shoulder stops (see Chapter 5, Trier).

Intent
- Activation of torso with hip and knee joint movement while maintaining force closure
- UE active continuity to the torso
- Heels gently press together activating LE to torso

Gait reasoning
- Pre-loading torso from feet on footbar with spring resistance
- UE activation to torso establishing midline connection to feet

Set-up
- 3–4 springs
- Non-skid rubberized mat on lower edge of Universal Reformer
- Footbar up

Starting position
- Sit on edge of Universal Reformer carriage, pelvis posteriorly rotated
- Hip joints externally rotated and abducted
- Metatarsals on footbar, calcanei touching
- Round Back
  - Hands placed and pressing into edge of carriage, torso in flexion
  - Eyes gazing toward abdominal wall
- Flat Back
  - Hands behind holding and pressing into shoulder stops
  - Extend thorax
  - Eyes gazing forward

Movement description
- Maintain Round Back position
  - Extend, externally rotate hip joints and knees moving carriage away from footbar
  - Dorsiflex ankles
  - Plantar flex ankles
  - Flex, externally rotate, abduct hip joints, flex knees moving carriage toward footbar
  - Repeat 10 times
- Maintain Flat Back position
  - Repeat same lower extremity sequence 10 times

CUES
- Eyes gazing downward with head balanced well with torso flexion
- Place feet on front frame with hands holding carriage, prior to placing feet on footbar to feel the continuous activation from hands and feet into torso
- Maintain continuous activation and place feet on footbar

Editor note
This specific client employs a standing movement strategy of excessive extension at the TLJ and end-range nutation with increased hip joint flexion. Round Back position is appropriate to restore the integrity of the TLJ with respect to the sacrum and force closure.

CUES: FLAT BACK
- Lean back with client's optimal organization for the movement task and maintaining force closure
- Pelvifemoral movement of extension and flexion

Editor note
The continuous activation from the hands pressing the shoulder stops facilitates a force vector that increases the tone of the torso extensors. To balance the force, a counter-reaction of posterior translation of the neck is necessary to balance the head on the vertical axis.

5. Ladder Barrel J. H. Pilates Swan Dive on Ladder Barrel (NPCE Study Guide 2021, p. 84)

Intent
- Activate the extensors stimulating force closure of the SIJ
- Active torso extension with uniform ROM and control of TL
- Feet pressing into wall to facilitate ground force
- UE movement of abduction to full flexion promotes extensor activity

Gait reasoning
- Establish proprioception of balanced torso extension and foot grounding
- Mobility of thorax for improved rotation

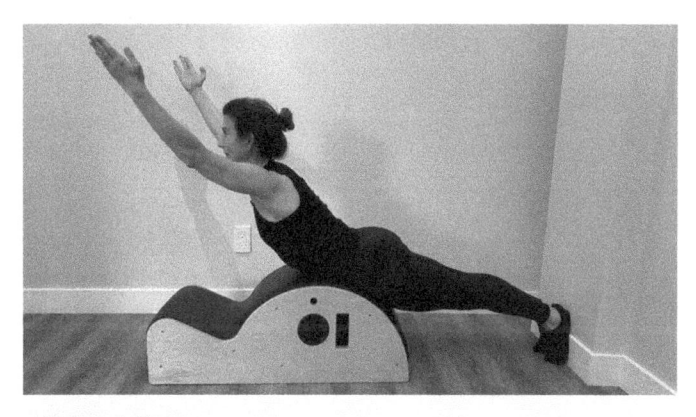

Figure 4.5
Derivative of J. H. Pilates "Swan on the Spine Corrector" (NPCE Study Guide p. 82)

Starting position
- Stand inside facing barrel, ladder to back
- Hold side of barrel to move into position
- Place anterior pelvis against the barrel
- Place metatarsals of both feet on lower rung of ladder
- Hip joints externally rotated and abducted
- Knees flexed
- Calcanei together
- Flex torso over the barrel
- Shoulders flexed overhead
- Elbows slightly flexed

Movement description
- Inhale, extend torso upright pressing pelvis into barrel and feet against rung
- Move into vertical torso position with arms overhead
- Exhale, move arms to 90 degrees abduction
- Inhale, simultaneously extend and externally rotate hip joints, extend knees, arms sweep overhead
- Exhale, flex over barrel returning to starting position

CUES

- Press feet into the ladder rung as the torso extends
- Let eyes follow the extension from the floor to the wall; choose an image such as "follow a ladybug crawling across the floor and up the wall in front of you"
- Feel your collarbones widen and rotate posteriorly with elevating arm movement
- Maintain torso length during descent phase, returning to starting position

Author note

It is important to cue the eyes to direct the movement from the head. When the thorax is immobile or excessively kyphotic, a possible compensation is for the upper cervical region to extend, placing the head forward of the COM. To counterbalance the head, the pelvis will posteriorly rotate causing the loss of SIJ force closure. Sustaining this compensation may cause strain of the posterior torso, specifically the ligamentous system that crosses the SIJ to the LE (Decker and Davidson 2017).

6. Backstroke on Universal Reformer

J. H. Pilates BackStroke on Universal Reformer (NPCE Study Guide 2021, p. 54)

Intent
- Proximal torso control with UE and LE movement
- Activation of torso flexors and extensors

Gait reasoning
- Torso control with limb motion

Set-up
- 2 springs
- Long box on Universal Reformer
- Hold handles

Starting position
- Supine on box
- Hips and knees flexed fully
- Feet in Pilates V
- Hold handles at forehead, forearms pronated (palms facing away)
- Trunk in upper abdominal curl

Movement description
- Inhale and reach UE and LE to ceiling
- Abduct UE and LE
- Circle LE back into adduction
- UE reach to thighs
- Exhale and return UE and LE back to starting position
- Reverse movement sequence

CUES
- Use the contact points on the long box to ensure optimal pelvic position for force closure, with weight at about S2
- Use tension of hands in straps and activation of the legs to stimulate torso activation
- Use the breath: exhale for drawing the thorax downward as the anterior thorax moves inferiorly while the posterior thorax moves superiorly and the abdominal wall moves posteriorly
- Important to maintain COM at S2 during flexion and limb movement

7. Teaser on Universal Reformer — J. H. Pilates Teaser on Universal Reformer (NPCE Study Guide 2021, p. 54)

Intent
- Challenging sagittal plane exercise
- Full-range torso movement on stationary LE and UE for developing balance of torso

Gait reasoning
- Reorganizing excessive TLJ rotation through torso control to enable improved midline for rotation during gait

Set-up — Information not recorded

Starting position — Information not recorded

Movement description — Information not recorded

CUES
- Movement occurs as one continuous motion, with the whole body moving from supine to teaser position
- Find the balance on the ischial tuberosities with sacral nutation and the TLJ posteriorly to sense the whole torso weight over COM

8. Long Stretch: Front on Universal Reformer — J. H. Pilates Long Stretch (NPCE Study Guide 2021, p. 55)

Intent
- Challenging whole-body exercise for torso control through distal activation
- Facilitating loading the UE, LE, and torso in a horizontal position while moving against resistance from springs

Gait reasoning
- Improving organization of TLJ to sacrum to assist in optimal rotational motion when standing

Chapter 4

Set-up   Information not recorded
Starting position   Information not recorded
Movement description   Information not recorded

CUES
- Maintain the torso organization from head to heels throughout the movement
- When pressing carriage away from footbar, use a sustained exhale to assist in maintaining client's optimal organization for the movement task

Author note
Client routinely does planks, push-ups, and TRX. This exercise helped her to improve axial elongation and stamina with optimal placement of torso.

9. Down Stretch on Universal Reformer

J. H. Pilates Down Stretch (NPCE Study Guide 2021, p. 55)

Intent
- Challenging whole-body exercise
- Maintain client's optimal organization for the movement task with LE extension and flexion
- Plantar flexion of feet, pressing on shoulder stops to stimulate posterior activation

Gait reasoning
- Stimulation of posterior activation from the feet to assist in push-off
- Encourages optimal extension strategy
- Adequate hip joint extension ROM allows for freedom of torso extension
- Decreasing excessive knee extension strategy during gait will decrease stress on patellofemoral joints

Set-up
- Springs: 1 medium and 1 light
- Footbar in high position

Starting position
- Springs: 1 medium and 1 light
- Footbar in high position

CUES
- Equal and opposite forces pressing into hands and feet
- Breathing pattern with inhale as carriage returns to facilitate torso extension
- Maintain the length between the pubic rami to xyphoid process
- Allow the eyes to follow the movement

Author note
It is typical of a hypermobile client to overextend the anterior hip joint, "hanging" rather than maintaining the sacral nutation (force closure) and congruent hip joints.

10. Knee Stretch Series on Universal Reformer

J. H. Pilates Knee Stretch (NPCE Study Guide 2021, p. 60)

Intent
- Integrate whole-body flexion and extension movement patterning
- Arched Back exercise increases SIJ stability via form closure

Gait reasoning
- Hip extension and plantar flexion necessary for push-off
- Hip extension strategy greater than knee flexion strategy

Set-up
- 2 springs
- Headrest and footbar up

Starting position
- Kneel on carriage with feet against shoulder stops
- Hold footbar, hands shoulder-width apart
- Torso flexion for Round Back and Knees Off versions
- Torso extension for Arched Back version

Movement description
- Press feet into shoulder stops
- Extend hip joints moving carriage away from footbar
- Maintain torso position
- Flex hip joints slowly returning carriage
- Repeat 10 times

11. Running on Universal Reformer

J. H. Pilates Running on Universal Reformer (NPCE Study Guide 2021, p. 60)

Intent
- Continuous activation from feet to torso
- Improve ankle articulation

Gait reasoning
- Improve stance phase with elastic recoil from the feet
- Dynamic dorsiflexion and plantar flexion articulating the feet to transfer weight in gait

Set-up
- 4 springs
- Headrest and footbar up

Starting position
- Supine on carriage
- Metatarsals on footbar, feet hip-joint-distance apart
- Hip joints flexed, adducted with knees flexed
- UE by sides pressing down on carriage

Chapter 4

Movement description
- Inhale, press feet into footbar extending hip and knee joints, moving carriage away from footbar
- Dorsiflex right ankle with knee extension
- Plantar flex left ankle while flexing left knee
- Alternate sides in a running motion
- Repeat 10 times

CUE
- Imagine almost jumping off the bar during the transitions between plantar flexion and dorsiflexion

Author note
The imagery of almost jumping off the bar activates proximally from the feet through the hip joints and torso—a whole-body activation.

12. Pelvic Lift on Universal Reformer

J. H. Pilates Pelvic lift (NPCE Study Guide 2021, p. 60)

Intent
- Initiating from pelvifemoral extension to aid in SIJ support
- Extension and flexion articulation for hip joint

Gait reasoning
- Improve hip joint extension for push-off phase
- Increase hip joint movement to decrease hypermobility of lumbar region improving overall quality of gait

Set-up
- 4 springs
- Headrest up

Starting position
- Supine on carriage
- Metatarsals on footbar
- Hip joints adducted, medial ankles together
- UE press down on carriage

Movement description
- Maintaining carriage at shoulder stops, begin hip joint extension
- Sequentially posteriorly rotate pelvis elevating pelvis 5 in. (12.7 cm)
- Maintain the lifted pelvis
- Extend hip and knee joints
- Repeat 6–8 times
- Finish at shoulder stops
- Sequentially lower pelvis from lumbar region to hip joints
- Return to starting position

CUES
* Move into the pelvic lift without moving the carriage
* Maintain the height of the pelvis throughout the movement to activate extensors in both directions of carriage movement

Author note
Years after birth, postpartum women lack strength and control of the LE and torso. The tendency is to posteriorly rotate the pelvis, either due to lack of lumbar lordosis, or because they are trying to support themselves by relying on the anterior position of the femoral joints that changes COM. Restoring the support of the torso over the COM equally weighted on both feet will help improve movement capacity and diminish pain.

13. Splits: Side on Universal Reformer

J. H. Pilates Splits: Side on Universal Reformer (NPCE Study Guide 2021, p. 61)

Intent
- Increase activation of hip joints to improve stance
- Activate the legs in external rotation, abduction, and adduction
- Improve glide of femoral head in acetabulum

Gait reasoning
- Improve ability and balance for one-leg stance phase
- Increase load in standing

Set-up
- 2 medium springs
- Footbar down, attach standing platform

Starting position
- Stand sideways on Universal Reformer with one foot on standing platform and one foot on carriage
- Externally rotate legs 45 degrees
- Knees extended

Movement description
- Inhale, pressing carriage out
- Exhale, resisting carriage closing
- Repeat 8 times
- Repeat on other side

Chapter 4

Author note
New mothers feel pressure to get their pre-baby body back very quickly after giving birth. The tendency is to exercise in ways that move the SIJ asymmetrically before there is adequate motor control support of the SIJ that can lead to chronic SIJ irritation and instability. It is wise to progress slowly to build client's control and confidence before moving to more challenging standing exercises that are splitting the legs in different directions, placing additional strain on the SIJ.

14. Jumping on Universal Reformer

Intent
- Dynamic torso control and support while jumping
- Gives client a sense of landing on their feet at end of session
- Dynamic, exhilarating exercise, particularly for those unable to jump or run post-injury or with a disability

Gait reasoning
- Initiate LE movement with hip strategy versus knee strategy
- Varying weight bearing
- Introduces pre-loading with single leg support while jumping on one leg while supine
- Motor control challenge for one-leg stance

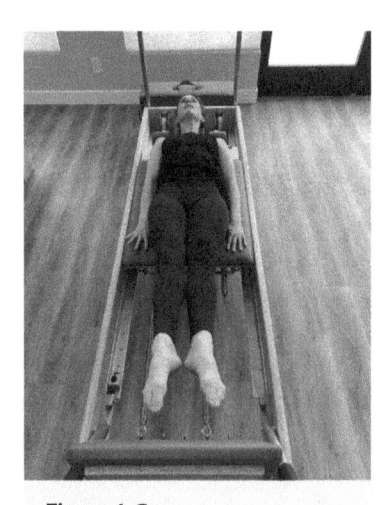

Figure 4.6

Set-up
- Jump board affixed to Universal Reformer
- 2 medium springs
- Headrest up

Starting position
- Supine on carriage
- UE by sides pressing down into carriage
- Feet parallel on jump board hip-joint-distance apart
- Hip and knee joints in flexion
- Carriage at shoulder stops

Movement description
- Press into feet
- Extend hip and knee joints, strongly plantar flexing to jump
- Land articulating through feet from forefoot to calcaneus
- Flex hip and knee joints and rebound for next jump
- Repeat 20 times
- Progress from bilateral to unilateral jumping

CUES
- Jump and land softly and quietly
- Imagine the jump board is like hot cement: you want to land and jump off it quickly!

Author note
The jump board is a terrific way to return to jumping with reduced load. Lying on the carriage provides sensory feedback of landing. The teacher easily observes the patterning of the entire body during dynamic movement, such as medial collapse (excess adduction and internal rotation of the femur and excessive pronation and collapse of the medial arch of the foot). For a more optimal strategy, use cues to guide the client to experience a change in their strategy.

The journey to Session 11

Session 4/12
Client self-report

- Fatigue scale 2
- Pain scale 1

Key changes observed

- Some hip joint "clicking" during Swan on the ball, which improved with changes of torso control
- Client did well with home program and is ready to progress

Reasoning behind choice of movements

- Discontinued fundamentals
- Client was not familiar with a classical sequence of exercises
- Balanced progression of all planes of motion (flexion, extension, rotation, and lateral flexion)
- Exercise sequence in accord with developmental sequence: supine, prone, sitting, standing

Session movement sequence
1. Hundred, modified

Chapter 4

2. Standing Footwork

3. Roll-Up with modification

4. Universal Reformer

- Footwork
- Hundred

5. Trapeze Table

- Roll-Down

6. Mat

- Single Leg Stretch
- Double Leg Stretch

7. Trapeze Table

- Push-Through Seated Front

8. Additional movements

- Swan with 26 in. (65 cm) ball
- Standing Footwork

Session 5/12
Client self-report

- Fatigue scale 4
- Pain scale 2

Key changes observed

- Decrease in anterior femoral tightness sensation due to improved connective tissue glide
- Noticed "pinchy" sensation in left anterior pelvifemoral area while doing the Hundred on the Universal Reformer, but not on the mat with wall for assistance

Reasoning behind choice of movements

- Balanced progression of torso movement
- Exercise progression via developmental sequence: supine, prone, sitting, kneeling, standing
- LE moving bilaterally, not unilaterally

Session movement sequence

1. Progressed from 5 small squats to Standing Footwork

2. Roll-Up

3. Spine Stretch

4. Standing Roll-Down at wall

5. Universal Reformer

- Footwork
- Hundred

6. Trapeze Table

- Roll-Down
- Leg springs with loops clipped together, hip joint extension/flexion only

7. Mat
- Roll Like a Ball

8. Additional movements

- Mat
  - Spine Stretch
  - Saw
- Trapeze Table
  - Parakeet, bilateral, legs only
- Mat
  - Swan with 22 in. (55 cm) ball
- Trapeze Table
  - Kneeling Mermaid, with partially deflated 9 in. (23 in.) ball between thighs at mid-femur

Session 6/12
Client self-report

- Fatigue scale 2
- Pain scale 1

Key changes observed

- Client gaining skill in force closure for support of SIJ, requiring fewer cues

Reasoning behind choice of movements

- Balanced progression of torso movements
- Progressed exercises according to developmental sequence
- LE moving bilaterally, not unilaterally
- One of client's goals was to be able to do a full workout on the Universal Reformer without pain; this session utilized the Universal Reformer almost exclusively in a classical order

Session movement sequence

1. Quadruped to kneeling on foam roller

2. Roll-Up without modification

3. Universal Reformer

- Footwork
- Hundred
- Short Spine Massage
- Coordination, with small, slow LE abduction/adduction
- Stomach Massage: Round Back, Flat Back

4. Additional movements

- Universal Reformer
  - Swan with 55 cm ball
  - Short Box Series
    - Round Back
    - Flat Back
  - Long Stretch Series
    - Long Stretch
    - Elephant
  - Knee Stretch Series
    - Round Back
    - Arched Back
  - Running and pelvic lift

> **Editor note**
> In Short Box Series Flat Back, the primary articulation occurs at the pelvifemoral joints. The spatial relationship of the thorax and pelvis is sustained throughout the pelvifemoral motion in the sagittal plane. Torso articulation is minimized.

Session 7/12
Client self-report

- Fatigue scale 8
- Pain scale 3
- Yoga, intensive all weekend, more tired than painful
- Able to do asymmetrical yoga poses with modifications, concentration, and without pain

Key changes observed

- Client seems tired but able to do exercises with good control and concentration

Reasoning behind choice of movements

- Decreased number and speed of exercises due to client fatigue

Session movement sequence

1. Rolling Like a Ball

2. Single Leg Stretch, Double Leg Stretch

Chapter 4

3. Saw

4. Stomach Massage on 22 in. (55 cm) ball, feet on wall

5. Universal Reformer

- Footwork
- Hundred
- Short Spine Massage
- Stomach Massage: Round Back, Flat Back

6. Swan on Spine Corrector

- Universal Reformer
  - Short Box Series
    - Round Back
    - Flat Back
  - Long Stretch Series
    - Long Stretch
    - Downstretch
    - Elephant
  - Knee Stretch Series
    - Round Back
    - Arched Back
  - Running and Pelvic Lift

Session 8/12
Client self-report

- Fatigue scale 6
- Pain scale 0

Key changes observed

- Client able to tolerate more yoga poses, with modifications and without pain
- Difficulty keeping pelvis from rotating to the right on Kneeling Mermaid

Reasoning behind choice of movements

- Utilized the Wunda Chair for personal workout variety and challenge
- Continued bilateral exercises
- Increased torso extension in home program, emphasizing lumbopelvic-femoral control

Session movement sequence
1. Single Leg Kick

2. Double Leg Kick

3. Wunda Chair

- Double Leg Pumps, all variations

4. Mat

- Hundred

5. Wunda Chair

- Washer Woman/Hamstring 2 (NPCE Study Guide 2021, p. 77)
- Spine Stretch Forward, Sitting Arm Push-Down
- Supine LE abduction/flexion with knee flexion and hip joint extension/flexion

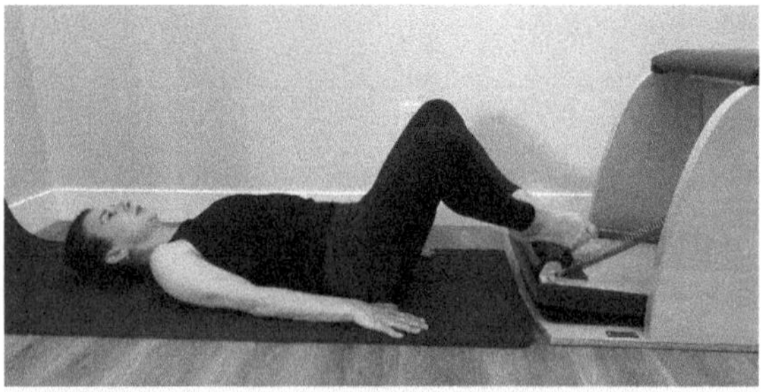

Figure 4.7

6. Additional movements

- Wunda Chair

Pilates and Sacroiliac Joint Dysfunction: Effect on Gait

- Swan Front and chest press
- Kneeling Mermaid/Side Arm Kneeling (Figure 4.8), with 9 in. (23 cm) partially deflated ball between the thighs at mid-femur
- Pull-Up
- Hamstring 3

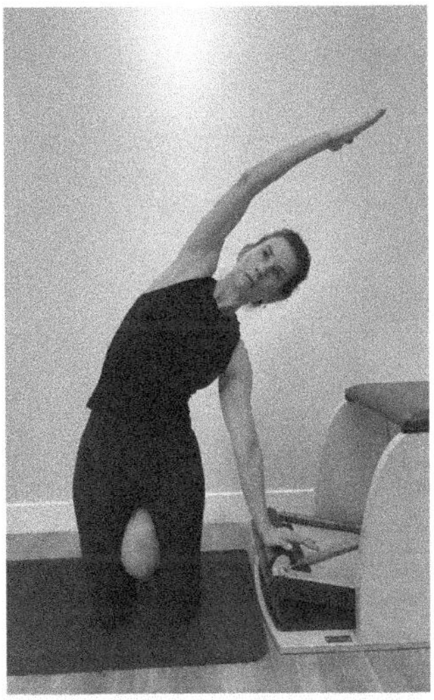

Figure 4.8

Session 9/12
Client self-report

- Fatigue scale 5
- Pain scale 1

Key changes observed

- Nothing noted

Reasoning behind choice of movements

- Discontinued Stomach Massage
- Continuation of building the session sequence

Session movement sequence
1. Rollover

2. Trapeze Table

- Hundred with springs attached low at one end of the frame
- Roll-Down
- Breathing (see Chapter 5 in Volume 1, Trier, Breathing coordination)
- Parakeet
- Magician

3. Additional movements

- Wunda Chair
    - Kneeling Mermaid
    - Swan
- Universal Reformer
    - Chest Expansion
    - Thigh Stretch
- Trapeze Table
    - Standing on floor (arm springs)
        - Punching
        - Butterfly

Session 10/12
Client self-report

- Fatigue scale 5
- Pain scale 1

Key changes observed

- Better initiation of femoral joint extension
- Less posterior pelvic tilt prior to hip joint flexion

Reasoning behind choice of movements

- Full Universal Reformer workout without pain
- Sessions 4–9 used the full suite of client's studio equipment

161

Chapter 4

- Session 10 utilized Universal Reformer at appropriate challenge level and pace

Session movement sequence
1. Full home program on mat

- Footwork
- Hundred
- Roll-Up
- Rollover
- Rolling Like a Ball
- Single Leg Stretch
- Double Leg Stretch
- Spine Stretch
- Corkscrew
- Saw
- Swan (with 22 in. [55 cm] ball)
- Single Leg Kick
- Double Leg Kick
- Bridge with variations
- Standing Footwork
- Wall

2. Universal Reformer

- Footwork
- Hundred
- Short Spine Massage
- Stomach Massage
  - Round Back
  - Flat Back
- Swan

3. Additional movements

- Long Box Series
  - Pulling Straps (Figure 4.9)
  - Backstroke
  - Teaser
- Short Box Series
  - Round Back
  - Flat Back
  - Side Bend (Figure 4.10)
  - Twist (Figure 4.11)

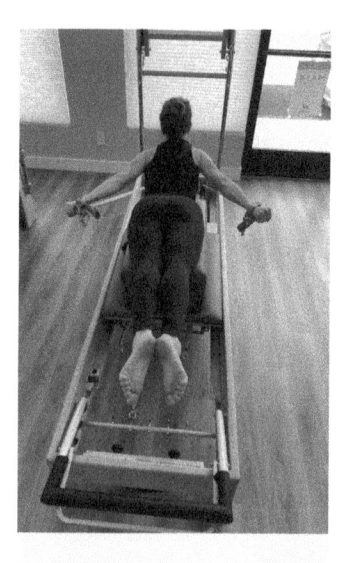

Figure 4.9

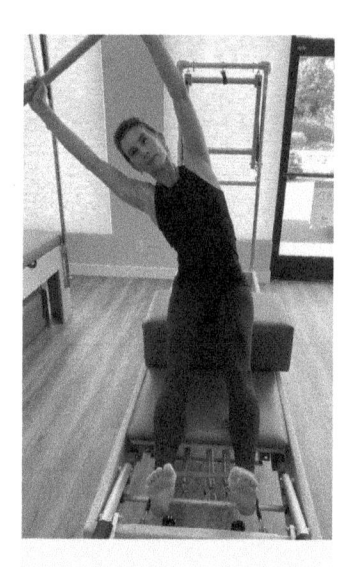

Figure 4.10

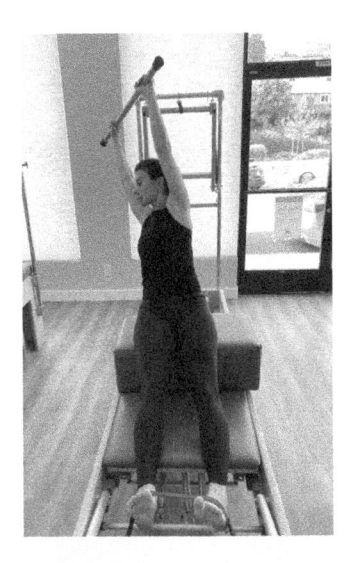

Figure 4.11

- Long Stretch Series
  - Long Stretch
  - Elephant
- Chest Expansion
  - Kneeling
  - Thigh Stretch
- Knee Stretch Series
  - Standing
  - Knees Off
- Pelvic Lift and Running
- Splits: Side

References

Ali, A., Andrzejowski, P., Kanakaris, N. K., and Giannoudis, P. V. (2020) "Pelvic girdle pain, hypermobility spectrum disorder and hypermobility-type Ehlers-Danlos syndrome: A narrative literature review." *Journal of Clinical Medicine, 9,* 12. DOI: 10.3390/jcm9123992.

Chuang, C. W., Hung, S. K., Pan, P. T., Kao, M. C. (2019) "Diagnosis and interventional pain management options for sacroiliac joint pain." *Tzu Chi Medical Journal, 31,* 4, 207–210.

Decker, M. J. and Davidson, B. S. (2017) "The ligamentous-myofascial system." In T. Liem, P. Tozzi, and A. Chila (Eds.) *Fascia in the Osteopathic Field.* Edinburgh: Handspring Publishing, p. 27.

Demmler, J., Atkinson, M., Reinhold, E., Choy, E., Lyons, R. A., and Brophy, S. T. (2019) "Diagnosed prevalence of Ehlers-Danlos syndrome and hypermobility spectrum disorder in Wales, UK: A national electronic cohort study and case–control comparison." *BMJ Open, 9.* DOI: 10.1136/bmjopen-2019-031365.

Enix, D. E. and Mayer, J. M. (2019) "Sacroiliac joint hypermobility biomechanics and what it means for health care providers and patients." *PM&R, 11,* Suppl. 1, S32–S39.

Falowski, S., Sayed, D., Pope, J., Patterson, D. *et al.* (2020) "A review and algorithm in the diagnosis and treatment of sacroiliac joint pain." *Journal of Pain Research, 13,* 3337–3348.

Gutke, A., Boissonnault, J., Brook, G., and Stuge, B. (2018) "The severity and impact of pelvic girdle pain and low-back pain in pregnancy: A multinational study." *Journal of Women's Health, 27,* 4, 510–517.

Hides, J. A., Donelson, R., Lee, D., Prather, H., Sahrmann, S. A., and Hodges, P. W. (2019) "Convergence and divergence of exercise-based approaches that incorporate motor control for the management of low back pain." *Journal of Orthopaedic & Sports Physical Therapy, 49,* 6, 437–452.

Jonely, H., Avery, M., and Desai, M. (2020) "Chronic sacroiliac joint and pelvic girdle pain and dysfunction successfully managed with a multimodal and multidisciplinary approach: A case series." *Orthopaedic Practice, 32,* 3, 154–160.

NPCE Study Guide (National Pilates Certification Exam Study Guide) (2021) Miami, FL: National Pilates Certification Program, Inc.

Page, P., Frank, C. C., and Lardner, R. (2010) "Assessment and Treatment of Muscle Imbalance: The Janda Approach." [E-book]. Human Kinetics, pp. 163–164. www.humankinetics.com. [Accessed August 8, 2023].

Rupert, M. P., Lee, M., Manchikanti, L., Datta, S., and Cohen, S. P. (2009) "Evaluation of sacroiliac joint interventions: A systemic appraisal of the literature." *Pain Physician, 12,* 399–418.

Schneider, B. J., Rosati, R., Zheng, P., and McCormick, Z. L. (2019) "Challenges in diagnosing sacroiliac joint pain: A narrative review." *PM&R, 11,* Suppl. 1, S40–S45.

Vleeming, A. and Schuenke, M. (2019) "Form and force closure of the sacroiliac joints." *PM&R, 11,* Suppl. 1, S24–S31.

Chapter 5

Pilates and Hip Joint Dysfunction: Effect on Gait

Glenn Withers

Hip joint pain is one of the most common complaints that presents in Pilates studios around the world. Pain in the hip joint region affects clients of all ages. In our clinic the range of ages with hip joint pain is 12 years of age and older. It is often considered that hip joint pain conditions are most commonly related to osteoarthritis. Current estimates of osteoarthritis pain in the hip joint and knee exceed 300 million cases worldwide (GBD study, 2015) however, hip joint pain is not confined to osteoarthritis. Labral tears, trochanteric bursitis, and gluteal tendinopathies are also associated with pain in this region. Among adults who play sports, the incidence of chronic hip pain is 30 to 40 percent (Thorberg et. a, 2017). Among all adults over 60, the incidence of hip pain is 12 to 15 percent (Christmas et al, 2002). In younger adults, hip pain related to labral injuries and synovitis are considered extremely common (Paoloni, 2020). .

Hip-related intra-articular overload injuries are common in young athletes. Most athletes can continue to train with pain for many months until eventually forced to withdraw from exercise due to pain. Continuing to train with pain can lead to development of non-functional movement patterns and compensation strategies which may further contribute to decreased function and performance.

Femoroacetabular impingement (FAI) has been defined as a motion-related clinical disorder with a triad of symptoms, clinical signs, and imaging findings. The primary symptoms are motion- or position-related pain in the anterior pelvifemoral or groin region, with potential clicking, catching, locking, stiffness, restricted hip range of motion (ROM), or the joint "giving way." There are two types of FAI—"cam" (osteophytes in the zone of the femoral head-neck junction) and "pincer" (osteophytes at the acetabular edges). A combination of both cam and pincer may be present.

Cam-type FAI has been shown to be common in young athletes resulting in sub-optimal function with effects on spinopelvic motion. Cam-type FAI impingement is characterized by a non-spherical femoral head or by an insufficient offset between the femoral head and neck.

This abnormal joint morphology combined with repetitive loading from the proximal femoral head abutting against the acetabulum may cause increased stress and damage to the articular cartilage during repetitive hip flexion and internal rotation.

Recent research has shown that the cam-type deformity may be linked to mechanical etiology emerging from the growth-plate-related scar of the proximal femoral head. This may have developed during adolescence as a response to vigorous sporting activity. Loading may impact long-term locomotor system.

In athletes, the most common complaint relating to FAI is groin pain exacerbated by intense activity, including repetitive hip flexion movements. Symptoms may be vague and diffuse, with pain often being referred medially toward the pubis symphysis, laterally toward the greater trochanter, or dorsally toward the gluteal muscles. Clinically, the most common finding with FAI examination relates to reduced ROM, specifically flexion and rotation.

Pilates movements that "grind" into the acetabulum or labrum can cause pain and dysfunction. The preferred movement plan develops proper loading of the torso-pelvic-lower extremity complex and improves hip joint glide. Key points for a Pilates practice include:

- Clarify which regions benefit from increased ROM
- Avoid rotational movements that may cause irritation

- Ascertain optimal loading for the condition
- Manage load to avoid discomfort
- Develop progressive loading for tissue conditioning

Client description: 45-year-old, identifies as male; Ironman athlete; 2-year history of anterior right hip joint pain

Dates of case report: Session 1: January 14, 2021; Session 12: March 3, 2021; in-person sessions biweekly then weekly

Studio apparatus and props
Pilates equipment

- Universal Reformer
- Wunda Chair with split pedal

Props used with equipment

- Mat
- Resistance band loop
- Resistance band, single length
- Foam roller

Home program props

- Mat
- Resistance band loop
- Resistance band, single length

- Foam roller
- Ankle weights

Methods and materials

Session 1/12
1. Health history interview

- 2019: identified anterior hip joint pain
- Initial pain during a run, felt a twinge, completed run
- Rested for a few days, felt better
- Returned to training and racing throughout 2019
- Continued to compete despite constant irritation
- Reduced training and racing load during 2020
- Pain increased when training resumed in September–October 2020

- Pain gradually increased September–December 2020
- Positive hip quadrant test (inner circle ++++)
- Positive FABER (flexion, abduction, external rotation) test
- Pain and lack of tissue glide in regions adjacent to site of lesion: medial groin, lateral thigh, lateral hemipelvis, superior to ilium, and adjacent to lumbar region
- Cleared lumbar region
- Sacroiliac joint dysfunction determined not to be a contributing factor
- Adductor tendinopathy determined not to be a contributing factor

2. Symptoms

- Pain in the anterior hip joint region
- Limited ROM of the anterior hip joint
- Occasional pain into the posterior hip joint region

3. Movement aids

- None

Final result of case report

Movement rehabilitation program led to full resolution of symptoms. The client returned to full pain-free activity and racing. The scheduled surgery was cancelled since it was no longer necessary.

Session 2/12: Initial assessment

1. General observations of gait

- Right: Trendelenburg movement strategy

- Lacks right hip joint extension on push-off phase of gait

- Bilateral increased foot/ankle pronation

- Limited right ankle dorsiflexion

Editor note
The Trendelenburg sign is most apparent during the gait cycle. When the leg supports the weight of the body on the lesioned side, the pelvis rises ipsilaterally. This presentation is more accurately a dipping of the pelvis toward the contralateral side. Since the region of the lesion cannot maintain the pelvis in a level plane the person falls toward the efficient side. Simultaneously, the torso translates and laterally flexes towards the lesioned side in an attempt to maintain balance (Gogu and Gandbhir 2022).

2. Standing tests

- Full torso rotation

- Observations of inefficient side: left
  - Decreased left rotation

- Hemipelvis inferior motion

- Observations of inefficient side: left
  - Significant dip of left hemipelvis when standing on right leg
  - Increased pronation of mid-foot when standing on right leg
  - Increased valgus of right knee when standing on right leg

Session 12/12: Post-assessment

1. General observations of gait

- Full, even weight bearing

- 5 degrees hip extension during push-off phase of gait

- No evidence of Trendelenburg strategy

- Efficient foot-ankle-knee movement relationships in gait and running

2. Standing tests

- Full torso rotation

- Observations of inefficient side: left
  - Improved left rotation

- Hemipelvis inferior motion

- Observations of inefficient side: left
  - No significant dip of left hemipelvis when standing on right leg
  - Thoracolumbar junction (TLJ) organizes to midline above sacrum
  - Improved bilateral stance

Editor note
The author describes how a Trendelenburg response presents in standing.

◆ Lateral pelvic shift

● Observations of inefficient side: right
  ■ Right hemipelvis elevates

3. Seated tests

◆ Thoracic rotation

● Observations of inefficient side: left
  ■ Reduced left rotation
  ■ Increased weight bearing on left ischial tuberosity

◆ Hip joint and knee flexion

● Observations of inefficient side: right
  ■ Limited ROM of right hip flexion accentuates right hemipelvis elevation
  ■ Tissue restriction in right hemipelvis region
  ■ Significant posterior pelvic rotation, on the right more than on the left

4. Sit and stand

◆ Lateral view

● Limited ability to transfer weight on ischial tuberosities anteriorly, on the right more than the left
● Visible pain response at weight-bearing initiation
● Asymmetrical weight-bearing on the left more than the right
● Full weight-bearing strategy of slight hip flexion on the right more than the left

3. Seated tests

◆ Thoracic rotation

● Observations of inefficient side: left
  ■ Improved left rotation
  ■ Decreased weight bearing on left ischial tuberosity

◆ Hip joint and knee flexion

● Observations of inefficient side: right
  ■ Improved ROM of right hip flexion
  ■ Slight right hemipelvis elevation
  ■ Posterior pelvic rotation diminished

4. Sit and stand

◆ Lateral view

● Improved ability of anterior weight transfer on ischial tuberosities
● No visible pain response at weight-bearing initiation
● Bilateral weight distribution improved

◆ Anterior view

● Organizes to midline
● No visible pain response
● Bilateral weight distribution improved

- ◆ Anterior view

- Left lumbopelvic weight shift
- Visible pain response
- Right lower extremity (LE): increased valgus knee tracking

5. Standing balance

- ◆ Two-leg stance, eyes open

- 60 seconds

- ◆ One-leg stance, eyes open

- Left leg: 60 seconds
- Unable to perform on right leg due to pain

5. Standing balance

- ◆ Two-leg stance, eyes open

- 60 seconds

- ◆ One-leg stance, eyes open

- Left leg: 60 seconds

- Right leg: able to balance on right leg

Session 3/12: Home program

Fatigue scale	8
Pain scale	9
Client self-report	• Anxious to avoid surgery—stressed that he may not be able to race again
Key changes observed by author at end of Session 3/12	• Ability to control load onto right LE • Improved hip joint extension • Decreased restriction from acetabular capsule region • Improved glide and activation of pelvifemoral tissues • Improved thoracic rotation due to a shared control of load throughout the torso • Improved foot-to-torso activation and force transfer through entire LE
Reason behind choice of sequencing	• Emphasize synergistic activation and integration of pelvic control structures • Stimulate lower limb activation in partial weight-bearing • Focus client attention on movement organization of proximal regions • Progressive controlled loading in full weight bearing • Improve anterior tissue glide and joint ROM in support of hip extension

Session movement sequence

1. Single Leg Stretch — Derivative of J. H. Pilates Single Leg Stretch (NPCE Study Guide 2021, p. 46)

Author note
This exercise is based on J. H. Pilates exercise Single Leg Stretch. Keeping the foot on the floor creates a closed kinematic context for optimal acetabular femoral congruency.

Intent	• Low load exercise that replicates the concept of reciprocal hip articulation differentiated from lumbopelvic region in efficient gait
Gait reasoning	• Improve control of lateral load transfer • Refine motions of pelvis and/or lumbar region

Starting position
- Supine on mat, knees flexed with feet in full contact with floor
- Feet hip-width apart
- Hands on anterior iliac spine for feedback of any pelvic motion
- Scapula in optimal placement on thorax
- Head and neck aligned to midline following sagittal torso contour

Movement description
- Inhale in preparation for movement to begin
- During exhalation slide left heel inferiorly along the floor ensuring that there is no drop of the left hemipelvis
- Toward the end of the LE movement ensure that no anterior pelvic rotation occurs
- During inhalation, slide left heel superiorly along the floor, filtering out anterior lumbopelvic rotation
- Return to starting position
- Repeat, alternating each LE, ensuring that the reciprocal LE movement does not disturb lumbopelvic midline organization

2. Scissors (See Chapter 5 in Volume 1, Gentry: Single Knee Folds)

Intent
- Low load patterning for gait reeducation

Gait reasoning
- Teach femur on pelvis movement articulating with low load in the sagittal plane

Starting position
- Supine on mat, knees flexed with feet in full contact with floor
- LE hip-width apart
- Scapula in optimal placement on thorax
- Head and neck following the contour of the torso

Movement description
- Inhale to prepare
- Exhale, sliding the right foot toward the ischial tuberosity prior to performing hip flexion, with knee flexion at 90 degrees
- Inhale, hold position
- Exhale, lower right foot to the mat
- Repeat on each side
- Repeat alternating on each side and ensuring that the reciprocal LE movement does not cause any pelvic or lumbar region movement

3. Shoulder Bridge
Derivative of J. H. Pilates Shoulder Bridge (NPCE Study Guide 2021, p. 49)

Intent
- Activate extensors
- Increase ROM of hip flexion and extension
- Articulate the lumbar region

Gait reasoning
- Manage the lack of hip joint extension
- Address imbalance and restriction of pelvifemoral tissues and joint glide

Starting position
- Supine on mat, knees flexed and feet in full contact with floor
- LE hip-width apart
- Scapula in optimal placement on thorax
- Head and neck follow contour of torso

Movement description
- Inhale to prepare
- During exhalation, perform posterior pelvic rotation with lumbar flexion
- Gently roll lumbar region into mat
- Continue to articulate the torso until scapulae are resting on mat
- Inhale and hold bridge position
- During exhalation slowly articulate down to starting position

4. Side lying hip joint abduction
Derivative of J. H. Pilates Side Kick (NPCE Study Guide 2021, p. 49)

Intent
- Lateral activation in low-load environment

Gait reasoning
- Address Trendelenburg gait pattern

Starting position
- Left side lying on mat
- Place a band around lower legs above the ankles
- LE extended
- Left upper extremity (UE) flexed and aligned with torso in midline orientation
- Right hand on floor for balance

Editor note
In resisted hip abduction the band location is significant. The closer the source of resistance is placed to the joint articulation the greater the concentration of force on the proximal tissues. When the source of resistance is located further away from the joint articulation, force vectors are distributed throughout the structure. In this exercise, applying the band above the ankles to impact hip loading also involves the knee.

Movement description	- Inhale to prepare - Exhale, abduct right LE in an arc, plantar flexing foot - Inhale, adduct right LE to starting position, dorsiflexing foot

5. Quadruped hip rotation

Intent	- Develop femur on pelvis ROM - Adaptation of torso to lateral LE movement - Refine motor control to improve pain management
Gait reasoning	- Diminish Trendelenburg sign
Starting position	- Quadruped on mat - Resistance band looped around right foot and fixed to stationary object posteriorly at the level of the foot - Right hip joint internally rotated to mid-ROM - Right lower limb hovering slightly above the mat
Movement description	- Inhale to prepare - Exhale, externally rotate and abduct right LE to mid-range - Sustain pelvic midline organization - Progress by increasing ROM

6. Swimming
Derivative of J. H. Pilates Swimming (NPCE Study Guide 2021, p. 50)

Intent	- Improve extension
Gait reasoning	- Increase extension for push-off
Starting position	- Prone on mat - Stack hands and rest forehead on hands - Use a cushion under the pelvis if necessary to reduce pain
Movement description	- Inhale to prepare - During exhalation extend left LE, hovering 1 in. (2.5 cm) off mat - During inhalation lower left LE to starting position - Repeat, alternating legs

7. Swimming: Variation
Derivative of J. H. Pilates Swimming (NPCE Study Guide 2021, p. 50)

Intent	- Activate contralateral patterning to support gait and function of Ironman sport

Gait reasoning	• Improve extension for push-off • Reinforce coordination of UE and contralateral LE activation • Improve contralateral movement for propulsion
Starting position	• Prone on mat • Use a cushion under the pelvis if necessary to reduce pain • Bilateral shoulder flexion resting UE on mat • Bilateral LE extension resting LE on mat
Movement description	• Inhale to prepare • During exhalation lift left UE and right LE off the mat hovering 1 in. (2.5 cm) • During inhalation return to starting position • Repeat with right UE and left LE • Alternate sides creating a swimming motion
8. Plank hold	Derivative of J. H. Pilates Leg Pull Front (NPCE Study Guide 2021, p. 50)
Intent	• Improve whole-body motor control in preparation for hip extension
Gait reasoning	• Improve midline organization
Starting position	• Quadruped on mat • Weight bearing on forearms • Torso in midline orientation
Movement description	• Exhale, extend right LE placing forefoot on mat in preparation to bear weight on foot • Extend left LE placing forefoot on mat in preparation to bear weight on foot • Organize in plank position • Hold plank breathing smoothly • Aim for 1 minute hold, progress to 5 minutes
9. Plank to Downward Dog	Derivative of J. H. Pilates Push-Up (NPCE Study Guide 2021, p. 51)
Intent	• Increase tolerance of loading UE together with torso integration • Induce posterior-anterior movement between UE and LE • Improve extension articulation and activation

Chapter 5

Gait reasoning	• Increase lower limb tissue glide around the rear foot • Linking lack of mobility of UE with hip joint limitations • Activate torso with limb loading
Starting position	• Quadruped on mat
Movement description	• Inhale to prepare • During exhalation shift weight to the feet with glenohumeral flexion and elbow extension, flexing at hip joints, extending knee joints, and lowering the heels to the mat (Downward Dog) • During inhalation sustain position • During exhalation shift body weight toward hands, extending the UE and hip and knee joints and lifting the heels • Return to plank position • Repeat up to ten times

10. Footwork on Universal Reformer: Dorsiflexion

Derivative of J. H. Pilates Footwork on Universal Reformer (NPCE Study Guide 2021, p. 52)

Intent	• Low loading for hip flexion and extension • Develop motor control without irritating the lesion
Gait reasoning	• Limb loading organization during flexion and extension
Set-up	• 3–4 medium springs
Starting position	• Supine on carriage • Feet dorsiflexed with heels on low footbar • Knee flexion less than 90 degrees • Heels aligned with the ischial tuberosities
Movement description	• Inhale to prepare • During exhalation extend hip and knee joints, pushing carriage away from footbar • Inhale, flex hip and knee joints as the carriage returns toward footbar • Maintain dorsiflexion throughout repetitions • Repeat 20 times towards fatigue

11. Footwork on Universal Reformer: External rotation

Derivative of J. H. Pilates Footwork on Universal Reformer (NPCE Study Guide 2021, p. 52)

Intent	• Improve the ROM of LE extension and flexion • Integrate activation from the foot to torso • Improve LE organization during flexion and extension

Pilates and Hip Joint Dysfunction: Effect on Gait

Gait reasoning	• Partial weight-bearing flexion/extension of the LE to improve ROM, avoiding compressive forces that may irritate the lesion and the capsule region
Set-up	• 3–4 medium springs
Starting position	• Supine on carriage • Feet dorsiflexed, heels on low footbar in external rotation • Knee flexion less than 90 degrees • External rotation of LE
Movement description	• Inhale to prepare • During exhalation extend hip and knee joints, pushing carriage away from footbar • During inhalation flex hip and knee joints as the carriage returns toward footbar • Maintain dorsiflexion throughout repetitions • Repeat 15–20 times toward fatigue

12. Footwork on Universal Reformer: Unilateral dorsiflexion

Derivative of J. H. Pilates Footwork on Universal Reformer (NPCE Study Guide 2021, p. 52)

Intent	• Improve ROM of LE extension and flexion • Integrate activation from foot to torso • Load unilateral LE
Gait reasoning	• Partial weight bearing, low load during flexion/extension • Refine motor control to adapt to ground forces
Set-up	• 2 medium springs
Starting position	• Supine on carriage • Right unilateral dorsiflexion, heel on low footbar in external rotation • Right knee flexion less than 90 degrees • Right external rotation of LE • Left non-weight-bearing LE at 90 degrees hip and knee flexion
Movement description	• Inhale to prepare • During exhalation, extend right hip and knee joint pushing carriage away from footbar • Inhale, flexing right hip and knee joint as carriage returns toward footbar • Maintain dorsiflexion throughout repetitions • Repeat 10 times • Change to left LE

Chapter 5

Session 11/12: Studio session

Key changes observed by author at end of Session 11/12
- Information not recorded

Reason behind choice of sequencing
- Information not recorded

Session movement sequence

1. Footwork on Universal Reformer: Ankle dorsiflexion and plantar flexion, bilateral and unilateral

Derivative of J. H. Pilates Footwork on Universal Reformer (NPCE Study Guide 2021, p. 52)

Intent
- Rear foot to forefoot articulation
- Lower limb motion
- Articulation of hip, knee, and ankle joints

Gait reasoning
- Increase loading of feet

Set-up
- 2 medium springs
- Left non-weight bearing LE at 90 degrees hip and knee flexion

Starting position
- Supine on carriage
- Metatarsals on low footbar
- Ankles plantar flexed
- Hip and knee joint flexion

Movement description
- Inhale to prepare
- During exhalation extend hip and knee joints pushing carriage away from footbar
- Maintain plantar flexion
- During inhalation dorsiflex ankle maintaining hip and knee joints in extension
- During exhalation flex hip and knee joints as carriage returns toward footbar
- Repeat 15–20 times
- Press carriage away from footbar
- Increase repetitions from 1 repetition to 10 with consistent ankle dorsiflexion and plantar flexion with hip and knee joints extended

CUES
- Control carriage return for continuous spring resistance (see Volume 1, Chapter 6)
- Accelerate plantar flexion

Author note
It is recommended to work the lower limbs to fatigue. This develops tissue endurance, a valuable aspect of Pilates training for high-level athletes.

2. Footwork on Universal Reformer: Running

Derivative of J. H. Pilates Running on Universal Reformer (NPCE Study Guide 2021, p. 60)

Intent
- Reciprocal LE flexion and extension
- Ankle-knee-hip joint articulation and timing

Gait reasoning
- Increase lower limb loading

Set-up
- 2–3 medium springs
- Low footbar

Starting position
- Supine on carriage
- Metatarsals on footbar, ankles in plantar flexion
- Feet aligned with center of hip joints
- Knee flexion less than 90 degrees
- Hip joint flexion, parallel LE

Movement description
- Inhale to prepare
- During exhalation extend hip and knee joints pushing carriage away from footbar
- Maintain plantar flexion
- Inhale, sustaining position
- During exhalation, dorsiflex ankle and lower right heel under footbar, keeping same-side knee extended
- Simultaneously, flex left hip and knee joint and plantar flex left ankle
- Inhale, change sides
- Repeat up to 20 times alternating sides in a reciprocal movement

Author note
This is a valuable exercise for retraining the reciprocal motions of the LE.

Chapter 5

3. Side lying flexion and extension on Universal Reformer

Intent	• Increase activation of pelvifemoral region in an orientation other than supine
	• Side lying accentuates activation of the lateral tissues
Gait reasoning	• To lessen the Trendelenburg response

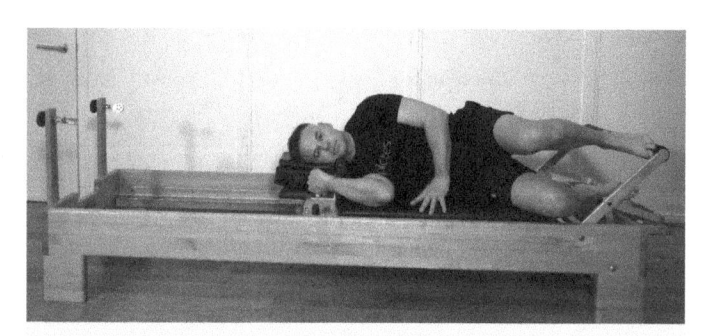

Figure 5.1

Set-up	• Springs: 1 heavy and 1 medium
	• Footbar down
Starting position	• Side lying on right side on carriage
	• Left metatarsals on footbar organized with center of hip joints
	• Knee flexion less than 90 degrees
	• Hip joint flexion, abducted maintaining parallel LE
	• Right LE hip and knee joint flexion resting on carriage
	• UE in front
	• Head supported
Movement description	• Inhale to prepare
	• During exhalation extend left hip and knee joints pushing carriage away from footbar
	• Lower left heel onto footbar as carriage moves away
	• Inhale, flex hip and knee joints as carriage returns toward footbar
	• Left heel may lift off footbar depending upon ROM of ankle
	• Maintain left LE abduction
	• Repeat 8–10 times on each side
	• Repeat exercise with LE in external rotation (Figure 5.2)

Author note
This is a valuable exercise for retraining the reciprocal motions of the LE.

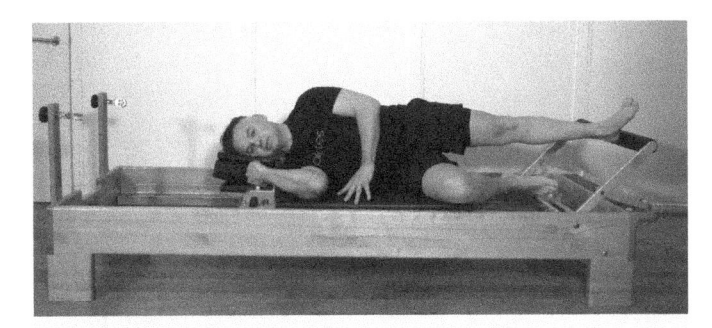

Figure 5.2

CUE
- Focus on articulation and organization of LE during flexion and extension

Author note
The side lying series accentuates activation of the lateral tissues and prevents the flexors from dominating the exercise compared with the supine series.

4. Side lying flexion and extension on Universal Reformer with foot strap

Intent
- Increased difficulty with decreased base of support
- Unilateral limb control, increasing lateral control
- Focus on pelvic control without the closed kinematic context of footbar support

Gait reasoning
- Improve motor control of limb under load

Chapter 5

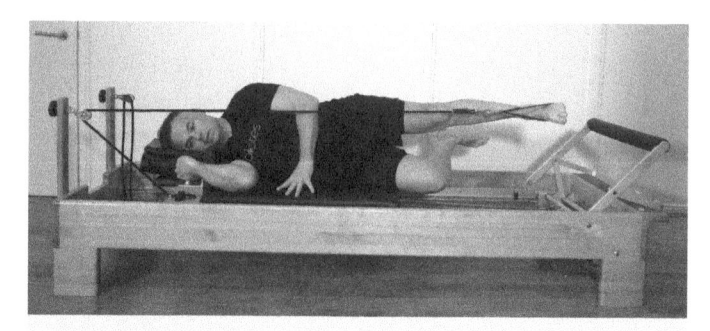

Figure 5.3

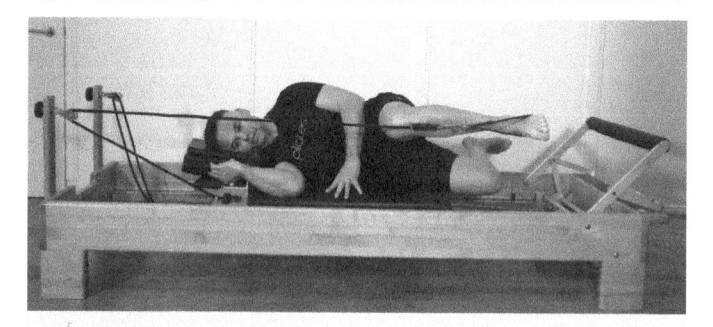

Figure 5.4

Set-up
- Footbar in down position
- 1–2 medium springs
- Foot strap
- Headrest lifted with 3 in. (8 cm) cushion on headrest

Starting position
- Side lying on right side on carriage
- Right LE hip and knee joint flexion resting on carriage
- Left foot placed in front foot strap
- Knee flexion less than 90 degrees organized with center of hip joints
- Hip joint flexion, abducted maintaining parallel LE
- Left hand on left hemipelvis
- Right UE resting on carriage
- Head supported

Pilates and Hip Joint Dysfunction: Effect on Gait

Movement description	- Inhale to prepare
- During exhalation, extend left hip and knee joints by pressing into the strap and moving carriage away from footbar
- Inhale, flex hip and knee joints as carriage returns toward footbar
- Maintain left LE abduction
- Repeat 8–10 times on each side
5. Side lying hip flexion and extension with knee extension on Universal Reformer	Derivative of J. H. Pilates mat Side Kick (NPCE Study Guide 2021, p. 49)
Intent	- Increased challenge to motor control
- Changes ROM of pelvic control with extended knee
Gait reasoning	- Increase limb load

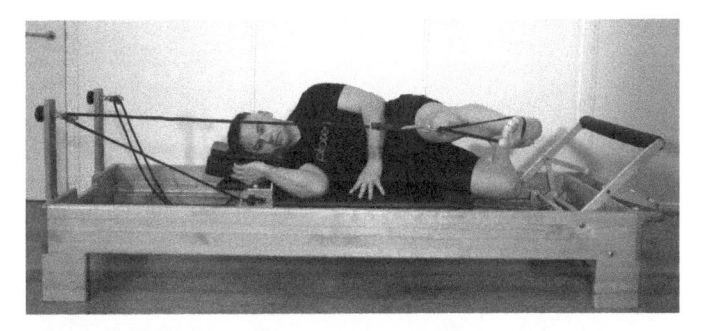

Figure 5.5

Set-up	- Footbar in down position
- 1–2 medium springs
- Foot strap
- Headrest lifted with 3 in. (8 cm) cushion on headrest
Starting position	- Side lying on right side on carriage
- Right LE hip and knee joint flexion resting on carriage
- Left hand on left hemipelvis
- Right UE resting on carriage
- Head supported
- Left foot placed in front foot strap
- Hip joint at 10–15 degrees flexion, with knee extension
- LE abducted to maintain parallel position

Chapter 5

Movement description
- Inhale, flex the left hip joint to approximately 90 degrees
- Exhale, extend the left hip joint
- Maintain abducted LE
- Repeat 8–10 times on each side

CUE
- Control the carriage movement during hip joint flexion

6. Prone knee flexion and extension on long box on Universal Reformer

Intent
- Increase load to LE in a different orientation, i.e., prone

Gait reasoning
- Improve limb control

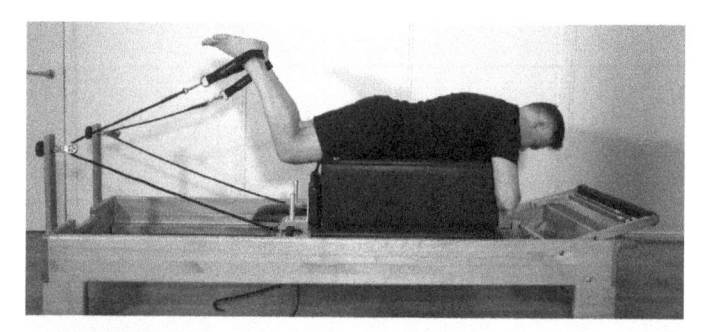

Figure 5.6

Set-up
- Footbar in down position
- 1–2 medium springs
- Headrest flat
- Box placed on carriage in "long" orientation
- Reduce the length of the pulley ropes

Editor note
The Universal Reformer box is placed on the carriage in one of two orientations. When the box is placed perpendicular to the long axis of the carriage it is called "short box." The other orientation, parallel to the long axis of the carriage, is called "long box" (see Appendix 3 in Volume 1).

Pilates and Hip Joint Dysfunction: Effect on Gait

Starting position	• Prone on long box • Head facing footbar • Patella positioned just off the back end of long box • Knees flexed to approximately 45 degrees • Foot straps looped around ankles • Arms by sides with hands lightly supporting sides of long box • Torso organized in midline and sagittal plane
Movement description	• Inhale to prepare • Exhale, flex the knees as far as control can be maintained • Inhale, extend the knees • Repeat 8–10 times

CUES
- Maintain prone position
- Exhalation prior to and throughout effort
- Knee flexion occurs without hip joint flexion

7. Straps: feet in loops, flexion and extension on Universal Reformer

Intent	• Improve hip ROM • Promote glide of acetabular femoral tissues
Gait reasoning	• Lower limb control
Set-up	• Low footbar position • 1/2 light spring to 2 medium springs • Appropriate head and neck support
Starting position	• Supine on carriage • Feet in foot straps • Hip joints extended to 45 degrees and knees fully extended • LE adducted, in parallel • Ankles in plantar flexion • UE resting beside the body
Movement description	• Exhale to prepare • Inhale, flex the hip joints to 90 degrees flexion • Knees remain extended • Exhale, extend the hip joints moving carriage away • Maintain LE adduction • Repeat 8–10 times

CUES
* Control carriage movement during hip joint flexion
* Move with control
* Avoid posterior rotation of pelvis

8. Quadruped hip flexion on Universal Reformer

Intent
- Improve pelvifemoral flexion and extension in quadruped orientation
- Challenge torso control

Gait reasoning
- Increase LE load in a different orientation in gravity

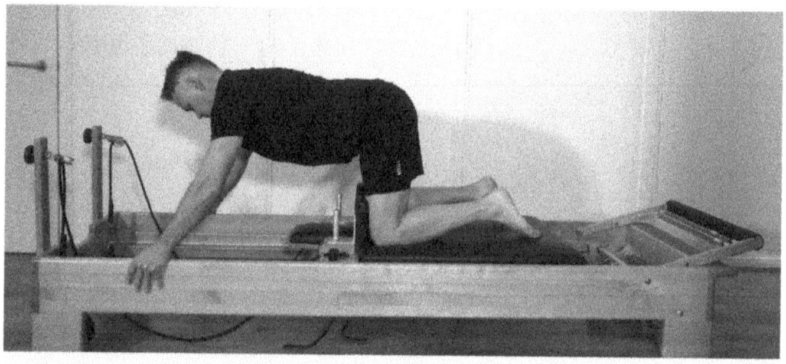

Figure 5.7

Set-up
- Footbar flat
- 1/2 light spring or no springs

Starting position
- Quadruped, facing toward the back of Universal Reformer
- Hands holding the sides of the frame
- UE at 110 degrees flexion, with elbows slightly flexed
- Knees against shoulder stops
- Hip joints at 15 degrees extension, moving carriage away from shoulder stops

Movement description
- Inhale to prepare
- During exhalation flex hip joints to approximately 90 degrees to move carriage away from footbar
- There should be no movement of the UE
- Inhale, extend the hips to move carriage toward footbar
- Repeat 10 times

Pilates and Hip Joint Dysfunction: Effect on Gait

CUES
- Starting position is important to establish ROM, moving femur on pelvis from extension into flexion
- Focus on glide of the knees moving under the torso

The journey to Session 11

Session 4/12
Client self-report

- Improving
- Feels less achy
- Night pain decreasing
- Pain scale 6
- Fatigue scale 6

Key changes observed

- Improving control, unilateral stance
- Increased LE extension to 0 degrees

Reasoning behind choice of movements

- Gradual increase of limb loading
- Progression from low load to increased load

Session movement sequence

1. Single Leg Stretch
2. Scissors
3. Shoulder Bridge
4. Side lying hip joint abduction
5. Standing wall squat
6. Universal Reformer

- Footwork
  - Heels parallel
  - External rotation
- Straps: feet in loops
  - Flexion and extension
  - Running
- Footwork
  - Unilateral on heels

7. Trapeze Table

- Standing torso flexion/extension for thoracic articulation

8. Additional movements

- Wunda Chair
  - Standing leg press
- Universal Reformer
  - Eve's Lunge

Session 5/12
Client self-report

- Improving
- Night pain intermittent only
- Beginning indoor bike with no pain
- Pain scale 3–4
- Fatigue scale 5

Key changes observed

- Improving lower limb loading
- Beginning to tolerate increased load
- Improved ROM in hip extension
- Improved Thomas Test

Chapter 5

> **Editor note**
> The Thomas test is a physical examination named after the Welsh orthopedic surgeon Hugh Owen Thomas (1834–1891). The client lies supine with the LE of the unaffected side flexed toward the torso and the LE of affected side extended. The test measures the ROM in extension to check for anterior or lateral capsular restrictions.

Reasoning behind choice of movements

- Continuing to progress limb loading

Session movement sequence

1. Single Leg Stretch into Scissors as combined movement

2. Shoulder Bridge

3. Standing wall squat to 90 degrees

4. Standing lunge with assistance of roller or pole

5. Universal Reformer

- Footwork
    - Heels parallel
    - External rotation
- Straps: feet in loops
    - Flexion and extension
    - Running
- Footwork, side lying, unilateral
    - On heels parallel
    - External rotation
- Overhead with elbow flexion and extension (derivative of J. H. Pilates Overhead/Jackknife, NPCE Study Guide 2021, p. 53)

6. Trapeze Table

- Standing torso flexion/extension for thoracic mobility, added thoracic rotation

7. Additional movement

- Wunda Chair
    - Standing unilateral LE, press hands on, hands off (Figure 5.8; derivative of J. H. Pilates Wunda Chair Standing Leg Pump Front, NPCE Study Guide 2021, p. 79)

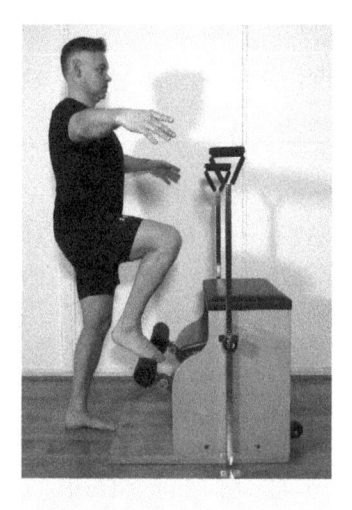

Figure 5.8

- Universal Reformer
    - Eve's Lunge

Session 6/12
Client self-report

- Improving
- Night pain resolved
- Indoor bike—no stiffness after 1 hour session
- Walk/run began—4 minute walk/1 minute run

Key changes observed

- Limb load acceptance improving
- Thomas test improving
- Unilateral stance improving

Reasoning behind choice of movements

- Gradual load retraining
- Improve torso adaptability to midline
- Extension control

Session movement sequence

1. Single Leg Stretch

2. Scissors

3. Shoulder Bridge

4. Quadruped thoracic rotation

5. Plank hold

6. Universal Reformer

- Footwork
   - Heels parallel
   - External rotation
   - Side lying flexion and extension, in parallel
   - Supine unilateral heel, increased spring load
- Shoulder Bridge with extension

7. Additional movements

- Wunda Chair
   - Standing, unilateral LE, press hands on, hands off
   - Standing reverse lunge (Figure 5.9; derivative of J. H. Pilates Forward Lunge/Straight Stand, NPCE Study Guide 2021, p. 77)

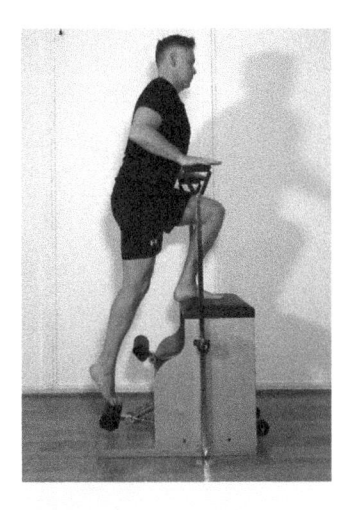

Figure 5.9

- Universal Reformer
   - Standing Splits: Side, reduced ROM
   - Standing Splits: Back
   - Eve's Lunge

Session 7/12
Client self-report

- No night pain
- Indoor and outdoor cycling for more than 1 hour
- Steady walk/run program
- Pain scale 3–4
- Fatigue scale 3–4

Key changes observed

- Improved gait with recognizable LE extension
- Sit to stand significantly improved with midline orientation
- One-leg stance improved

Reasoning behind choice of movements

- Continue gradual load increase
- Focus on thoracic mobility
- Increase pelvifemoral activation

Chapter 5

Session movement sequence
1. Single Leg Stretch

2. Scissors

3. Shoulder Bridge, added lateral shift and unilateral LE stance

4. Swimming

5. Wall squat and wall sit

6. Standing lunge

7. Resistance band around tibias

- Walking lunge
- Lateral walking

8. Universal Reformer

- Footwork
  - Heels parallel
  - External rotation
- Side lying flexion and extension, in parallel
  - Supine unilateral heel, increased spring load
- Footwork, side lying, unilateral
  - On heels parallel
  - External rotation
- Straps: feet in loops
  - Flexion and extension
- Side lying flexion and extension with knee extension
  - Side lying flexion and extension with foot strap
- Eve's Lunge

9. Additional movements

- Wunda Chair
  - Standing unilateral LE, press hands on, hands off with increased spring load
  - Standing reverse lunge with decreased spring load
  - Standing reverse lunge with knee flexion (Figure 5.10; derivative of J. H. Pilates Backward Step Down/Running Start, NPCE Study Guide 2021, p. 75)

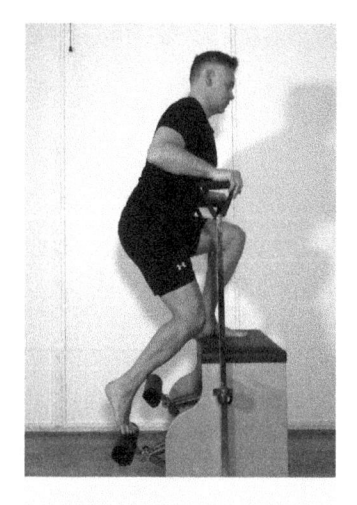

Figure 5.10

Session 8/12
Client self-report

- Reports no pain since last session
- No night pain
- Bike increasing with no concern
- Walk/run—increased to 2 minute run/3 minute walk repeated 4 times

Key changes observed

- Thomas test improving
- Unilateral stance—very little translation
- Improved sit to stand

Reasoning behind choice of movements

- Continuing previous goals

Session movement sequence
1. Universal Reformer

- Footwork
  - Heels parallel
  - External rotation
  - Side lying flexion and extension, parallel
  - Supine unilateral heel, increased spring load
- Footwork, side lying, unilateral, increased spring load and repetitions
  - On heels parallel
  - External rotation
- Straps: feet in loops
  - Flexion and extension
  - Side lying flexion and extension with knee extension
  - Side lying flexion and extension with foot strap
- Quadruped unilateral hip flexion and extension using jump board

2. Wunda Chair

- Standing unilateral LE, press hands on, hands off with increased spring load
- Standing reverse lunge with decreased spring assistance
- Standing reverse lunge with knee flexion

Session 9/12
Client self-report

- Feels good
- No pain reported
- No night pain
- Cycling, no pain
- Running—maintaining walk/run program
- Note—swimming not included, due to lockdown pools all closed

Key changes observed

- No Trendelenburg noted in unilateral stance
- Unilateral hopping pain-free

Reasoning behind choice of movements

- Gradual progression of previous goals

Session movement sequence
1. Universal Reformer

- Footwork
  - Heels parallel
  - External rotation
  - Side lying flexion and extension, in parallel
  - Supine unilateral heel, increased spring load
- Footwork, side lying, unilateral increased spring load and repetitions
  - On heels parallel
  - External rotation
- Straps: feet in loops
  - Flexion and extension
  - Side lying flexion and extension with knee extension
  - Side lying flexion and extension with foot strap
- Quadruped unilateral hip flexion and extension using jump board

2. Wunda Chair

- Standing unilateral LE, press hands on, hands off with increased spring load
- Standing reverse lunge with decreased spring assistance
- Standing reverse lunge with knee flexion

3. Additional movement

- Straps: feet in loops on Universal Reformer, added abduction/extension/adduction/flexion for full ROM of hip joints

Chapter 5

Session 10/12
Client self-report

- Feels strong
- Pain scale 0
- Fatigue scale 0

Reasoning behind choice of movements

- Technique reviewed and advice given on performance
- Progression of previous goals

Session movement sequence
1. Universal Reformer

- Footwork
  - Heels parallel
  - External rotation
  - Side lying flexion and extension, in parallel
  - Supine unilateral heel, increased spring load
- Footwork, side lying, unilateral increased spring load and repetitions
  - On heels parallel
  - External rotation
- Straps: feet in loops
  - Flexion and extension
  - Side lying flexion and extension with knee extension
  - Side lying flexion and extension with foot strap
- Quadruped unilateral hip flexion and extension using jump board

2. Wunda Chair

- Standing unilateral LE, press hands on, hands off with increased spring load
- Standing reverse lunge with decreased spring load
- Standing reverse lunge with knee flexion

3. Trapeze Table

- Standing torso flexion/extension for thoracic rotation

4. Additional movement

- Thomas test using springs off side of Trapeze Table
  - Client supine on edge of table with head at spring attachment on vertical side pole
  - Assume Thomas Test position placing loop of foot strap around mid-foot
  - Hold spring to control tension and pull on LE
  - Avoid hyperextension at TLJ

References]
Christmas C, Crespo CJ, Franckowiak SC, Bathon JM, Bartlett SJ et al. (2002) How common is hip pain among older adults? Results from the Third National Health and Nutrition Examination Survey. *J Fam Pract* 51: 345-348.

Dawson, J., Linsell, L., Zondervan, K. et al. (2004) "Epidemiology of hip and knee pain and its impact on overall health status in older adults." *Rheumatology, 43,* 497–504.

Gogu, S. and Gandbhir, V. N. (2022) Trendelenburg Sign. [Updated 2022, Nov 14]. In: StatPearls [Internet]. Treasure Island, FL: StatPearls Publishing; 2023 Jan-. www.ncbinlmnihgov/books/NBK555987. [Accessed August 31, 2023].

Lancet. (2016) "Global, regional, and national incidence, prevalence, and years lived with disability for 310 diseases and injuries, 1990-2015: a systematic analysis for the Global Burden of Disease Study 2015". *Lancet.* 388 (10053): 1545–1602.

NPCE Study Guide (National Pilates Certification Exam Study Guide) (2021) Miami, FL: National Pilates Certification Program, Inc.

Paoloni, J. A. (2020). *Approach to the adult with unspecified hip pain.* In J. L. Melvin (Ed.), UpToDate.

Segal, N. A., Felson, D. T., Torner, J. C. et al. (2007) "Greater trochanteric pain syndrome: Epidemiology and associated factors." *Archives of Physical Medicine and Rehabilitation, 88,* 988–992.

Thorborg K, Rathleff MS, Petersen P, Branci S, Holmich P (2017) Prevalence and severity of hip and groin pain in sub-elite male football: a cross-sectional cohort study of 695 players. *Scand J Med Sci Sports* 27: 107-114.

Chapter 6

Pilates for Arthroscopic Knee Meniscus Repair Post-Surgery: Effect on Gait

William Li

Meniscal cartilage plays an essential role in the function and biotensegral organization of the knee. The meniscus functions in load bearing, load transmission, shock absorption, joint stability, joint lubrication, and joint congruity. It is the most injured structure in the human knee. A traumatic meniscus tear is defined by the history of a sudden onset of joint-line pain generally associated with significant knee injury.

Meniscal tear rates are reported at around 60 per 100,000. However, the true incidence is likely grossly underestimated since multiple studies demonstrate asymptomatic meniscal tears. Increased exposure to athletic activity increases the risk of injury to the meniscus. Today individuals are more active in later decades of life. Tears are more common in the third, fourth, and fifth decades of life.

Treatment consists of partial meniscectomy, complete meniscectomy, meniscal repair, meniscal transplantation, and tissue regeneration using stem cell therapy. Arthroscopic meniscectomy is still one of the most common orthopedic procedures. However, long-term results after major meniscectomy reported the degradation of underlying cartilage and subsequent development of early osteoarthritis. Meniscal repair has become more common to prevent joint degeneration. In traumatic tears, the first-line choice is repair or non-removal. Current guidelines recommend management of acute inflammation (rest, ice, compression, and elevation), anti-inflammation medications, and physiotherapy in the early stages, prior to potential surgical intervention.

Several factors may influence meniscal healing post-surgery. The most important may be the meniscal blood supply. The timing and type of meniscal tear may also impact healing. Peripheral meniscal tears are thought to have better healing potential. Acute, traumatic tears tend to have higher healing rates than chronic tissue degeneration. Age is another topic for consideration. Preserving meniscal tissue is particularly important for the long-term health of young athletes. Younger patients may have a higher healing potential.

Meniscal healing following surgical repair is influenced by post-operative range of motion (ROM), weight-bearing status, and biotensegral factors (Scarr 2018). Many rehabilitation programs propose avoiding weight-bearing forces as an important goal in the immediate post-operative period to protect the repair from high compressive and shear forces.

An accelerated protocol with immediate weight bearing at tolerance and early motion during non-weight bearing with partial immobilization for up to six weeks post-operatively is reported. Accelerated rehabilitation protocols are not associated with higher failure rates following meniscal repair.

Chapter 6

Client description: 32-year-old female, identifies as female; Zumba teacher

Dates of case report: Session 1: September 6, 2019; Session 12: October 24, 2019; all in-person sessions

Studio apparatus and props
Pilates equipment

- Universal Reformer
- Wunda Chair
- CoreAlign®

Props used with equipment

- Footplate for Universal Reformer
- Universal Reformer box
- Rotator disc, no resistance
- Mat

Home program props

- Foam roller, 36 in. (90 cm) long, 6 in. (15 cm) in diameter
- Balance pad (foam pad or air cushion disc)
- BOSU® ball
- Resistance band
- Marbles
- Rubber balls, 1 in. (2.5–3 cm) in diameter
- Mat

Methods and materials

Session 1/12
1. Health history interview

- Pain in right knee after Zumba class, early June 2019
- MRI showed right knee medial meniscus tear
- Arthroscopic meniscus repair surgery, end of July
- Began gait-focused Pilates training, early September

2. Symptoms

- Sharp pain in medial right knee, more pronounced when weight bearing or walking
- Inflammation of right knee joint
- Knee exam with manual pressure applied, first medially then laterally, to patella demonstrated a positive medial "bulge sign" consistent with a moderate amount of fluid
- Limited ROM of right knee in flexion and extension

3. Movement aids

- 2 canes used when walking

Final result of case report
Client demonstrated efficient gait. She resumed teaching Zumba.

Session 2/12: Initial assessment

1. General observations of gait

- ◆ Walked with assistance of 2 canes

2. Standing tests

- ◆ Full torso rotation

- ● Observations of inefficient side: both
- ● Right
  - ■ Weight shifted to left leg
  - ■ Minimal pelvifemoral rotation
- ● Left
  - ■ Weight shift to right leg
  - ■ No limitation of thoracic rotation
  - ■ Left foot: excessive supination
  - ■ Right foot: no adaptation

- ◆ Hemipelvis inferior motion

- ● Observations of inefficient side: right
  - ■ Inability to lower the right hemipelvis
  - ■ Limited left lateral lumbar flexion due to lumbar region onset of right lateral flexion

- ◆ Hemipelvis superior motion

- ● Observations of inefficient side: left
  - ■ Inability to transfer pelvis over right leg
  - ■ Insufficient left ankle plantar flexion

- ◆ Lateral pelvic shift

- ● Observations of inefficient side: right
  - ■ Thorax excessively translates to the left when pelvis shifts right
  - ■ Feet do not adapt
  - ■ Limited left femoral abduction

Session 12/12: Post-assessment

1. General observations of gait

- ◆ No canes
- ◆ Walked smoothly with right thoracic rotation more limited than left

2. Standing tests

- ◆ Full torso rotation

- ● Observations of inefficient side: right
  - ■ Weight slightly shifted to the left leg
  - ■ Improved pelvis on femur rotation
  - ■ Bilateral foot adaptation

- ◆ Hemipelvis inferior motion

- ● Observations of inefficient side: right
  - ■ Right hemipelvis lowering slightly improved
  - ■ Limited left lateral lumbar flexion due to lumbar region onset of right lateral flexion

- ◆ Hemipelvis superior motion

- ● Observations
  - ■ Able to transfer pelvis over right leg
  - ■ Left heel lift with normal ability to plantar flex

- ◆ Lateral pelvic shift

- ● Observations
  - ■ Pelvis shifts bilaterally right and left
  - ■ Thorax rotates symmetrically during lateral shift of pelvis to each side
  - ■ Bilateral foot and ankle adaptation

3. Seated tests

◆ Thoracic rotation

● Observations of inefficient side: right
  ■ Limited right rotation

◆ Hip joint and knee flexion

● Observations of inefficient side: right
  ■ Weight shifted to left ischial tuberosity
  ■ Increased torso flexion with right thoracic translation

Author note
Included dorsiflexion and knee flexion test. Right was inefficient due to limited knee flexion.

4. Sit and stand

◆ Lateral view

● Accomplished primarily by the left leg
● Excessive forward leaning of torso

◆ Anterior view

● Weight bearing greater on left side than right
● Right knee maintains flexion, avoiding full extension in standing

5. Standing balance

◆ Two-leg stance, eyes open

● 60 seconds
● Weight shifts to left leg

◆ One-leg stance, eyes open

● Only able to balance on the left leg: 60 seconds
● Unable to balance on right leg: 0 seconds

3. Seated tests

◆ Thoracic rotation

● Observations
  ■ Symmetrical thoracic rotation

◆ Hip joint and knee flexion

● Observations
  ■ Symmetrical bilateral hip joint and knee flexion
  ■ Slightly limited knee flexion when heel slides up opposite leg

Author note
Included dorsiflexion and knee flexion test. Both sides were efficient but right was less efficient due to limited knee flexion.

4. Sit and stand

◆ Lateral view

● Symmetrical right and left hip flexion and extension
● Torso maintains midline organization during sit and stand

◆ Anterior view

● Accurate right and left ankle dorsiflexion
● Patellae track over 2nd toes

5. Standing balance

◆ Two-leg stance, eyes open

● 60 seconds
● No difficulty in two-leg stance with eyes open

◆ One-leg stance, eyes open

● Left leg: 60 seconds
● Right leg: 50 seconds

Session 3/12: Home program

Fatigue scale	5
Pain scale	5
Client self-report	• Anxious, excited, hesitant to shift weight to right leg and to flex right knee
Key changes observed by author at end of Session 3/12	• No indications of avoiding right knee weight bearing • Accurate physical response to verbal cues • Improvement in midline organization during standing weight bearing
Reason behind choice of sequencing	• Improve stability, control, and coordination of right lower limb • Improve knee ROM in non-weight bearing and partial weight bearing • Facilitate proprioceptive awareness of feet-torso connections • Develop gradual improvement in weight-bearing endurance

Session movement sequence

1. Side lying hip joint abduction with knee flexion (Clam)	Derivative of J. H. Pilates Side Kick (NPCE Study Guide 2021, p. 49)
Intent	• Practice abduction in non-weight bearing in preparation for weight bearing • Refine lumbopelvic control • Refine control of external rotation of hip joint
Gait reasoning	• Refine pelvic control during internal rotation and external rotation of hip joint • Refine control of knee in flexion during leg movement
Starting position	• Side lying on mat with torso organized to midline in three planes • Hip and knee flexion to 90 degrees • Lower hand supports head • Upper hand on floor in front of the chest
Movement description	• Keeping the big toes touching, inhale during slow external rotation of the ceiling leg in the acetabular femoral joint • Exhale during return to starting position • Maintain torso stability throughout the movement

2. Bridge

Intent
- Activate extension and flexion of pelvis on hip joint
- Develop torso control during lower extremity (LE) extension
- Increase midline control of torso during sagittal movement of the lumbopelvic region

Gait reasoning
- Reinforce lumbopelvic-femoral organization in gait
- Lumbopelvic-femoral motion for stance and swing phases of gait
- Develop torso control during stance phase of gait

Starting position
- Supine, knees in flexion, feet flat on mat
- Arms by sides

Movement description
- Activate abdominals, lift lumbopelvic region off mat, toward ceiling
- Avoid lumbar extension
- Avoid hyperextension of thoracolumbar junction (TLJ)
- Return lumbopelvic region to mat

3. Lateral LE abduction/adduction

Derivative of J. H. Pilates Side Kick (NPCE Study Guide 2021, p. 49)

Intent
- Develop torso control in side lying
- Develop torso control in all planes
- Activate lateral torso stabilizers
- Develop control, ROM, and endurance required for LE abduction/adduction

Gait reasoning
- Support lumbopelvic-femoral control in gait
- Optimize whole-body weight shift during walking

Starting position
- Lying on side, place the lower hand under the head and the top hand on mat in front of xiphoid process
- Organize torso in sagittal midline
- Organize torso to midline in transverse and coronal planes
- The floor leg may be in parallel or in external rotation with the floor ankle and toes in dorsiflexion

Movement description
- During inhalation abduct ceiling leg, preserving torso organization to the midline in all three planes
- During exhalation return to starting position
- Throughout the movement organize the whole body to midline in all planes

4. Side lying LE flexion/ abduction/adduction

Derivative of J. H. Pilates Side Kick (NPCE Study Guide 2021, p. 49)

Intent
- Increase control of hip joint in flexion, abduction, adduction
- Refine whole-body organization to midline in side lying during movement of the ceiling leg

Gait reasoning
- Articulate the acetabular femoral motion required for gait cycle
- Refine adaption of torso during lower limb movement

Starting position
- Lying on side, place lower hand under head and top hand on mat in front of xiphoid process
- The floor leg may be in parallel or in external rotation
- Floor ankle and metatarsophalangeal (MTP) joints in dorsiflexion provide stabilizing contact with floor

Movement description
- In a continuous motion, move ceiling leg in flexion, abduction/external rotation, adduction
- Repeat 5 times
- Change direction
- Inhale during flexion and abduction
- Exhale during external rotation, adduction
- Organize whole body to the midline in all planes throughout movement

5. Single Leg Kick

Derivative of J. H. Pilates Single Leg Kick (NPCE Study Guide 2021, p. 48)

Intent
- Activate extensors and flexors of the torso and LE

Gait reasoning
- Stimulate non-weight-bearing flexion/extension of knees
- Improve knee ROM without high force compressive and shear forces to the meniscus
- Practice relative movement of tibia and femur in non-weight-bearing, open kinematic context

Starting position
- Prone on mat
- Support thoracic extension with elbows, forearms, and hands in contact with the mat
- Legs and feet aligned to the midline

Movement description
- During staccato inhalation rapidly flex right knee twice
- During exhalation extend right knee to starting position
- Repeat with left leg
- Alternate knee flexion and extension 10 times
- Sustain thoracic extension throughout the movement of the legs
- Support extension of the TLJ
- Avoid hyperextension of the TLJ
- Minimize tibial external rotation

6. Standing lateral weight shifting on BOSU ball

Derivative of J. H. Pilates Side Kick (NPCE Study Guide 2021, p. 49)

Editor note

Although J. H. Pilates did not have access to the BOSU ball he did include in his repertoire movement sequences standing on dynamic surfaces. For example, Universal Reformer Splits (NPCE Study Guide 2021, pp. 61–62) and Wunda Chair Forward Lunge, Side Lunge (NPCE Study Guide 2021, p. 77). The BOSU ball augments the Pilates equipment environment by stimulating gait-relevant movement vectors, including lumbosacral lateral flexion.

The BOSU ball is an air-filled half sphere. The client can stand on the convex surface with the flat surface on the mat. In contrast, the client can stand on the flat surface with the convexity on the mat. Each orientation provides unique challenges to standing balance, requiring integration of proprioception and vestibular and visual information.

Intent
- Develop whole-body proprioceptive acuity
- The BOSU ball challenges balance
- Develop dynamic whole-body balance on a dynamic surface
- Standing on the flat surface of the BOSU ball amplifies lateral weight shifts

Gait reasoning
- Stimulate torso control during lateral flexion
- Stimulate medial and lateral glide of the acetabular femoral joint
- Stimulate torso adaptability to standing on a dynamic surface

Starting position	• Stand on the flat side of the BOSU ball • LE in parallel • Arms by sides
Movement description	• Maintaining the midline orientation, shift weight to forefeet without flexing hip joints • Shift laterally between right and left • Focus the eyes forward to the horizon • Practice adapting to midline stance

7. Single-leg stance on the balance pad

Derivative of J. H. Pilates Side Kick (NPCE Study Guide 2021, p. 49)

Editor note

Although J. H. Pilates did not have access to a balance pad, he did include movement sequences standing on dynamic surfaces in his repertoire. For example, The Foot Corrector (NPCE Study Guide 2021, pp. 89–90) and Wunda Chair Standing Leg and Foot Press (NPCE Study Guide 2021, p. 76). The balance pad augments the Pilates equipment environment by stimulating gait-relevant movement vectors, including foot-ankle adaptability in pronation and supination.

Intent	• Stimulate foot and ankle proprioception • Stimulate foot and ankle adaptability in pronation and supination • Stimulate whole-body movement adaptability • Challenge integration of vestibular, proprioceptive, and visual systems to support balance
Gait reasoning	• Ability to transfer weight between right and left sides • Integrate LE proprioception with torso adaptability
Starting position	• Stand on balance pad • LE in parallel • Arms by sides
Movement description	• Refine balance on right and left sides, organizing to midline in all planes • Stand on right leg • Flex right hip joint and knee to above 90 degrees • Alternate right and left LE movements • Observe for deviations from midline including exaggeration of lateral flexion

8. Supine ankle series

Intent
- Change orientation to gravity for articulation of talotibial joint
- Improve control throughout ROM in dorsiflexion

Gait reasoning
- Reinforce adequate articulation of dorsiflexion and plantar flexion required for gait
- Improve adaptability of stance

Starting position
- Supine on mat with right hip joint flexion and knee extension, facing plantar surface of foot toward ceiling
- Slight flexion of knee is appropriate to achieve an optimal position for the client
- Left knee flexion with foot on mat

Movement description
- Articulate the foot and ankle through all ROM
- Plantar flex and move the foot into inversion and eversion
- Dorsiflex and move the foot into inversion and eversion

9. Seated plantar flexion and dorsiflexion

Intent
- Articulation and activation of dorsiflexion and plantar flexion
- Improve LE push-off and foot loading
- Stimulate proprioception in new organization

Gait reasoning
- Decrease ground forces through seated position for improved foot responses
- Enhance proprioception of the plantar side of the foot with the ground

Starting position
- Seated on a chair in an optimal position for the client
- Feet planted on floor
- Knees slightly lower than hip joints
- LE abduction

Movement description
- Articulate from the rear foot to the phalanges into plantar flexion
- Return to starting position
- Articulate the foot from the forefoot to the calcaneus into dorsiflexion
- 10 repetitions

10. Marble pickup

Intent
- Improve articulation and activation of the foot-LE

Gait reasoning
- Improve foot sensory input for adapting to varied ground surfaces

Starting position
- Seated on a chair in an optimal position for the client
- Feet planted on floor
- Knees slightly lower than hip joints
- Place marbles on floor at the forefoot

Movement description
- Pick up one marble at one time beginning with the phalanges
- Place marble in the box
- Pick up 10–15 marbles
- Repeat with the other foot

11. Foot articulation with resistance band

Intent
- Improve ROM and articulation of feet
- Challenge endurance of foot and ankle control

Gait reasoning
- Improve foot adaptability to ground forces

Starting position
- Seated on a chair in an optimal position for the client
- Feet planted on floor
- Knees slightly lower than hip joints
- Place band on the floor vertically in line with the forefoot

Movement description
- Place the right forefoot on the end of the band
- Pull the band toward the rear foot
- Repeat 5 times with each side

12. Single leg arcs maintaining single-leg stance

Intent
- Increase proprioception and coordination
- Improve lumbopelvic dynamic stability

Gait reasoning
- Adaptability to weight transfer from one side to the other
- Integrate proprioception with torso activation

Starting position
- Stand in parallel in optimal position
- Progress to standing in external rotation

Movement description
- Maintaining midline orientation, abduct right LE
- Move the right LE in a variety of directions to challenge balance
- Change sides
- 8 repetitions for each side

Session 11/12: Studio session

Fatigue scale 2

Pain scale 0

Client self-report
- After previous session, less fatigue and more energy
- No pain during one hour of medium-intensity training

Key changes observed by author at end of Session 11/12
- Fluid integration of leg swing with lumbopelvic-femoral rhythm during flexion, bringing knee and foot forward to heel strike without a lateral shift
- Lower closed kinematic chain coordination facilitated ankle plantar flexion in push-off gait phase
- Sacrum, TLJ, and occiput organized to midline in all three planes resulting in upright torso

Reason behind choice of sequencing
- With normal function of the body, perform advanced exercises in the session
- Build client confidence in her capacity for activities of daily living and exercise

Session movement sequence

1. Footwork on Universal Reformer Derivative of J. H. Pilates Footwork on Universal Reformer (NPCE Study Guide 2021, p. 52) and Running (NPCE Study Guide 2021, p. 60)

Intent
- Improve ROM of LE extension and flexion
- Integrate activation from foot to torso
- Awareness of LE organization during flexion and extension

Gait reasoning
- Non-weight-bearing flexion/extension of knees to improve ROM without high compressive and shear forces to the meniscus

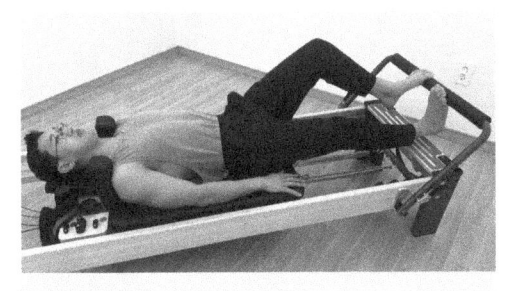

Pilates for Arthroscopic Knee Meniscus Repair Post-Surgery: Effect on Gait

Figure 6.1

Set-up
- Springs: 2 medium and 1 light or 2 medium
- Footbar supports 75 degrees hip joint flexion
- Option to use Universal Reformer footplate

Editor note
The Universal Reformer footbar supports greater ROM of ankle dorsiflexion when the forefoot is in contact with the footbar and the rear foot is in open kinematic context. The footplate provides greater contact for the plantar surface of the foot. This may increase proprioceptive information for knee tracking.

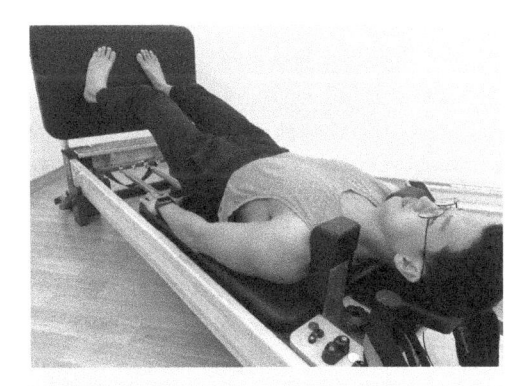

Figure 6.2

Starting position
- Supine on carriage
- Heels on footbar aligned with ischial tuberosities
- Knee flexion less than 90 degrees

Chapter 6

Movement description
- Exhale, extend hip and knee joints pushing carriage away from footbar
- Inhale, flex hip and knee joints as the carriage returns toward footbar
- Foot and leg positions on footbar
  - Heels
  - Forefoot
  - 30 degrees external rotation
- Internal rotation
- Tendon stretch
- Running
- 5–10 repetitions for each position

CUES
- Inhalation and exhalation activate the torso throughout movement
- Organize torso to the midline in all planes throughout movement
- Integrate optimal position of the torso and LE throughout the movement

Author note
Reduce the force of the spring in the early stage of recovery in order to avoid shear forces on the meniscal repair region (see Volume 1, Chapter 6).

2. Straps: feet in loops on Universal Reformer

Derivative of J. H. Pilates Footwork on Universal Reformer (NPCE Study Guide 2021, p. 52) and Running (NPCE Study Guide 2021, p. 60)

Intent
- Experience full excursion of hip joint ROM
- Improve proprioception and articulation of hip joint movement
- Improve bilateral rotational symmetry

Gait reasoning
- Supine position for ease of focusing on hip joint ROM for leg swing
- Improve external rotation of hip joint
- Improve stride length
- Facilitate activation of dorsiflexion with knee extension

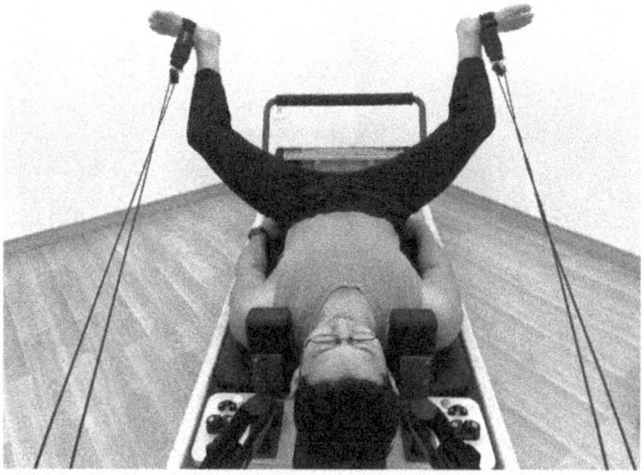

Figure 6.3

Set-up
- Springs: 1 or 2 medium and 1 light
- Low footbar

Starting position
- Supine
- Feet in straps
- Hip flexion to 60–70 degrees
- Knees extended
- Hands by sides, palms down

Movement description
- Movement variations
  - Pull straps into extension and flexion, LE adducted
  - Abduction, adduction
  - Full ROM extension, abduction, flexion, adduction
  - External rotation, knee flexion with heels together, extend and flex knees
  - External rotation, knee flexion with heels together, hip joint flexion and extension with no change of knee flexion
- 6–10 repetitions for each variation

CUES
- Observe optimal position for the client's torso throughout movement variations
- Cue client to emphasize the weaker leg for symmetrical movement
- Do not hyperextend the knees

Author note

Reduce the force of the spring in the early stage of recovery in order to avoid shear forces on the meniscal repair region (see Volume 1, Chapter 6).

3. Eve's Lunge on Universal Reformer

(See Chapter 5 in Volume 1, Gentry, Eve's Lunge)

Intent
- Dynamic torso organization during hip joint flexion and extension
- Vary forces acting on hip joint to promote coactivation of flexors and extensors

Gait reasoning
- Increase the ability to coordinate acetabular femoral flexion and extension
- Torso midline organization during LE movements

Set-up
- Springs: 1 medium and 1 light
- Footbar on high setting

Starting position
- Stand on left side of Universal Reformer
- Left foot on floor in line with bottom of carriage
- Left foot aligned with hip joint
- Left knee is flexed
- Right foot against shoulder stop
- Right knee flexion, hovering off the carriage
- Two hands on footbar

Movement description
- Press the carriage away from footbar extending right hip and knee joints while maintaining the position of torso and head
- Flex right hip and knee joints while returning the carriage toward the frame

CUES
- Maintain position of the torso
- Observe optimal organization of LE and torso
- Organize the head and neck regions to the midline in all planes

4. CoreAlign ankle plantar flexion with dorsiflexion of metatarsophalangeal joints

Derivative of J. H. Pilates Side Kick (NPCE Study Guide 2021, p. 49)

Editor note

Although J. H. Pilates did not have access to the CoreAlign, he did include movement sequences standing on dynamic surfaces in his repertoire. For example, Universal Reformer Splits (NPCE Study Guide 2021, pp. 61–62). The CoreAlign augments the Pilates equipment environment by supporting gait-relevant movement skills including reciprocal flexion and extension of the acetabular femoral joints.

The CoreAlign is a recent addition to the Pilates environment (2000). Its inclusion in Pilates studios follows the trends since the early 1980s, noted in Volume 1, Chapter 2 (see CoreAlign exercises in Volume 2 Chapters 8 and Volume 1, Chapter 14). The CoreAlign, invented by physiotherapist Jonathan Hoffman, consists of two carts sliding in parallel within a frame. A ladder at one end of the frame provides attachments for the hands and for cords with handles. The carts attach via elastics to either or both ends of the frame. The CoreAlign augments the Pilates apparatus environment by supporting a variety of vectors and balance assistance not available on the Universal Reformer. Challenges to standing balance, requiring integration of proprioception and vestibular and visual information, can be gradually introduced, calibrated to client tolerance.

Intent
- Develop lower leg alignment in push-off phase of gait
- Develop coordination required for reciprocal leg movement
- Develop whole-body organization while moving on a dynamic surface
- Refine upright standing posture
- Train coordination and balance

Gait reasoning
- The CoreAlign is a useful environment for addressing gait because it develops the ability to perform reciprocal leg movements with resistance from different directions
- Hands holding the ladder rung support balance while client adapts to the novel training environment
- Adjustable resistance provided by elastic cords supports progressive strength and endurance training

Chapter 6

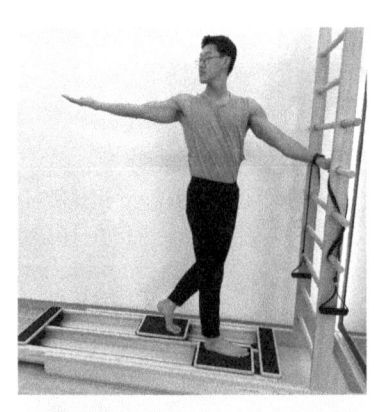

Figure 6.4

Set-up
- Face the ladder, one cart aligned in left lane, the other aligned in right lane
- 1 or 2 light elastic tubes attach each cart to ladder end of the frame
- Calibrate elastic resistance for client safety in upright stance
- If the resistance is too light, the client is at risk for instability
- If the resistance is too heavy, shear forces will compromise meniscus repair region

Starting position
- Stand facing the ladder
- One foot in each cart
- Hands hold ladder at waist height
- Upright stance organized to midline in all planes
- Gaze at horizon level

Movement description
- Movement variations
- Flex one knee and plantar flex the same-side ankle, raising the heel to push the cart backwards as if showing the bottom of the foot to someone behind you
- Maintain thighs parallel to each other
- Maintain torso upright during LE articulation
- Return to the starting position by lowering the heel and returning the carts to the starting position beside the ladder
- Alternate each leg during desired number of repetitions

CUES
- Align the head, thorax, and pelvis to the midline on all planes throughout movement
- Keep the knee in place directly below the hip joint
- Keep the center of the heel aligned with the 2nd metatarsal during ankle plantar flexion throughout cart movement
- Organize the shoulder girdle during hand contact with ladder rungs
- Minimize dependence on hand-ladder contact to maintain balance
- Gradually progress to maintaining balance without holding the ladder with hands

Author note
This movement stimulates integration of distal-to-proximal and proximal-to-distal proprioception. Connections between the foot, ankle, LE, pelvis, and torso translate into accurate gait coordination.

5. CoreAlign sagittal lunge
Derivative of J. H. Pilates Splits on Universal Reformer (NPCE Study Guide 2021, pp. 61–62)
(See Editor note above)

Intent
- Integrate leg strength and power with pelvis and torso
- Strengthen the legs for functional movements such as lowering to the ground and bending down to reach for an object behind
- Integrate torso rotation with coordination of reciprocal LE movements

Gait reasoning
- Lunges are powerful functional exercises that develop whole-body synergistic strength, endurance, and coordination
- Synergistic activation of the neuromyofascial system connecting the LE with the torso is critical for developing power and endurance for activities such as hiking, running, and biking
- Knee joint integrity requires the coordination, strength, and endurance of these tissue continuities

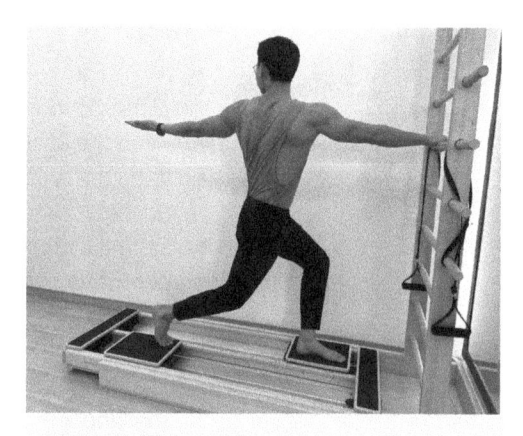

Figure 6.5

Set-up
- Facing the ladder, one cart aligned in left lane, the other aligned in right lane
- 1 or 2 light elastic tubes attach each cart to ladder end of the frame
- Calibrate elastic resistance for client safety in upright stance
- If the resistance is too light, the client is at risk for instability
- If the resistance is too heavy, shear forces will compromise tissue integrity of meniscus repair region

Starting position
- Stand facing the ladder
- One foot in each cart
- Hands hold ladder at waist height
- Upright stance organized to midline in all planes
- Gaze at horizon level

Movement description
- Press one cart back during bilateral knee flexion to 90 degrees
- Torso and head also move back away from ladder, aligning with movement of cart back from ladder
- Simultaneously extend both knees, returning the whole body to starting position at ladder
- The LE that moves cart back away from ladder maintains knee alignment with torso and head
- Alternate left and right sides throughout the repetitions
- Progress by adding torso rotation
- Torso rotation may be toward the side of the LE that is sliding the cart away from the ladder
- Or, torso rotation may be toward the side of the LE that is keeping the cart at the ladder

CUES
- Visualize a straight line from the head to the back of the knee
- Avoid hyperextension of the TLJ
- Keep the front knee aligned with or behind the 2nd metatarsal
- Organize the shoulder girdle during hand contact with ladder rungs
- Minimize dependence on hand-ladder contact to maintain balance
- Gradually progress to balance without holding ladder with hands

Author note
Limit ROM so the client can sustain motor control throughout the movement. Lower the torso only as far as is comfortable or appropriate for the client's motor control. The elastic bands that attach each cart to the frame require synergistic activation of LE and whole-body tissues responsible for concentric and eccentric movement.

6. CoreAlign Splits: Side
Derivative of J. H. Pilates Splits on Universal Reformer (NPCE Study Guide 2021, pp. 61–62)

Intent
- Develop motor control, strength, endurance, and tissue glide during LE adduction
- Develop motor control, strength, endurance, and tissue glide during LE abduction
- Develop balance and coordination required to sustain upright organization in a dynamic environment, standing with each foot on a moving cart

Gait reasoning
- Synergistic activation of the tissues and structures required for LE abduction and adduction varies according to the elastic resistance that attaches each cart to the frame
- Light-to-no resistance emphasizes adduction
- Increased resistance emphasizes abduction

Set-up
- 1 cart placed in each lane of track
- Elastic tubes attach each cart to ladder end of frame
- Calibrate elastic resistance for client safety in upright stance
- If the resistance is too light, the client is at risk for instability
- If the resistance is too heavy, shear forces will compromise meniscus repair region
- Emphasize adduction by using light elastic or no elastic
- Emphasize abduction by using stronger elastics

Starting position
- Stand upright with side to ladder, one foot on stable standing platform, other foot on cart
- Hand closest to the ladder holds the rung below shoulder height in the plane of scaption
- Organize the whole body to midline in all planes

Movement description
- Abduct the LE standing on the cart—the central axis of the whole body adjusts to maintain the torso and head centered between the two feet
- Adduct the LE standing on the cart, returning to the starting position—the central axis of the whole body adjusts to maintain the torso and head centered between the two feet
- As balance improves, increase ROM of abduction and let go of the ladder hand grip
- Progress by adding a squat
  - Knee flexion, abduction, knee extension, adduction

CUES
- Organize the torso and head to midline throughout each exercise
- Press the plantar surface of the big toes, the 1st ray, into the cart, creating a ground force that stimulates activation of the adductor region and tissues of the pelvic outlet
- Calibrate the forces of LE abduction and adduction to maintain torso equidistant between the feet

Author note
CoreAlign Splits: Side and Universal Reformer Splits: Side are similar. The CoreAlign ladder offers an accessible hand grip for clients who lack standing balance in a dynamic environment.

7. Wunda Chair Leg Pumps
Derivative of J. H. Pilates Standing Leg Pump: Front on Wunda Chair (NPCE Study Guide 2021, p. 79) and Double Leg Pumps on Wunda Chair (NPCE Study Guide 2021, p. 72)

Intent
- Increase load of LE to improve flexion and extension
- Challenge dynamic stability during LE activation

Gait reasoning
- Improve distribution of load forces through the LE

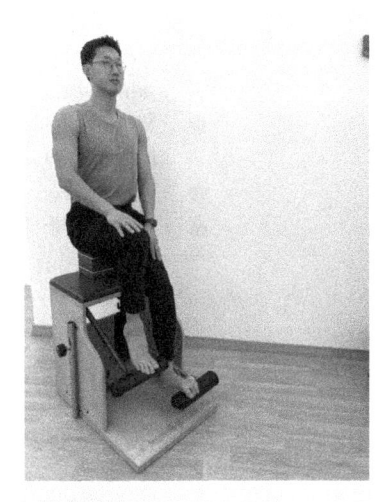

Pilates for Arthroscopic Knee Meniscus Repair Post-Surgery: Effect on Gait

Figure 6.6

Set-up	• 2 heavy springs
Starting position	• Seated on Wunda Chair with ischial tuberosities at front edge of chair seat • One foot on each foot pedal • Hands hold front edge of chair seat

Movement description	Double Leg Pumps
	• Exhale, pressing the pedals down maintaining optimal position of torso and LE
	• Inhale, returning the legs to the starting position
	• Foot position variations
	  ■ Rearfoot on the pedals with LE parallel
	  ■ Forefoot with heels slightly raised in ankle plantar flexion
	  ■ Midfoot parallel with LE
	  ■ External rotation with forefoot on pedals, slight plantar flexion
	  ■ Hip joint abduction, with heels on pedals
	  ■ Forefoot with legs parallel, plantar flex and dorsiflex without LE flexion or extension
	  ■ Split pedal with rearfoot on pedal alternating hip flexion and extension, 5 repetitions for each variation

Single Leg Pumps
- Unilateral movement: place one foot on pedal and extend knee of other leg
- Exhale, pressing the pedal down maintaining optimal position of torso and LE
- Inhale, returning the legs to the starting position
- Foot position variations
    - Rearfoot on pedal with LE parallel
    - External rotation with forefoot on pedal, slight plantar flexion
    - 10 repetitions each side

CUES
- Maintain weight evenly distributed on ischial tuberosities
- Observe optimal LE alignment
- Single Leg Pump: hold the free extended straight LE as high as possible without posterior pelvic rotation

Author note
In early stages of recovery, use a small box to decrease hip and knee flexion in starting position.

8. Wunda Chair lunges
Derivative of J. H. Pilates Wunda Chair Forward Lunge/Straight Stand (NPCE Study Guide 2021, p. 77)

Intent
- Increase load of LE to improve flexion and extension
- Challenge dynamic stability during LE activation

Gait reasoning
- LE loading to increase push-off and leg swing
- Increase endurance
- Reorganize dynamic stability of knee joint
- Develop integrity of tissues in knee region

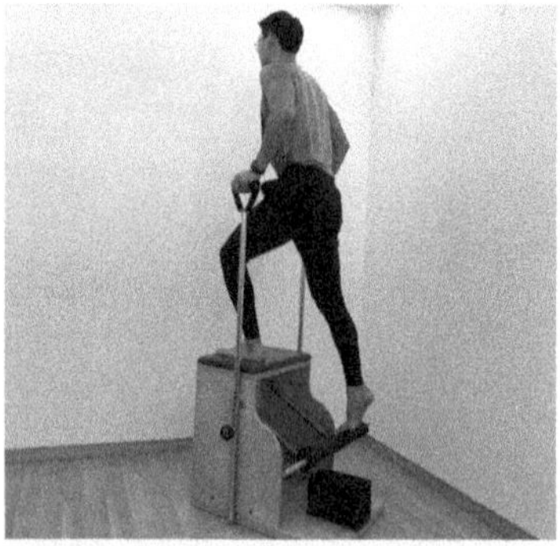

Figure 6.7

Set-up	• 2–4 heavy springs
Starting position	• Stand in front of Wunda Chair • Press pedal down with right foot • Place left foot on top of chair • Use handles for assistance, build up to cross-arm position
Movement description	• Inhale, transfer weight to left LE, lifting the pedal • Exhale, lower the pedal partially in the direction of the floor • 10–15 repetitions • Change sides

CUES
- Maintain pelvic orientation in the sagittal plane
- Observe LE optimal organization: do not allow the knee to move anterior of forefoot

Author note
If the knee adducts, or the pelvis unlevels, place hand at lateral pelvis to cue abduction. Discontinue if client experiences pain or discomfort.

9. Wunda Chair bridge Derivative of J. H. Pilates Single Leg Pump: Lying Flat (NPCE Study Guide, p. 76)

Intent	• Articulate from feet to torso • Activate extensors
Gait reasoning	• LE motion for stance and swing phases • Improved stance phase

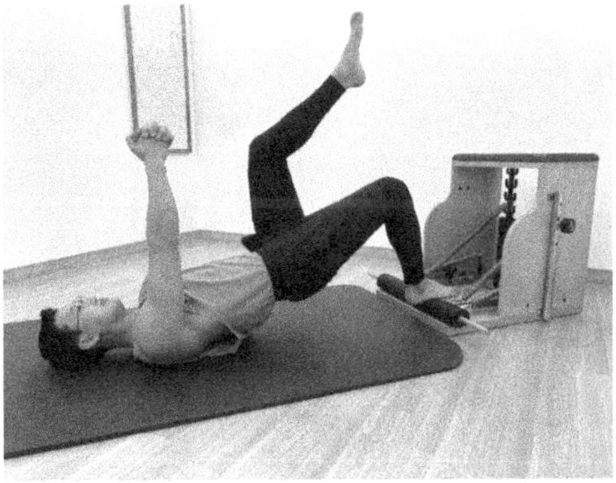

Figure 6.8

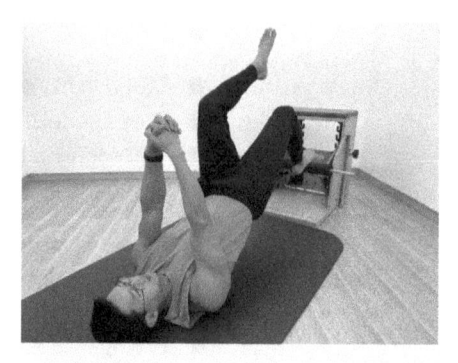

Figure 6.9

Set-up
- Springs: 1 heavy and 2 light

Starting position
- Supine on mat with rearfoot placed on foot pedal
- LE parallel with knees flexed
- Press the foot down without pelvis elevating
- Arms by sides on floor, arms off the floor to increase difficulty

Movement description
- Exhale, articulate into a bridge position initiating from the coccyx
- Inhale, articulate down returning to starting position
- Repeat 5 times
- Move into the bridge hold
- Maintaining the pedal down, lift right foot off the pedal
- Right hip joint and knee flexion
- Alternate right and left 5 times
- Advance to unilateral bridge position, lifting pedal up and down
- Alternate right and left
- Repeat reciprocal motion

CUES
- Observe optimal position for the client
- Maintain pelvis orientation during the movement
- Maintain thorax and pelvis relationship in the midline
- Press the upper arms into the mat to assist hip joint extension
- Move the pedal smoothly and with control

Author note
Place a non-skid rubberized mat under the chair to avoid sliding or place the chair against a wall. Discontinue if client experiences pain or discomfort.

The journey to Session 11

Session 4/12
Client self-report

- Less apprehensive to shift weight to right LE
- Fatigue scale 4
- Pain scale 4–5

Key changes observed

- Reduced tendency to supinate during ankle plantar flexion.

Reasoning behind choice of movements

- Improve ground force contact during push-off phase of gait, contributing to gait efficiency.

Session movement sequence
1. Side lying hip joint abduction with knee flexion

2. Lateral LE abduction/adduction

3. Supine ankle series

4. Standing weight shifting on the floor

5. Universal Reformer

- Footwork (springs: 1 medium and 1 light)
  - Rearfoot, external rotation on forefoot
- Straps: feet in loops (springs: 1 medium and 1 light)
  - Flexion and extension, knees extended

Session 5/12
Client self-report

- Felt soreness at lateral right femur
- Fatigue scale 3
- Pain scale 4

Key changes observed

- R lumbar stability improved in the frontal/coronal plane during knee flexion and extension

Reasoning behind choice of movements

- Knee flexion and extension during all phases of gait ought not impair lumbar-pelvic organization to the midline in all three planes

Session movement sequence
1. Standing weight shifting on the floor

2. Seated plantar flexion and dorsiflexion

3. Side lying hip joint abduction with knee flexion

4. Lateral LE abduction/adduction

5. Side lying LE flexion/abduction/adduction

6. Universal Reformer

- Footwork (springs: 1 medium and 1 light)
  - Rearfoot, external rotation on forefoot, dorsiflexion and plantar flexion
- Straps: feet in loops (springs: 1 medium and 1 light)
  - Flexion and extension, knees extended
  - Abduction/adduction
  - External rotation with feet together, hip flexion and extension

Session 6/12
Client self-report

- Standing weight between the center of pelvis without pain in the right knee

Chapter 6

- Fatigue scale 3
- Pain scale 2

Key changes observed

- Smooth distal to proximal transfer of force from foot to ankle to knee to hip

Reasoning behind choice of movements

- Smooth distal to proximal transfer of force from foot to ankle to knee to hip

Session movement sequence
1. Standing weight shifting on balance pad

> **Editor note**
> A balance cushion or pad may be an air cushion disc or foam pad.

2. Single-leg stance

3. Bridge

4. Standing leg lifts

5. Foot articulation with resistance band

6. CoreAlign

- Ankle plantar flexion with dorsiflexion of MTP joints
- Torso upright arm jumps

7. Universal Reformer

- Eve's Lunge
- Straps: feet in loops

Session 7/12
Client self-report

- Standing weight distributed evenly without right knee pain
- Fatigue scale 3
- Pain scale 0

Key changes observed

- Improved left thoracic rotation organized to the midline

Reasoning behind choice of movements

- Symmetry of thoracic rotation contributes to gait efficiency

Session movement sequence
1. Standing leg lifts

2. Standing weight shifting on BOSU ball

3. Lateral LE abduction/adduction

4. Side lying LE flexion/abduction/adduction

5. Marble pickup

6. CoreAlign

- Splits: Side
- Reciprocal hip flexion and extension

7. Wunda Chair

- Bridge

8. Ladder Barrel

- Facing the ladder, foot on barrel with knee flexion

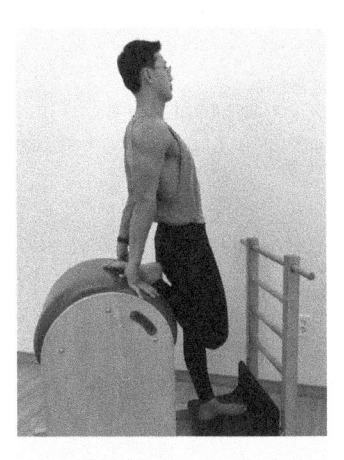

Figure 6.10

- Facing the barrel with LE extended on barrel
- Standing side to barrel, extended leg on barrel

Session 8/12
Client self-report

- No fear of flexing right knee
- Soreness of the anterior tibia area
- Fatigue scale 2
- Pain scale 0

Key changes observed

- Improved R foot-ankle-knee-hip tracking during hip extension

Reasoning behind choice of movements

- Efficiency of push-off phase of gait contributes to stride length

Session movement sequence
1. Seated plantar flexion and dorsiflexion

2. Supine ankle series

3. Unilateral stance on the balance pad

4. Add LE movement in many directions

5. Universal Reformer

- Footwork (springs: 1 medium and 1 light)
  - Rearfoot, external rotation on forefoot, dorsiflexion and plantar flexion
- Straps: feet in loops (springs: 1 medium and 1 light)
  - Flexion and extension, knees extended
  - Abduction/adduction
  - External rotation with feet together, hip flexion and extension
- Eve's Lunge

6. CoreAlign

- Ankle plantar flexion with dorsiflexion of MTP joints
- Sagittal lunge with ankle plantar flexion

7. Additional movements

- Rolling ball on plantar surface of foot
- Foam roller on anterior and posterior lower limb

Session 9/12
Client self-report

- Walking without canes
- Fatigue scale 2
- Pain scale 0

Key changes observed

- Improved R foot-ankle-knee-hip tracking during hip extension

Reasoning behind choice of movements

- Control of lateral pelvic stability protects the lumbar-pelvic region from tissue irritation caused by compensations for knee disorganization

Session movement sequence
1. Bridge

2. Side lying hip joint abduction with knee flexion

3. Lateral LE abduction/adduction

4. Side lying LE flexion/abduction/adduction

5. Standing leg lifts on the balance pad

6. Wunda Chair

- Leg Pumps
- Lunges
- Bridge

7. CoreAlign

- Ankle plantar flexion with dorsiflexion of MTP joints

Session 10/12
Client self-report

- Feels normal in daily life
- Fatigue scale 1
- Pain scale 0

Key changes observed

- Right leg matches left leg initiation of hip extension rather than lagging behind left leg extension

Reasoning behind choice of movements

- Symmetrical hip extension contributes to gait efficiency and reduced wear of hip-lumbo-sacral region

Session movement sequence
1. Single Leg Kicks

2. Bridge, added unilateral

3. Squat on the BOSU ball

4. CoreAlign

- Splits: Side
- Lunges
- Reverse lunge
- Hip abduction/adduction with knee flexion/extension
- Single leg side lean

References

Abrams, G. D., Frank, R. M., and Gupta, A. K. (2013) "Trends in meniscus repair and meniscectomy in the United States, 2005–2011." *American Journal of Sports Medicine, 41*, 2333–2339.

Allen, P. R., Denham, R. A., and Swan, A. V. (1984) "Late degenerative changes after meniscectomy: Factors affecting the knee after operation." *The Journal of Bone and Joint Surgery (Br), 66*, 5, 666–671.

Arnoczky, S. P. and Warren, R. F. (1982) "Microvasculature of the human meniscus." *The American Journal of Sports Medicine, 10*, 2, 90–95.

Chambers, H. G. and Chambers, R. C. (2019) "The natural history of meniscus tears." *Journal of Pediatric Orthopaedics, 39*, 6, Suppl. 1, S53–S55.

De Carlo, M. and Armstrong, B. (2010) "Rehabilitation of the knee following sports injury." *Clinics in Sports Medicine, 29*, 1, 81–106.

Hede, A., Jensen, D. B., Blyme, P., and Sonne-Holm, S. (1990) "Epidemiology of meniscal lesions in the knee: 1215 open operations in Copenhagen 1982–1984." *Acta Orthopaedica Scandinavica, 61*, 5, 435–437.

Huckell, J. R. (1965) "Is meniscectomy a benign procedure? A long term follow up study." *Canadian Journal of Surgery, 8*, 254–260.

Jorgensen, U., Sonne-Holm, S., Lauridsen, F., and Rosenklint, A. (1987) "Long-term follow-up of meniscectomy in athletes: A prospective longitudinal study." *The Journal of Bone and Joint Surgery British Volume, 69*, 1, 80–83.

Kurosawa, H., Fukubayashi, T. and Nakajima, H. (1980) "Load-bearing mode of the knee joint: Physical behavior of the knee joint with or without menisci." *Clinical Orthopaedics and Related Research, 149*, 283–290.

Levy, I. M., Torzilli, P. A., and Warren, R. F. (1982) "The effect of medial meniscetomy on anterior-posterior motion of the knee." *Journal of Bone and Joint Surgery American Volume, 64*, 6, 883–888.

Mintzer, C. M., Richmond, J. C., and Taylor, J. (1998) "Meniscal repair in the young athlete." *American Journal of Sports Medicine, 26*, 5, 630–633.

NPCE Study Guide (National Pilates Certification Exam Study Guide) (2021) Miami, FL: National Pilates Certification Program, Inc.

Philippe, B. and Roland, B. (2017) "The knee meniscus: Management of traumatic tears and degenerative lesions." *EFORT Open Reviews, 2,* 5, 195–203.

Rockborn, P. and Messner, K. (2000) "Long-term results of meniscus repair and meniscectomy: A 13-year functional and radiographic follow-up study." *Knee Surgery Sports Traumatology Arthroscopy, 8*, 1, 2–10.

Scapinelli, R. (1968) "Studies on the vasculature of the human knee joint." *Acta Anatomica, 70,* 305–331.

Scarr, G. (2018) *Biotensegrity: The Structural Basis of Life.* 2nd Ed. Edinburgh: Handspring Publishing.

Spang, R. C., III, and Nasr, M. C. (2018) "Rehabilitation following meniscal repair: A systematic review." *BMJ Open Sport Exercise Medicine, 4*, 1. DOI: 10.1136/bmjsem-2016-000212.

Venkatachalam, S., Godsiff, S. P., and Harding, M. L. (2001) "Review of the clinical results of arthroscopic meniscal repair." *Knee, 8,* 129–133.

Chapter 7

Pilates and Ankle Dysfunction: Effect on Gait

Ann McMillan

The ankle is the most frequently injured joint in the body. More than 20,000 ankle sprains occur each day in the United States (Burke 2018).

Foot pain is reported as common in the general population with prevalence estimates from population surveys ranging from 17 to 30 percent. Ankle disorders can result from damage to bone, muscle, or soft tissue. Common ankle disorders include: sprains (injury to ligaments), fractures, tendonitis (inflammation of the tendons), impingement, arthritis (chronic inflammation of joints) (Hendry *et al.* 2018). Disorders of the foot and ankle can be associated with pain and dysfunction of other joints, especially the knees (Cooper *et al.* 2011).

Common symptoms are inflammation involving any of the bones, ligaments, or tendons in the foot that can cause foot pain (Mayo Clinic Staff 2021).

Sprains and strains can lead to reduced ankle motion predominantly in dorsiflexion. Functional rehabilitation exercise programs can prevent loss of articulation. Soft tissue goes through three phases as it heals: inflammation, repair (also called proliferation), and remodeling. Inflammation is necessary for normal healing and can last up to 5 days; exercise is not recommended during this phase. The repair phase allows for the replacement of tissues that are no longer viable following injury and can last from one to two months. Remodeling strengthens the tissue produced during the repair phase and can last up to one year (Houglum 2005).

Once the swelling subsides, exercise to restore range of motion (ROM) can start. When ROM is recovered, muscle strengthening can begin with isometric leaning exercises that progress to isotonic open chain exercise. The process can continue with proprioceptive training and specific exercises aimed at return to occupation which mimic the desired sport or activity (Wolfe *et al.* 2001). Respect your scope of practice and always check with the acting physician, physiotherapist, or athletic therapist for clear exercise objectives, guidelines, and limitations.

Anterior impingement syndrome of the ankle affects many athletes and can be due to inflammation and scar tissue or bone spurs that form in the anterior ankle at the talocrural joint. It limits ROM and can cause pain (Stanford Medicine Health Care 2021). Repeated micro-traumas can cause inflammation. Due to inflammation the soft tissue will swell and have reduced elasticity, leading to an impingement (Cerezal *et al.* 2003).

This syndrome is also called footballer's ankle or athlete's ankle, because these sports are responsible for creating pressure on the ankle's cartilage. Despite the name, this can happen in many different types of sports, including soccer, football, and basketball, and in dancers.

Limitation of activity to allow inflammation to recede, soft tissue massage, taping, and physiotherapy management can help. In some cases, surgery might be required. Physical therapy follows similar guidelines to sprain and strain recovery. As always, check with the acting physician, physiotherapist, or athletic therapist for exercise guidelines and limitations.

A diagnostic is performed through the following methods: patient reported outcome measures (PROMs), clinical examination, static foot structure and alignment, joint ROM, muscle performance, footwear assessment, dynamic assessment of foot motion (including gait analysis), dynamic assessment of plantar load distribution, and provocational tests (Rao, Riskowski, and Hannan 2012).

Various medical interventions are available. Results can improve when combining treatment methods such as manual therapy of the foot and ankle, application of Kinesio® tape, and functional rehabilitation. Also, prescribed foot orthotics (devices that are worn inside the shoes) designed with the intent to correct foot misalignment and gait can be beneficial.

Client description: 20-year-old biological female, identifies as female; elite international level ice dance athlete

Dates of case report: Session 1: December 17, 2019; Session 12: April 4, 2020. Interruption due to subject participating in ice dance competitions. Due to COVID, Session 12, final assessment, was an online Zoom session

Studio apparatus and props
Pilates equipment

- Universal Reformer
- Trapeze Table
- Wunda Chair with split pedal

Props used with equipment

- Mat
- Soft balls, 4 in. (10 cm)
- Half roller
- Jump board
- Heavy resistance 12 in. (30 cm) rotator discs
- Small box

Home program props

- Mat
- Roller
- Half roller

- Strap
- Soft balls, 4 in. (10 cm)

Methods and materials

Session 1/12
1. Health history interview

- 2018: anterior ankle impingement syndrome on right ankle
- Swelling of the capsule was regulated through rest, manual therapy, and anti-inflammatory drugs
- Pain decreased
- Mobilization, strength, and proprioceptive training reestablished function
- Ankle dorsiflexion is still limited; following coaches' request to maintain consistency in training movement, sequences are optimized for lower extremity function

- Concussions in 2011 and 2017, condition now stable

2. Symptoms

- Intense ankle pain decreased gradually
- Currently pain is occasional and linked to intense workload
- Occasional neck pain
- Rigorous training creates generalized tension, frequent bruising, and connective tissue strain

3. Movement aids

- None

Final result of case report
Gait is well organized with improved coordination of synchronized pelvic and thorax rotation, the feet less externally rotated, and increased dorsiflexion. Coaches recognized changes in her gait patterning: improved lower extremity (LE) organization, increased knee flexion, improved midline organization, and improved performance on the ice.

Session 2/12: Initial assessment

1. General observations of gait

- Feet externally rotated
- Heel strike on lateral aspect of feet, tibias externally rotated
- No toe push-off and resupination
- Swing phase limited, dorsiflexion brings feet in lateral rotation
- Anterior pelvic tilt
- Excessive lumbar and thoracic extension at push-off
- Limited hip joint extension
- No thoracic rotation, arm swing propels the torso
- Limited spring action and shock absorption of arch of foot
- Overall stiffness

2. Standing tests

- Full torso rotation
- Observations of inefficient side: left
  - Thorax in right lateral translation at onset
  - Limited left femur adduction
  - Limited ankle adaptation in pronation or supination
  - Shift of weight to the right on end range
  - Torso extension to achieve end range rotation

Session 12/12: Post-assessment

1. General observations of gait

- Reduction of externally rotated feet
- Heel strike migrated back to lateral heel
- Improved push-off and resupination
- Improved dorsiflexion
- Slight reduction of anterior pelvic tilt
- Excessive torso extension still present
- Slight hip joint extension improvement
- Pelvis transfers laterally and thorax rotates
- Improved spring action and shock absorption through arch of foot
- Reduction of overall stiffness, fluid gait

2. Standing tests

- Full torso rotation
- Observations of inefficient side: both
  - Thorax in right lateral translation at onset
  - Limited left femur adduction
  - Bilateral feet pronation and supination synchronized with torso rotation
    - Reduction of shift of weight to the right on end range
    - Reduced torso extension rotation to achieve end ROM

- ◆ Hemipelvis inferior motion

- ● Observations of inefficient side: right
  - ■ Translates pelvis to left
  - ■ Limited lumbar movement
  - ■ Limited left hip joint adduction and internal rotation

- ◆ Hemipelvis superior motion

- ● Observations of inefficient side: left
  - ■ Limited left hemipelvis elevation
  - ■ No right lumbar translation
  - ■ Right thorax translations
  - ■ Limited plantar flexion

- ◆ Lateral pelvic shift

- ● Observations of inefficient side: left
  - ■ Limited right hemipelvis inferior motion
  - ■ Right thoracic translation
  - ■ Left hip joint limited adduction

3. Seated tests

- ◆ Hip joint and knee flexion

- ● Observations of inefficient side: left
  - ■ Weight shifts to the right ischial tuberosity to flex left hip joint

Author note
Included dorsiflexion and knee flexion test. Both were efficient bilaterally. Included hip abduction with external rotation. Right was efficient, left was inefficient. On left inefficient side, subject shifted weight to the right ischial tuberosity.

4. Sit and stand

- ◆ Lateral view

- ◆ Hemipelvis inferior motion

- ● Observations of inefficient side: both
  - ■ Improved right hemipelvis inferior motion
  - ■ Lateral lumbar movement present
  - ■ Improved left hip joint adduction and internal rotation

- ◆ Hemipelvis superior motion

- ● Observations of inefficient side: left
  - ■ Improved hemipelvis elevation
  - ■ Right lumbar translates minimizing thoracic right translation
  - ■ Improved plantar flexion

- ◆ Lateral pelvic shift

- ● Observations of inefficient side: left
  - ■ Right hemipelvis lowers
  - ■ Reduced right thoracic translation
  - ■ Improved left hip joint adduction

3. Seated tests

- ◆ Hip joint and knee flexion

- ● Observations of inefficient side: left
  - ■ No weight shifting

Author note
Included dorsiflexion and knee flexion test. Both were efficient bilaterally. Included hip abduction with external rotation. Both were efficient. No shift of weight.

4. Sit and stand

- ◆ Lateral view

- Torso leans forward excessively
- Torso forward lean in response to limited ankle dorsiflexion
- Increased tone of torso extensors

◆ Anterior view

- Shifts weight to the right
- Thorax rotates and translates right
- Bilateral knee valgus both to standing and sitting
- Left foot pronates
- Right foot supinates

5. Standing balance

◆ Two-leg stance, eyes open

- Both sides: 60 seconds

◆ One-leg stance, eyes open

- Right leg: 60 seconds
- Left leg: 60 seconds

◆ One-leg stance, eyes closed

- Right leg: 10 seconds
- Left leg: 7 seconds

- Reduced torso lean forward
- Improved dorsiflexion
- Increased tone of torso extensors

◆ Anterior view

- Weight evenly distributed
- Reduced right thoracic rotation and translation
- Slight bilateral knee valgus
- Decreased pronation of left foot
- Decreased supination of right foot

5. Standing balance

◆ Two-leg stance, eyes open

- Right leg: 60 seconds
- Left leg: 60 seconds

◆ One-leg stance, eyes closed

- Right leg: 10 seconds
- Left leg: 5 seconds

Session 3/12: Home program

Fatigue scale	3
Pain scale	0
Client self-report	● Tired from a long day of skating, but feeling good
Key changes observed by author at end of Session 3/12	● Subject aware of externally rotated feet during gait ● Enthusiastic to improve LE and torso relationship ● Medially rotating tibia and keeping foot/ankle in neutral reduced knee pain
Reason behind choice of sequencing	● Increase ankle dorsiflexion and pronation ● Promote LE awareness and alignment ● Activate LE continuity through torso

Session movement sequence

1. Prone rolling anterior LE on mat	This exercise has three variations using either a roller or 1 or 2 small, soft balls (see exercises 2 and 3 below for variations)
Intent	● Stimulate connective tissue of femur ● Increase hip glide to address anterior pelvis and reduce excessive lordosis
Gait reasoning	● Improve the contralateral patterning of the pelvis and torso
Starting position	● On roller ■ Lying prone, with anterior femurs on roller and elbows supporting torso on mat
Movement description	● Roller on femurs ● Roll central medial and lateral aspects of femurs on roller ● 8 repetitions
2. Prone rolling anterior LE on mat, variation 1	
Intent	● Stimulate connective tissue of femur ● Increase hip glide to address anterior pelvis and reduce excessive lordosis
Gait reasoning	● Improve the contralateral patterning of the pelvis and torso
Starting position	● With 1 small ball ■ Lying prone on mat, with forehead resting on hands, with ball under right femur, knee flexed softly

Movement description	• With small ball under right thigh
	▪ Hold pressure for 1 minute
	▪ Slowly move tibia from right to left, crossing the ball
	▪ Repeat with ball under left thigh
	▪ 8 repetitions

3. Prone rolling anterior LE on mat, variation 2

Intent	• Stimulate connective tissue of femur
	• Increase hip glide to address anterior pelvis and reduce excessive lordosis
Gait reasoning	• Improve the contralateral patterning of the pelvis and torso
Starting position	• With 2 small balls
	▪ Lying prone on mat, with forehead resting on hands
	▪ Place the 2 balls on the anterior pelvis inside each iliac crest, keeping both knees flexed
Movement description	• With 2 small balls
	▪ Hold pressure and breathe for 1 minute
	▪ Slowly move tibia from right to left, crossing the balls
	▪ Repeat on the left side
	▪ 8 repetitions

4. Side lying hip glides using strap

Intent	• Improve hip joint ROM
	• Stimulate extensor activation
	• Rebalance forces acting on the hip joint
Gait reasoning	• Improve LE adaption to ground forces and transfer of weight
	• Develop awareness of cause-effect relationship between extensors and flexor activation

Starting position   Medial side
- Side lying on left side
- Left hip extension and knee flexion
- Right hip and knee flexion
- Strap around left ankle, straddling over the right shoulder
- Hold strap with both hands in front of the chest

Lateral side
- Side lying on right side
- Left hip extension and knee flexion
- Right hip and knee flexion
- Strap around left ankle, straddling over the left shoulder
- Hold strap with both hands in front of the chest

Movement description   Medial side
- Gently pull on strap to increase extension
- Keep forefoot perpendicular to tibia
- Anchor right foot to the floor
- 16 repetitions, holding the last stretch for 4 slow breaths

Lateral side
- Small range of left LE flexion/extension motion
- Rock the pelvis posteriorly and anteriorly
- Adduct the thigh as the LE extends
- Keep forefoot square to tibia
- Anchor right foot to the floor
- 16 repetitions, holding the last stretch for 4 slow breaths

5. Standing Mermaid against wall

Intent
- Develop ease in global lateral movement
- Develop kinesthetic awareness by providing contrasting left and right tissue sensations

Gait reasoning
- Ease lateral connective tissue to address anterior pelvic tilt and excessive lumbar extension
- Improve weight distribution and foot loading in standing

Chapter 7

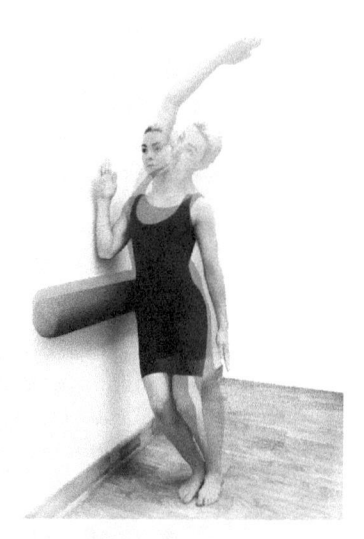

Figure 7.1

Starting position
- Stand laterally with feet about 1 ft (30 to 40 cm) from wall
- Lean one hemipelvis into horizontal roller, just above greater trochanter
- Knees flexed
- LE parallel
- Flex elbow of upper extremity (UE) closest to wall, keeping other UE by side

Movement description
- Exhale, simultaneously extending the knees as the torso laterally flexes away from the wall
- Reach the wall side UE overhead
- Inhale, return to starting position
- UE close to wall articulates to extend
- Create opposition between the outside foot pressing into the ground and the hemipelvis pressing into the roller
- Create opposition between UE close to wall extending diagonally away from the wall and UE by sides reaching for the ground
- 8 repetitions
- Pause to sense differences on left and right side before starting the second side
- Pause to sense overall effect after completing both sides

6. Scissors keeping head on the floor

Intent
- Coordinated LE and UE motion in flexion and extension
- Develop contralateral patterning

Gait reasoning
- Encourage torso activation in contralateral movement

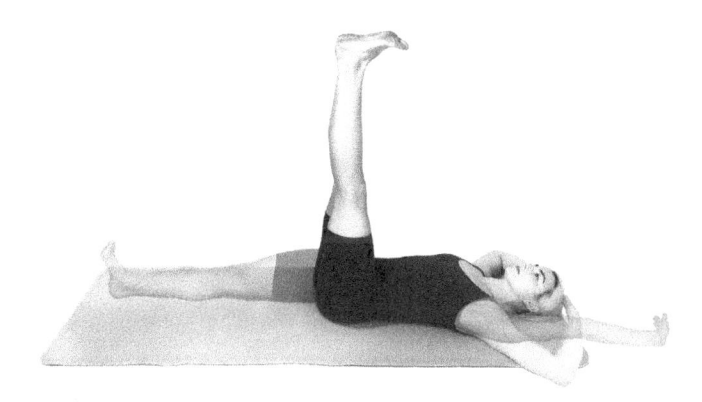

Figure 7.2

Starting position
- Supine on mat
- Knees extended, hip joint at 90 degrees flexion, ankle in dorsiflexion
- UE on floor, elbows flexed at ear level with back of the hands touching the top of the head
- Shoulders and elbows flexed

Movement description
- Exhale, simultaneously bringing right LE to the floor in extension, as the left elbow extends and the left hand reaches overhead
- Inhale, reversing the motion to return to the starting position
- Repeat for the other side
- 8 repetitions

7. Side Kick on roller

Intent
- Activate the continuity of the LE to the torso from a LE medial organization
- Activate medially to counter tendency to abduct/flex
- Improve pelvifemoral adaptation

Gait reasoning	• Improve leg swing
Starting position	• Lie on right side on mat • Head resting on right humerus, left hand on mat • Left hip joint at 90 degrees flexion, knee extended, ankle resting on roller • Right hip joint at 0 degrees, knee extended • Align forefoot perpendicular to tibia, both feet dorsiflexed
Movement description	• Press right LE into mat for lateral activation • 10 repetitions • Lift left LE off the roller, perform abduction/external rotation/extension/adduction/flexion of femur • 10 circles in each direction

8. Hip joint articulation supine on half roller

Intent	• Provide a pendulum motion for oscillation of hip joint from flexion/abduction to extension/adduction • Increase torso and hip joint extensor activation
Gait reasoning	• Increase hip joint extension • Coordinate the movement of hip joint and torso

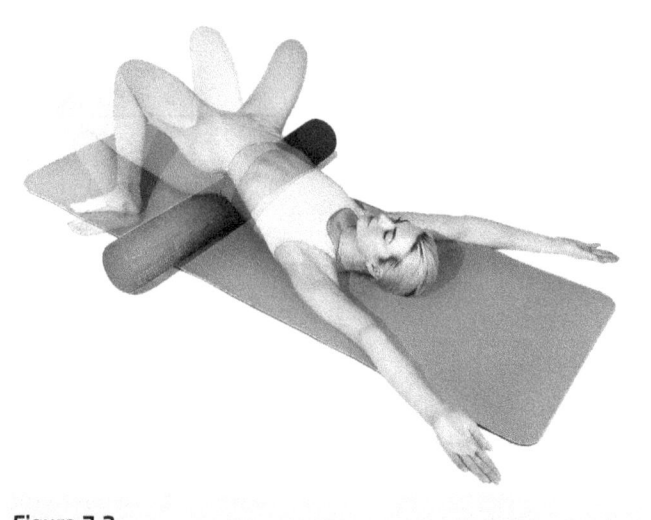

Figure 7.3

Pilates and Ankle Dysfunction: Effect on Gait

Starting position	• Lie supine on half roller with posterior pelvis at sacrum level perpendicular on roller • Feet flat on mat • LE abducted with full knee flexion, feet close to roller • UE resting on floor, shoulders flexed and abducted
Movement description	• Slowly exhale pressing right foot into floor • Articulate right hip joint in extension as pelvis rotates left • Inhale into posterior lateral thorax • Return to starting position • 8 repetitions • Hold final hip joint extension for 4 breaths

9. Half Kneeling Mermaid

Intent	• Improve hip joint adaptation to force • Place hip joint in a disadvantaged position to activate extensors
Gait reasoning	• Promote extensor activation in gait

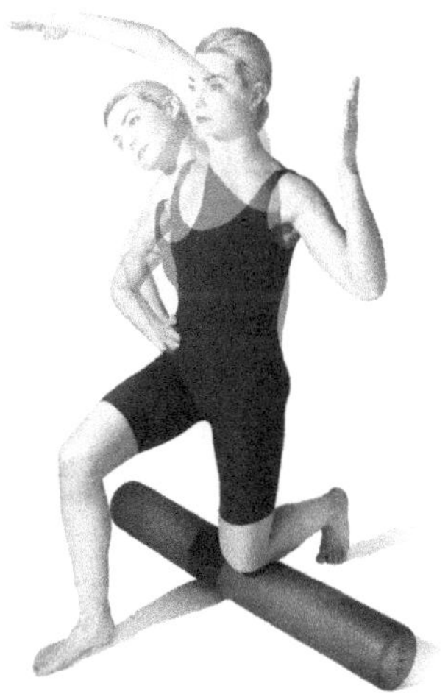

Figure 7.4

Starting position	• Half kneeling with right knee on floor • Right hand next to right shoulder, elbow flexed • Left hand on superior aspect of hemipelvis

Movement description	• Exhale, left lateral flexion as right hand reaches overhead
• Inhale, return to starting position
• 8 repetitions
• Create opposition by pressing right knee into the ground and flex right UE diagonally overhead
• Aim left ischial tuberosity to the ground
• 8 repetitions
• Option: thorax small flexion rotation and extension rotation
• Repeat for the other side

10. Dorsiflexion with roller

Intent	• Promoting myofascial gliding
• Stimulate articulation and awareness in dorsiflexion and pronation
Gait reasoning	• Promote fluidity of foot motion
• Increase ankle dorsiflexion
• Develop adaptable foot pronation
Starting position	• With 2 small balls
• Quadruped position
• Kneel on roller
Movement description	• With 2 small balls
• Squat pre-test: note sensation and depth of squat
• Roll on center, medial, lateral aspects from toes to mid shin on right tibia for 60 seconds
• Stand, repeat squat test and compare left to right sides
• Repeat for the left side
• Repeat squat test and observe the side-to-side balance

11. Adapted Mulligan dorsiflexion

Editor note
Brian Mulligan, FNZSP(Hon), DipMT, is a physiotherapist who developed the Mulligan™ Manual Therapy Concept—manual therapy techniques utilizing mobilization with movement (MWM)—to relieve pain and increase ROM (Mulligan 2023).

Intent	• Improve talocrural dorsiflexion
• Promote medial tibial rotation
• Promote centration of acetabulum

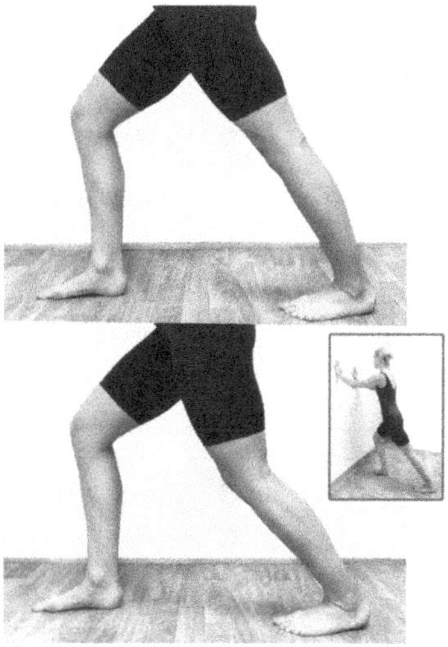

Pilates and Ankle Dysfunction: Effect on Gait

Figure 7.5

Gait reasoning	• Promote ankle dorsiflexion in swing phase • Promote foot pronation • Increase ankle and foot awareness • Stimulate spring motion foot arches
Starting position	• Leaning forward, hands on wall • Right hip extension, right ankle dorsiflexed, knee extended • Left hip and knee flexion
Movement description	• Walk to be aware of feet sensation • Flex right knee in available range, maintaining hip joint extension • Track the patella over 2nd and 3rd toes • Feel tibia move toward forefoot • Allow the plantar vault to flatten and elongate as knee bends (Kapandji 2019) • Extend the knee, pressing rear foot into floor • 20 repetitions • Repeat walk around to feel difference of right to left • Repeat on left side • Repeat walk around, observing balance

Author note
Imagery for the foot as a trampoline as the knee bends is that the trampoline flattens (Kapandji 2019).

12. Standing ankle articulations

Intent
- Increase ankle joint ROM
- Replicate gait ankle motion

Gait reasoning
- Increase ankle proprioception
- Develop pronation
- Reduce tibial lateral rotation
- Change weight distribution during heel strike to lateral aspect of calcaneus
- Promote fluidity in foot motion

Starting position
- Standing in front of mirror
- Hands on superior ilia
- Left foot anterior
- Right foot posterior

Movement description
- Move right rear foot in motion inversion and eversion
- Heads of metatarsals remain in contact with ground
- Gait awareness: compare right and left
- 20 repetitions
- Change sides

13. Standing proprioception

Intent
- Improve proprioception and organization of standing

Gait reasoning
- Incorporate global optimal articular congruency to gait pattern

Starting position
- Standing with feet parallel
- Soft ball between medial malleoli
- UE by sides

Movement description
- Standing, feel the opposing forces of the feet pressing into the ground and the crown of the head upward
- Gently press 1st metatarsals and calcanei into ground
- Internally rotate the feet in opposition to externally rotating femurs
- Hold stance for a few breaths
- Relax and walk to notice sensation of spiral

14. Standing vertical rear foot raise

Intent	● Challenge control of global articular congruency ● Link the role of the LE to whole-body organization from the floor up
Gait reasoning	● Efficient use of ground forces that is integrated into the whole structure
Starting position	● Stand and promote organization as in exercise 13, "Standing proprioception" ● Soft ball placed between medial malleoli
Movement description	● Shift weight posteriorly and anteriorly on feet ● Notice sensation of pressure increase on metatarsals as weight goes forward ● Find the weight centered on foot ● Without moving, recreate pressure under metatarsals, feel activation travel up LE into torso ● Keep increasing pressure on metatarsals until calcaneus comes off floor into plantar flexion ● Intend on elevating without forward body translation ● 4 repetitions ● On last repetition, half lower the feet and hold gaze to right then left twice ● Finish standing to take moment to feel the feet's whole-body sensation

Session 11/12: Studio session

Fatigue scale	0
Pain scale	0
Client self-report	● Increased energy since ice rinks are closed due to COVID and training off ice ● Experiences a sense of "everything works" that made exercises harder
Key changes observed by author at end of Session 3/12	● Embodied movement sequences ● Demonstated fluidity of movement in transitions ● Improved distribution of ground forces through feet ● Pelvis transfers laterally, thorax rotates ● Hip joints and tibial plateau organized to midline of LE

Chapter 7

Reason behind choice of sequencing	- Use supine torso contact on the Universal Reformer for kinesthetic and proprioceptive response to better organize movement
- Focus on dorsiflexion and pronation promoting resilience needed for fluid gait pattern
- Recalibrate the forces around the hip joints and center the pelvis out of anterior tilt
- Rebalance extensors and flexors to minimize excessive extension
- Create optimal body organization on two feet and reproduce skating force vectors to encourage transfer to sports

Author note
COVID restrictions forced the class to be held at a different location. Push-through bar was not available for this session. Washer Woman on chair replaced the Push-Through Seated Front Series.

Session movement sequence

1. Footwork on Universal Reformer	Derivative of J. H. Pilates Footwork on Universal Reformer (NPCE Study Guide 2021, p. 52)
Intent	- Ankle articulation and control
- Medially rotate tibial plateau on femoral condyles
- Control lower limb and foot in parallel and in external rotation
- Coordinate breathing during footwork
Gait reasoning	- Stimulate optimal transmission of ground forces through the body
- Improve resilience in the foot and ankle
- Decrease tibial torsion
Set-up	- 3 medium springs
- Lighter springs
- Jump board
- Half roller
- Soft ball between malleoli for all parallel work
Starting position	- Supine on half roller with flat surface down, feet on jump board
- Feet parallel in center of jump board
- Hip joints at 0 degrees of flexion when knees extended
- Soft ball placed between malleoli

Movement description
- LE parallel
- Rear feet in contact with jump board, knees slightly flexed
- 8 repetitions
- LE parallel
- Hip and knee flexion, rear feet off jump board
- 8 repetitions
- Repeat with feet at 45 degrees with hip joints in external rotation
- 8 repetitions

Variation of LE sequence
- Knees flex in parallel
- No carriage movement as rear feet lift to plantar flexion
- Knees extend as carriage moves
- Keep knees extended, lowering rear feet to dorsiflexion
- Reverse LE sequence
- Repeat both directions of LE sequence in external rotation

CUES
- Keep pressure on soft ball between malleoli, especially during final degrees of knee extension
- Maintain 1st metatarsophalangeal (MTP) joint in contact with jump board, particularly during knee extension
- Patella in line with 2nd toe in internal rotation, especially with extended knees
- Cue feet parallel for tibial internal rotation in opposition to LE external rotation

Author note
This client has marked tibial external rotation which brings the feet into an externally rotated stance. When placing the feet parallel in Footwork, the legs compensate resulting in valgus knee. Cueing feet parallel as the hip joints externally rotate facilitated relative internal rotation of the tibia.

2. Preparation side lying on Universal Reformer

Intent
- Activation around the hip joints to rebalance the flexors and extensors

Gait reasoning
- Activate extensors for push-off

Chapter 7

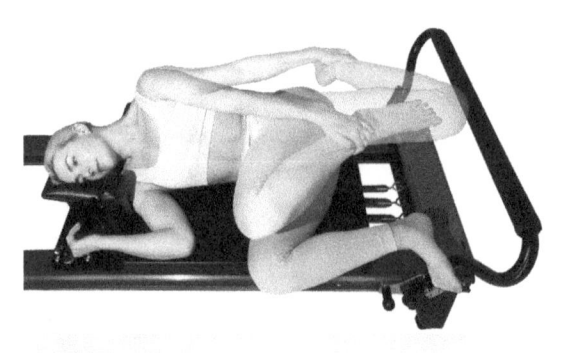

Figure 7.6

Set-up	• Adjust bar to accommodate knee movement for preparation • All springs to stabilize carriage
Starting position	• Side lying on Universal Reformer, knees into chest • Head on headrest • Top hand holding top ankle
Movement description	• Move hip joint into flexion and extension • 8 repetitions • Hold final extension position for three breaths

CUES
- Maintain pelvis position while swinging leg anteriorly and posteriorly
- Do not allow lumbar extension to increase

3. Pelvic lift/bridge on Universal Reformer

Intent	• Internally rotate tibia relative to femoral external rotation • Control LE in parallel
Gait reasoning	• Improve adaptability to ground forces • Rebalance hip flexors and extensors • Reorganize the pelvis to reduce anterior tilt • Reduce lumbar and thoracic extension for improved rotation
Set-up	• High bar • Springs: 2 medium and 1 light • Headrest down • Soft balls between malleoli and between 1st MTP joints

Pilates and Ankle Dysfunction: Effect on Gait

Starting position	• Lying supine • Rear feet on footbar, LE parallel • UE by sides
Movement description	• Hold final extension position for three breaths

Variation 1
- Articulate from the pelvis through the torso into Bridge position without carriage movement
- Articulate down to starting position
- 3 repetitions

Variation 2
- Flex elbows to 90 degrees
- Lift pelvis off carriage and hold
- Press elbows into carriage
- Alternate right and left hip joints in flexion/extension with knees flexed
- Keep carriage stable

Variation 3
- Lift pelvis off carriage in Bridge and hold
- Move carriage away and toward footbar
- Knee extension and flexion

CUES
- Pelvis lifts to height for activation avoiding thoracolumbar extension
- Cue feet parallel in opposition to hip external rotation
- Activate the extensors by pressing opposite elbow and foot downward prior to flexing hip joint

Author note
This is a great opportunity to address multiple issues in a supine environment for continuity of foot with a derotated tibia and sagittal plane organization. Practicing in supine prepares the body for standing work.

4. Quadruped, head facing back of Universal Reformer

Derivative of J. H. Pilates Knee Stretch Series on Universal Reformer (NPCE Study Guide 2021, p. 60)

Intent	• LE and UE articulation on stationary torso • Motor control of hip flexion and extension

Chapter 7

Gait reasoning	• Encourage sagittal plane organization to midline
Set-up	• Medium spring • High bar
Starting position	• Quadruped position • Hands on frame, knees and feet on carriage
Movement description	• With stable torso flex and extend hip joints • 8 repetitions

CUE
- Press the hands against the frame as rear foot presses into bar

Editor note
The hands on the frame facilitate reorganizing tension and compression throughout the body for improved articulation of the hip joints.

5. Quadruped, head facing back of Universal Reformer, unilateral LE extension

Derivative of J. H. Pilates Knee Stretch Series on Universal Reformer (NPCE Study Guide 2021, p. 60)

Intent	• Contralateral movement of UE/LE on torso • Activate torso during hip extension
Gait reasoning	• Promote hip extension maintaining sagittal torso control

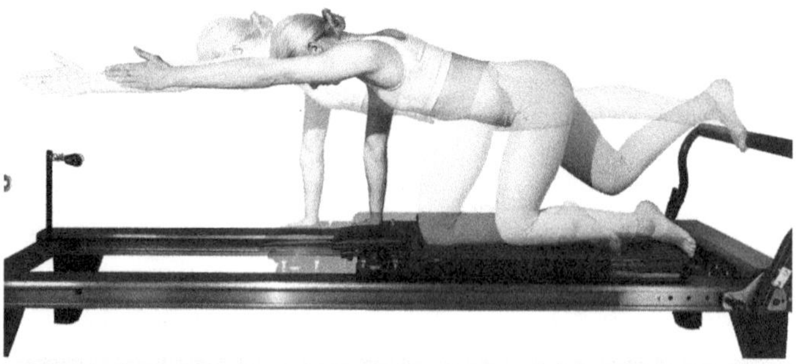

Figure 7.7

Set-up	• Medium spring
	• High bar
Starting position	• Quadruped position
	• Place hands on carriage, unilateral rear foot on high bar
Movement description	• Maintaining one hand contact on frame, flex contralateral shoulder
	• Press foot into bar
	• Extend hip joint and knee
	• Return carriage to starting position
	• 8 repetitions
	• Repeat for the other side

CUE
- Proactively press into supportive hand and knee before extending right knee and hip joint

Editor note
The hands on the frame facilitate reorganizing the tension and compression throughout the body for improved articulation of the hip joints.

6. Tendon Stretch and running on Universal Reformer

Derivative of J. H. Pilates Footwork on Universal Reformer: Tendon Stretch (NPCE Study Guide 2021, p. 52) and Running on Universal Reformer (NPCE Study Guide, p. 60)

Intent	• Increase ROM dorsiflexion on LE optimal organization
	• Increase foot adaption in pronation and supination
	• Increase foot resiliency
Gait reasoning	• Improve dorsiflexion
	• Increase supination to pronation and resupination through foot between heel strike and toe push-off
	• Improve feet adaption of ground forces
Set-up	• 3 medium springs
	• Footbar supports hip joints at 30 degrees flexion when carriage is out and knees are extended
Starting position	• Supine on carriage
	• LE in parallel, metatarsals on footbar

Movement description
- Press the carriage away and extend the hip joints and knees
- In extension, unilaterally roll rear foot from pronation to supination while maintaining foot in dorsiflexion
- 8 repetitions
- Repeat for the other foot
- Unilaterally press the carriage away as if standing on one LE
- Flex and extend the knee with ankle in dorsiflexion
- 8 repetitions
- Repeat for the other foot
- Bilaterally, alternate knee flexion "running in place"
- 16 repetitions

Author note
The dorsiflexion with unilateral knee flexion can be seen as a Universal Reformer adapted Mulligan dorsiflexion mobilization.

CUES
- Maintain all metatarsals in contact with footbar as foot rolls in and out
- Imagery of "going on edges" of skate blades
- In knee flexion track the patella over 2nd and 3rd metatarsals

Author note
This sequence provides foot articulation in all planes.

7. Straps: feet in loops on Universal Reformer

Derivative of J. H. Pilates Leg Springs: Supine on Trapeze Table (NPCE Study Guide 2021, pp. 67–68)

Intent
- Articulate hip joints in all end ROM to replicate sport requirement
- Motor control of femur on pelvis
- Finish series with LE adduction to reduce anterior pelvic tilt and torso extension

Gait reasoning
- Promote torso organization to reduce lumbar and thoracic extension
- Rebalance and reduce anterior pelvic rotation

Set-up
- 2 medium springs
- Foot straps attached to ropes

Pilates and Ankle Dysfunction: Effect on Gait

Starting position	• Lying supine on carriage
	• Feet placed in straps
	• Hip joints abducted/externally rotated, knees flexed, rear feet together and forefeet apart
	• UE by sides
Movement description	This exercise has a four-movement progression:
1. Alternating knee flexion/extension	• Extend knees and hip joints to 30 degrees flexion, LE parallel
	• Return to starting position
	• Extend knees and hip joints to 90 degrees flexion, LE parallel (or maximum hip joint flexion maintaining sacrum on carriage)
	• Return to starting position
	• 8 repetitions
2. Abduction to maximal range	• From starting position move to maximal hip abduction and knee extension
	• Return to starting position
	• 8 repetitions
3. Dynamic multi-planar pelvifemoral mobilization	

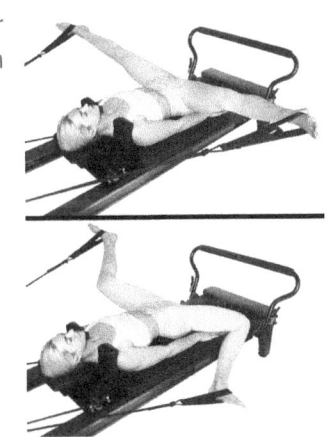

Figure 7.8

- Start with hip joints fully abducted, knees slightly flexed
- Roll pelvis right as left femur internally rotates and both knees increase flexion
- Bring left hip joint into full extension and right hip joint into flexion
- Reverse motion to the other side
- Lumbopelvic motion accommodates the position of the femoral head which reduces medial knee torque
- 20 repetitions

Chapter 7

4. Adduction mini-beats in parallel
- Maintain knees extended with 0 degree hip joint flexion in parallel
- Perform very small range quick abduction/adduction, abducting no wider than the shoulders
- Isometric hold of legs together for 20 seconds

CUES
- Knee flexion/extension, maintaining sacrum contact with carriage
- Maximal abduction with external rotation with relative internal rotation of tibia, minimizing tibial external rotation

Author note
Technical, artistic sports athletes have a propensity to achieve great hip joint end ROM which produces movement compensations. Observing and cueing for reorganization helps minimize compensations.

8. Scooter on Universal Reformer (See Chapter 5 in Volume 1, Gentry: Eve's Lunge)

Editor note
"Eve's Lunge" and "Scooter" often refer to similar exercises. In this case, the author focused on the torso relationship to movement of the LE in the sagittal plane to facilitate proprioception of standing with optimal foot loading.

Intent
- Rebalance the forces acting on the hip joint to promote the coactivation of flexors and extensors
- Training in proprioception of standing with optimal foot loading

Gait reasoning
- Increase stance leg extension input for forward propulsion

Set-up
- Springs: 1 medium and 1 very light
- High bar

Starting position
- Stand on left side of Universal Reformer
- Left foot on floor in line with bottom of carriage
- Knee is extended
- Left foot in line with femoral joint
- Right foot against shoulder stop on ipsilateral side
- Right knee flexion, hovering off the carriage
- Both hands on footbar

Movement description	• Press the carriage away with right hip joint extension and left hip and knee flexion
	• Carriage returns home as right hip joint and knee flex and left hip joint and knee extend
	• 8 repetitions
	• On final repetition, rest knee on pushed out carriage, gently rock pelvis left to right
	• Change to 1 medium spring
	• Stand upright
	• Hands off footbar
	• Both knees are flexed and both elbows are at 90 degrees flexion
	• Push carriage back as left shoulder flexes and moves front and right shoulder extends
	• Return carriage to starting position
	• 20 repetitions
	• Switch to other side

CUES
- Press rear foot of extending hip joint into shoulder stop to promote extensor activation
- Create opposing force vectors between foot on shoulder stop and standing leg knee
- Allow UE to swing as in gait patterning

Author note
Scooter facilitates transferring the organization practiced in supine to standing through proprioception.

9. Wunda Chair: Washer Woman	Derivative of J. H. Pilates Washer Woman Over the Chair/Hamstring 2 (NPCE Study Guide 2021, p. 77)
Intent	• Sagittal plane torso motion
	• Rebalance anterior and posterior forces acting on the torso
Gait reasoning	• Improves thoracolumbar fascia resiliency to promote overall gait rhythm
Set-up	• 2 light springs in high position
Starting position	• Stand in front of foot pedal, knees extended in parallel

Movement description
- Articulate from the head through the torso in flexion to press the pedal down
- Keeping hands on pedal and torso in flexion, bring the pedal up
- 8 repetitions
- Finish articulating the torso into extension to stand upright

CUE
- Feet rotate in opposition to hip joints while moving torso

10. Wunda Chair: Standing leg extension

Derivative of J. H. Pilates Achilles Stretch on Wunda Chair (NPCE Study Guide 2021, p. 79)

Intent
- Promotes hip joint articulation in flexion while standing
- Internally rotates head of tibia on femoral condyles
- Controls lower limb and foot alignment in parallel in standing

Gait reasoning
- LE motor control and standing balance for optimal transfer of ground forces to the torso

Set-up
- Heavy spring in high position
- If split chair with no dowel, handles attached
- Handles in place

Starting position
- Stand on a wooden platform, with right foot on platform, left rear foot on pedal
- Spring is in tension as pedal is already down
- Hands on handles

Movement description
- Knee and hip joint flexion to lift the pedal mid-range
- Knee and hip extension to push pedal back to ground
- Hands let go of handles after 2 to 4 repetitions
- Repeat without hands on handles for 20 repetitions
- Repeat for the other side

CUES
- Push pedal, feeling foot to head
- Imagine chewing gum stuck under rear foot as pedal rises
- Aim ischial tuberosity while moving LE inferiorly

Author note
Emphasis on the downward motion of the pedal is a prodigious tool to help perceive the action of ground forces through the pelvis and torso.

11. Standing leg extension on Wunda Chair

Derivative of J. H. Pilates Standing Leg Pump: Side on Wunda Chair (NPCE Study Guide 2021, p. 79)

Intent
- Enhance torso control and improve balance in response to ground forces
- Lateral force transmission is prevalent in skating

Gait reasoning
- Develop awareness against lateral forces
- Activate hip joint for adaptive control
- Induce lateral pronation supination force vectors to stimulate the force transmission on the ice

Set-up
- 2 light springs in high position
- If split chair, dowel in place
- Small box in front of pedal
- High handles in place

Starting position
- Stand to side of Wunda Chair pedal with LE parallel, knees extended
- Place left foot on small box
- Right foot on pedal
- Right hand on handle
- Left hand on left hemipelvis

Movement description
- Right knee/hip flexion and extension
- 8 repetitions
- Gradually lift hand an inch away from handle
- 8 repetitions
- Add left lateral torso flexion as pedal is pushed down to right lateral flexion as the pedal moves up
- Gradually lift hand an inch away from handle

CUES
- Coordinate the foot action with torso activation for controlled motion of pedal
- Imprint sole of foot into small box to stimulate activation of standing side

Author note
Standing Wunda Chair exercises can progress to adding a rotator disc for standing LE various degrees of rotation. This provides the multiple force vectors necessary for skating skills.

Chapter 7

12. Standing internal/external rotation on resisted rotator discs

Intent
- Improve ankle motor control with LE internal and external rotation
- Increase awarenss of how the foot relates to the whole body
- Internally rotate tibia relative to femur

Gait reasoning
- Increase proprioception of lumbar-pelvic-femoral adaptation to feet
- Produce a force vector to stimulate tibial internal rotation relative to hip joint external rotation
- Rebalance the foot-pelvis organization for improved verticality

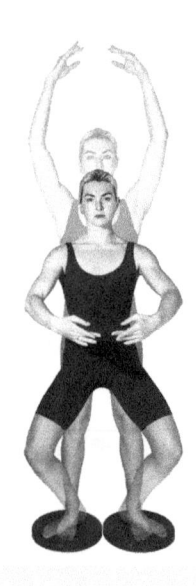

Figure 7.9

Set-up
- Heavy resistance 12 in. (30 cm) rotator discs

Starting position
- Stand on discs, feet at 45 degrees external rotation
- Hip and knee extension
- Shoulders at 90 degrees flexion
- Palms face each other, fingertips touch
- Elbows flexed

254

Movement description
- Pivot discs from external to internal rotation
- 20 repetitions
- Flex and extend hip joints and knees remaining in parallel
- Discs stationary
- 10 repetitions
- Flex and extend hip joints and knees
- Simultaneously, perform shoulder flexion/extension as discs pivot
- Start in knee flexion, LE in 45 degrees external rotation
- Shoulders at 90 degrees flexion
- Extend knees, LE parallel
- Shoulders at 180 degrees flexion
- Return to starting position
- 10 repetitions

CUES
- Initiate disc rotation by imprinting your full foot on the disc
- Place extra pressure under the rear foot
- Organize to midline orientation

Author note
The force vectors of resisted internal rotation in standing create a unique environment for the client by balancing forces to produce optimal movement for the task.

The journey to Session 11

Session 4/12
Client self-report

- "Back feels looser at end of session"
- Fatigue scale 3
- Pain scale 0

Key changes observed

- Improved congruency of hip joint and tibia in parallel during Footwork
- Receiving sensory feedback to difference of left and right strides in home program review
- Balls between the malleoli and 1st metatarsals promote tibial medial rotation during knee flexion and extension

Reasoning behind choice of movements

- Footwork in parallel develops motor control for femur-tibia-ankle coordination
- Reduce lumbar region extension and anterior pelvic rotation through flexion

Session movement sequence
1. Standing portion of home program

- Gait awareness: take a few steps, notice sensations
- Adapted Mulligan dorsiflexion, right
- Gait awareness: compare right and left
- Adapted Mulligan dorsiflexion, left
- Gait awareness
- Right standing ankle articulations
- Gait awareness: compare right and left

- Left standing ankle articulations
- Final gait awareness and integration

2. Universal Reformer

- Footwork
- Tendon stretch ankle roll
- Running
- Straps: feet in loops
  - Adduction mini-beats in parallel
  - High LE angle
  - Abduction
  - Dynamic multi-planar pelvifemoral mobilization

3. Trapeze Table

- Roll-Down
- Push-Through Seated Front

Session 5/12
Client self-report

- "Back feels looser and longer at end of session"
- Fatigue scale 3
- Pain scale 0

Key changes observed

- Improved congruency of hip joint and tibia in parallel during Footwork
- Good MTP contact on the footbar and improved hip joint centration
- Standing foot-torso not as organized as in supine

Reasoning behind choice of movements

- Increasing adaptability for smoother gait rhythm
- Home program gait awareness to improve proprioception
- To improve dorsiflexion for stance

Session movement sequence
1. Standing portion of home program

- Gait awareness and integration
- Adapted Mulligan dorsiflexion, right
- Standing ankle articulations, right and left
- Gait awareness: compare right and left
- Adapted Mulligan dorsiflexion, left
- Final gait awareness and integration

2. Universal Reformer

- Footwork
  - Parallel balls between malleoli and 1st metatarsals
  - On calcaneus
  - On MTPs, plantar and dorsiflexion
- Tendon stretch ankle roll
- Running
- Leg arcs
  - Adduction mini-beats in parallel
  - Low LE angle
  - High LE angle
  - Abduction
  - Dynamic multi-planar pelvifemoral mobilization

3. Trapeze Table

- Roll-Down
- Push-Through Seated Front
- Mermaid

Session 6/12
Client self-report

- "I felt I was able to get more mobility in my ankles"
- Very sore all over from return to training after a week off
- Neck discomfort upon waking up, but fine after training

- Fatigue scale 6
- Pain scale 3

Key changes observed

- Diminished valgus knee
- Ankle articulations difficult
- Used mirror for client to correlate seeing and feeling movement

Reasoning behind choice of movements

- Addition of rotator discs enhances LE control during internal and external rotation
- Continue proprioception of feet to torso
- Increase ankle and foot articulation
- Acetabular femoral articulation and motor control in end ranges related to sport-specific requirements

Session movement sequence
1. Standing portion of home program

- Gait awareness and integration
- Adapted Mulligan dorsiflexion, right
- Ankle articulations: inversion/eversion
- Gait awareness: compare right and left
- Repeat on left
- Final gait awareness and integration

2. Universal Reformer

- Footwork on jump board and rotator discs
  - Parallel, external rotation
  - On metatarsals, plantar flexion and dorsiflexion in external rotation
  - Alternate between LE internal and external rotation in knee flexion on a stable carriage, repeat with extended knees
- Straps: feet in loops
  - Adduction mini-beats in parallel
  - High arcs
  - Abduction
  - Dynamic multi-planar pelvifemoral mobilization
- Tendon stretch ankle roll
- Running

3. Trapeze Table

- Roll-Down
- Push-Through Seated Front
- Mermaid, thoracic translation hand on tower bar, no springs

Session 7/12
Client self-report

- "I feel I am walking straighter at end of session. I also feel less tired"
- Left latissimus dorsi area painful upon contraction, reason unknown
- Fatigue scale 7
- Pain scale 3

Key changes observed

- Ankle articulation is gaining suppleness, especially on left foot
- Client consciously walks with feet parallel
- Observing improved gait patterning

Reasoning behind choice of movements
- Supine lying on half roller facilitates a greater midline organization challenge than lying directly on carriage

Session movement sequence
1. Standing portion of home program
done at end of session

- Leg spiral in standing
- Gait awareness and integration
- Adapted Mulligan dorsiflexion, right
- Gait awareness: compare right and left

Chapter 7

- Right ankle articulation: inversion and eversion
- Gait awareness: compare right and left
- Repeat on left
- Final gait awareness and integration

2. Universal Reformer

- Footwork on jump board lying on half roller
    - Knee flexion/extension in parallel
    - Add rotator discs
    - Knee flexion/extension in external rotation
    - On metatarsals, plantar flexion and dorsiflexion in external rotation
    - Alternate between internal and external rotation in knee flexion on stable carriage, repeat with knees extended
- Straps: feet in loops
    - Adduction mini-beats in parallel
    - High LE angle
    - Abduction
    - Dynamic multi-planar pelvifemoral mobilization
- Tendon stretch ankle roll
- Running

3. Trapeze Table

- Roll-Down lying on half roller
- Push-Through Seated Front
- Mermaid

4. Additional movement

- Imagery of the bones of the spine and pelvifemoral model was used to teach the motion of the hip joints during Footwork on the Universal Reformer. A skeletal model was placed on the subject's torso to facilitate a sensory motor experience to embody the coordination of the LE

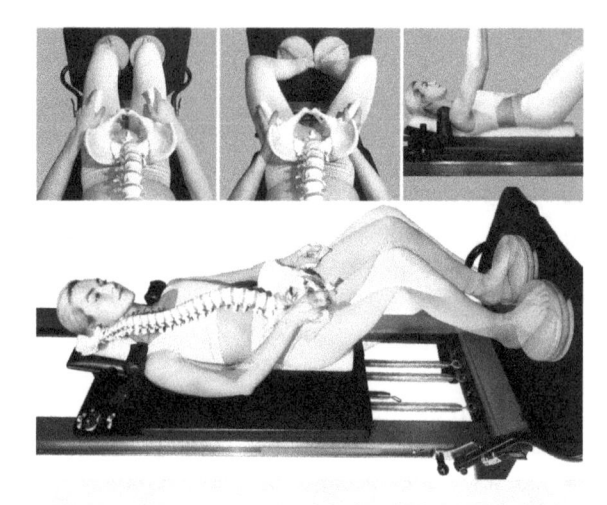

Figure 7.10

Session 8/12
Client self-report

- "For the first time, I can easily walk with feet in a natural fashion. I was so tired from training when we started, but now I feel energized by the Pilates session"
- Pain from post-training fatigue, previously reported mid-thorax pain, is gone
- Fatigue scale 7
- Pain scale 2

Key changes observed

- Significant gait improvement observed by fluid motion with feet in parallel

Reasoning behind choice of movements

- Repeating sequence provides opportunity for integration
- Introduction of standing work on rotator discs to integrate from the feet up
- Produce a force vector using discs, stimulating

tibial internal rotation relative to hip joint external rotation

Session movement sequence
1. Prone rolling anterior LE

- Divided between Trapeze Table and standing rotator disc work

2. Universal Reformer

- Footwork on jump board lying on half roller
    - Knee flexion/extension in parallel
    - Add rotator discs: partial knee flexion in parallel and external rotation
    - End range knee flexion in external rotation
    - On metatarsals, plantar flexion and dorsiflexion in external rotation
    - Alternate between LE internal and external rotation in knee flexion on a stable carriage; repeat with knees extended
- Straps: feet in loops
    - Adduction mini-beats in parallel
    - High arcs
    - Abduction
    - Dynamic multi-planar pelvifemoral mobilization
- Tendon stretch ankle roll
- Running

3. Trapeze Table

- Roll-Down lying on half roller
- Push-Through Seated Front
- Mermaid
- Prone rolling anterior LE

4. Standing on resisted rotator discs

- 45 degrees external rotation, disc resists internal rotation
- Final gait integration

Session 9/12
Client self-report

- "I feel peaceful, I feel stretched, I feel at peace and upper back is now at 2 out of 10"
- Woke up feeling sick with a sore throat, but felt fine after training
- Fatigue scale 8
- Pain scale 3

Key changes observed

- Still a conscious effort to organize feet, tibia, and femur in standing

Reasoning behind choice of movements

- To continue building foot resiliency
- Shortened Footwork Series to leave time for additional home program for feet
- Scooter on Universal Reformer to promote extension in standing
- Push-Through Seated Front with rotation to facilitate reciprocal rotation of thorax and pelvis

Session movement sequence
1. Standing portion of home program

- Observe torso flexion in standing
- Ball rolling for right foot
- Repeat, observe torso flexion, notice changes
- Ball rolling for left foot
- Repeat torso flexion test, notice changes
- Standing in parallel, plantar flexion and dorsiflexion with minimal forward shift of weight
- Gait awareness and integration

2. Universal Reformer

- Footwork with footbar lying on half roller
    - Parallel on calcaneus
    - On metatarsals, dorsiflexion and plantar flexion

Chapter 7

- Running
- Straps: feet in loops
    - Adduction mini-beats in parallel
    - High LE angle
    - Abduction
    - Dynamic multi-planar pelvifemoral mobilization
- Scooter

3. Trapeze Table

- Roll-Down lying on half roller
- Push-Through Seated Front
- Mermaid
- Push-Through Seated Front with twist

4. Standing on resisted rotator discs

- Feet at 45 degrees external rotation, disc resists internal rotation
- Gait awareness and integration

Session 10/12
Client self-report

- "It felt great to move, as I am not presently skating due to the coronavirus pandemic, since all the arenas are closed. I was feeling sore in my legs from yesterday's private ballet class but now I feel less mental fatigue and less soreness at end of session"
- "I am surprised by the strong mental work that goes into the standing work at the chair!"
- Fatigue scale 5
- Pain scale 0

Key changes observed

- Range of hip extension in bridging is limited
- Increased ROM of hip joints and reduced lateral flexion in Wunda Chair observed in hip and knee flexion/extension facing pedal

- Focusing on hip joint, externally rotating in opposition to tibia and internally rotating to achieve optimal LE organization

Reasoning behind choice of movements

- To promote equipment management efficacy, Washer Woman on Wunda Chair will substitute for Push-Through Seated Front
- To promote torso and LE continuity and activation
- Low resistance Footwork replaces rotator discs on jump board since discs were not available for Footwork
- Bridging in preparation for standing work at Wunda Chair and on resisted discs

Session movement sequence
1. Universal Reformer

- Footwork on jump board
    - Lying on half roller
    - On metatarsals, plantar flexion and dorsiflexion in parallel and external rotation
    - Minimal spring resistance to challenge torso control
    - Side lying
- Bridging series
- Straps: feet in loops
    - Alternate with LE at low angle and high angle
    - Adduction mini-beats in parallel
    - Abduction
    - Dynamic multi-planar pelvifemoral mobilization
- Running
- Scooter

2. Wunda Chair

- Washer Woman
- Hip and knee flexion/extension facing pedal

3. Standing on resisted rotator discs

- Feet at 45 degrees external rotation, disc resists internal rotation

References

Burke, D. (2018) Ankle disorders: Causes, symptoms and diagnosis. Healthline. [Online]. www.healthline.com/health/ankle-disorders. [Accessed August 18, 2023].

Cerezal, L., Abascal, F., Canga, A., Pereda, T. et al. (2003) "MR imaging of ankle impingement syndromes." *American Journal of Roentgenology*, 181, 2, 551–559. www.ajronline.org/doi/full/10.2214/ajr.181.2.1810551. [Accessed August 18, 2023].

Cooper, B., Omori, D., Ritter, J., and Sessums, L. (2011) Disorders of the foot and ankle for the internist. Walter Reed Army Medical Center. [Online]. www.sgim.org/file%20library/sgim/resource%20library/meeting%20handouts/sgim/2011/we02-handout-1-.pdf. [Accessed August 18, 2023].

Hendry, J. G., Fenocchi, L., Woodburn, J., and Steultjens, M. (2018) "Foot pain and foot health in an educated population of adults: Results from the Glasgow Caledonian University Alumni Foot Health Survey." *Journal of Foot and Ankle Research*, 11, 48. DOI: 10.1186/s13047-018-0290-1.

Houglum, P. A. (2005) *Therapeutic Exercises for Musculoskeletal Injuries*. 2nd Ed. Champaign, Il: Human Kinetics.

Kapandji, A. I. (2019) *The Physiology of the Joints – Volume 2: The Lower Limb*. 7th Ed. Edinburgh: Handspring Publishing, p. 242.

Mayo Clinic Staff (2021) Symptoms: Foot pain. [Online]. www.mayoclinic.org/symptoms/foot-pain/basics/causes/sym-20050792. [Accessed August 18, 2023].

Mulligan, B. (2023) Mulligan Manual Therapy Concept. [Online]. https://bmulligan.com. [Accessed August 18, 2023].

NPCE Study Guide (National Pilates Certification Exam Study Guide) (2021) Miami, FL: National Pilates Certification Program, Inc.

Rao, S., Riskowski, J., and Hannan, M. (2012) "Musculoskeletal conditions of the foot and ankle: Assessments and treatment options." *Best Practice and Research in Clinical Rheumatology*, 26, 3, 345–368.

Stanford Medicine Health Care (2021) Anterior ankle impingement (footballer's ankle). [Online]. https://stanfordhealthcare.org/medical-conditions/bones-joints-and-muscles/ankle-anterior-impingement.html. [Accessed August 18, 2023].

Wolfe, M. W., Uhl, T. L., Mattacola, C. G., and McCluskey, L. C. (2001) "Management of ankle sprains." *American Family Physician*, 63, 1, 93.

Chapter 8

Pilates and Spinal Cord Injury: Effect on Gait

Stephanie Behrendt Comella

Spinal cord injury (SCI) occurs from trauma, compression, or disease which disrupts normal function of the spinal cord (USI 2019). Between 250,000 and 500,000 people suffer an SCI annually worldwide (WHO 2013).

SCI causes partial to complete loss of movement and sensation. Individuals are assessed with a level of injury corresponding to the location of damage in the spinal cord (e.g., C6): cervical (C) injuries affect all four limbs (tetraplegia/quadriplegia), while thoracic (T), lumbar (L), and sacral (S) injuries affect two limbs, usually the legs (paraplegia). An ASIA (American Spinal Injury Association) score also indicates the severity of paralysis: ASIA A indicates *complete* "paralysis," and ASIA B–D indicates varying degrees of *incomplete* "paresis" (ASIA 2019).

In addition to impairment of the limbs, most individuals struggle with torso and hip joint control: Most C-level injuries are challenged in simply sitting upright while T- and L-level injuries are challenged in quadruped, kneeling, and standing positions. Individuals may use a wheelchair or ambulate with a walker or crutches.

Sensation impairments include the graded ability to feel touch, heat and cold, and painful stimuli. Insidious neurological pain can be extremely debilitating.

With impaired sensation, discomfort (e.g., full bladder) may manifest with autonomic dysreflexia—most prevalent in C-level SCI—which is characterized by flushed skin, cold sweat, and hypertension (Blauwet and Donovan 2021; Christopher & Dana Reeve Foundation 2021). Immediate removal of the stimulus usually stabilizes the situation. If symptoms persist for more than 2–5 minutes, call 911.

Complete SCI leads to severe muscle atrophy everywhere below the level of injury, resulting in hypermobile joints which should be supported during exercises. Use extra padding on equipment and under straps to avoid pressure sores and skin shearing resulting from reduced tissue padding and circulation.

Incomplete injuries tend to preserve muscle size due to hypertonic muscle activity and involuntary muscle spasms, which are triggered by changes in position, lack of sleep, infection, and stress.

Several autonomic body functions are impacted, including body temperature regulation and continence control (Blauwet and Donovan 2021). Adjust room temperature accordingly or have hot or cold pads available. Some individuals use semi-permanent catheters with urine collection bags (usually attached to their leg) for continuous drainage. Trainers should avoid positions that compromise tubes or bags.

Some individuals may need pressure on the abdomen to facilitate full breath cycles (especially full exhalation) when sitting or standing. Induce gradual positional changes and/or manually squeeze leg muscles to increase venous return to avoid fainting from orthostatic hypotension.

Lack of whole-body movement increases the risk for cardiovascular disease, early onset osteoporosis, and muscle wasting, all of which can be deferred with weight-bearing activities and exercise. ER visits can be common due to a revolving door of urinary tract infections, skin sores, and pain episodes. Many individuals are diagnosed with depression due to the abrupt change in lifestyle (Bombardier 2021).

Editor note
Any movement impairment from an SCI may be accompanied by responses of emotion such as post-traumatic stress. For additional information please read the introduction of Chapter 30.

Individuals with a traumatic SCI may have spinal fusions and/or hardware to stabilize vertebral fractures, which contraindicates spinal segmentation exercises. Be aware of hypermobility above and below fusions. In traumatic SCI, other areas of the body may have also been injured (ribs, pelvis, head concussion) and are only sometimes addressed appropriately.

Client description: 23-year-old biological female, identifies as female; student of sociology

Dates of case report: Session 1: July 28, 2020; Session 12: September 1, 2020; continuous, in-person sessions

Studio apparatus and props
Pilates equipment

- Trapeze Table
- Universal Reformer
- CoreAlign
- Wunda Chair with split pedal

Props used with equipment

- 9 in. (23 cm) ball, one-third deflated
- Non-skid rubberized mat, 7.5 in. x 14 in. x 0.5 in. (19.05 cm x 35.56 cm x 1.27 cm)
- Sling
- Foam roller
- Spinal corrector/arc
- Rotator discs for Universal Reformer jump board
- Rotator discs for CoreAlign
- Large 15 in. (38 cm) rotator disc

Home program props

- Mat

- 9 in. (23 cm) ball, one-third deflated
- Pillow or bolster

Methods and materials

Session 1/12
1. Health history interview

- In January 2016, the client suffered an L1–L4 incomplete SCI from a 35 ft (10.5 m) fall, along with multiple other orthopedic injuries including left elbow fracture, right knee fracture, and multiple fractures in both feet and ankles
  - Surgery: an L1–L4 fusion and metal rods T5–L5
  - Bilateral external fixators on upper leg-pelvis sustained for 4 months
  - Lower leg fixators sustained for 8 months
  - 11 of the 16 initial surgeries were foot reconstruction
  - The degree of denervation below the knee (including foot drop) may be a result of the

initial injury and/or as a result of surgeries and reconstruction
- Completed urethral bladder sling surgery in March 2020 to address incontinence during movement: involves C-section like incisions and fascial graft on the urethra
- Prescribed methadone for pain management

2. Symptoms

- Decreased blood flow in lower leg and foot, resulting in cold calves and feet and susceptibility of pressure sores on feet
- Toe contractures (toes no longer lay flat), greater on the right than the left
- Concerns for incontinence and prolapse, particularly during movement and bearing down
- Chronic back pain which is general relieved with stretching and massaging lower extremity (LE) flexors
- Tendency to overheat during exercise, possibly due to methadone side effects

3. Movement aids

- Primarily uses a wheelchair when outside of the home and a rolling walker to maneuver inside the home
- AFOs (ankle-foot orthoses to address foot drop)
- Two Lofstrand crutches
- For this study used only crutches unless noted otherwise

Final result of case report
The client increased in confidence and efficiency and improved posture in gait with decreased weight bearing through crutches. She was also able to perform sit-to-stands without using one hand to push off from her chair. In addition, the client experienced relative decreases in anxiety and pain.

Session 2/12: Initial assessment

1. General observations of gait

- Used bilateral Lofstrand crutches and ankle-foot orthoses (AFOs)
- Relies on crutches for support and balance, especially during right stance phase
- Excessive scapular movement from moving and loading through crutches
- Although crutch placement mimics a reciprocal gait pattern, LE and upper extremity (UE) move unilaterally (minimal thoracic rotation relative to pelvis)
- Excessive right internal rotation upon right heel strike and during stance phase
- Excessive lateral shift and pelvic rotation when transferring weight from foot to foot
- Limited propulsion through extension and plantar flexion
- 5 steps plus hops through crutches to turn around, favoring right turn

2. Standing tests

- Full torso rotation

- Observations of inefficient side: both
    - Minimal sequential thoracic rotation in either direction
    - Right rotation
        - Weight shift into left leg
    - Left rotation
        - Initiated rotation with pelvis instead of head

Session 12/12: Post-assessment

1. General observations of gait

- Used bilateral Lofstrand crutches and AFOs
- Decreased reliance on crutches observed in taller upright posture
- Improved shoulder girdle organization and movement strategies
- Slight increase in differentiation between thoracic and pelvic rotation, but still relatively uniform
- Decreased right internal rotation upon heel strike and during stance phase
- Decreased lateral weight shift and pelvic rotation in transferring weight from foot to foot
- Increased propulsion through extension and plantar flexion
- 4 steps to turn around without hopping through crutches
- Improved confidence and proprioception, does not need to look at feet

2. Standing tests

- Full torso rotation

- Observations of inefficient side: left
    - Both sides
        - Improved thoracic rotation preceding hip joint rotation
        - Dramatically increased range of motion (ROM) of hip joints
    - Left rotation
        - Still wants to initiate with pelvis

- ○ Lack of external rotation in right femur
  - Feet and ankles did not adapt during rotation, maintained in defaulted pronation

◆ Hemipelvis inferior motion

● Observations of inefficient side: both
  - No lumbar lateral flexion on either side resulting in contralateral rib translations and shoulder elevation
  - Inability to lower the left innominate, adapted with left pelvic translation/weight shift and right pelvic rotation

◆ Hemipelvis superior motion

● Observations of inefficient side: both
  - Minimal lumbar lateral flexion on either side resulting in contralateral rib translation and shoulder elevation
  - No plantar flexion on either side

◆ Lateral pelvic shift

● Observations of inefficient side: right
  - Isolated pelvic shift is not possible due to hardware and spinal fusions, adapted with full body weight shift
  - Right shift: lumbopelvic rotation rather than coronal plane motion
  - Feet and ankles did not adapt

3. Seated tests

◆ Hip joint and knee flexion

● Observations of inefficient side: both
  - Bilaterally performed similarly
  - Hip joint external rotation/abduction with contralateral torso rotation and thoracic translation

- ○ Increased external rotation of right hip joint
  - Feet and ankles did not adapt

◆ Hemipelvis inferior motion

● Observations of inefficient side: both
  - Bilateral innominate lowering with improved lumbar lateral flexion bilaterally
  - Decreased contralateral rib translation and shoulder elevation
  - Weight distribution improved

◆ Hemipelvis superior motion

● Observations of inefficient side: left
  - Improved but limited lumbar lateral flexion, adapted with smaller weight shift
  - Increased left plantar flexion

◆ Lateral pelvic shift

● Observations of inefficient side: left
  - Improved right lateral pelvic shift with torso adapting with right thoracic translation over pelvis
  - Decreased right lumbopelvic rotation due to improved lateral flexion and femoral abduction/adduction
  - Feet and ankles did not adapt

3. Seated tests

◆ Hip joint and knee flexion

● Observations of inefficient side: right
  - Left side had improved femoral centration and gliding
  - Less weight shift and torso rotation

Chapter 8

Author note
Included dorsiflexion and knee flexion test. Both were inefficient bilaterally. Bilaterally performed similarly, with paired external rotation. Weight shift to same side ischial tuberosity. Contralateral torso rotation; strategy of increased hip joint flexion rather than dorsiflexion. Included hip abduction with external rotation. Both were inefficient bilaterally. Client leaned back to initiate movement.

4. Sit and stand

◆ Lateral view

- Uses right hand to push-off seat with left hand in crutch
- Maintains good torso organization

◆ Anterior view

- Observable right bias in initiation with weight shift left to complete the stand
- Significant internal rotation and adduction (valgus) throughout movement, more significant on right side
- Right foot shifts medially during stand

5. Standing balance

◆ Two-leg stance, eyes open

- Started with 2 crutches but quickly dropped right crutch and only used left crutch for balance feedback
- 22 seconds
- Held a relatively wide stance, valgus alignment with knee flexion

◆ One-leg stance, eyes open

- Used 2 canes
- Similar on both sides (about 23 seconds)—needed crutches more on right leg
- Sought balance by adducting lifted knee

Author note
Included dorsiflexion and knee flexion test. Able to keep heel on ground. Maintained torso organization, no leaning or rotation. Improved left dorsiflexion maintaining heel on floor. Plantar flexion was not available; however, client understood the motor pathway and maintained foot on floor. Included hip abduction with external rotation. Maintained torso organization, no leaning or rotation.

4. Sit and stand

◆ Lateral view

- Held both crutches, but did not push off seat, no AFOs
- Much smoother transition off the seat
- Increase in confidence and speed
- Good control on descent

◆ Anterior view

- Decreased weight shifting throughout stand
- Decreased internal rotation and adduction (valgus) on right
- Right foot stays grounded

5. Standing balance

◆ Two-leg stance, eyes open

- No crutch support
- 20 seconds

◆ One-leg stance

- Less reliant on crutches
- Right leg: 20 seconds
- Left leg: 12 seconds
    - Did not use crutches to readjust
    - Was able to hold lifted leg slightly abducted

Session 3/12: Home program

Fatigue scale	4
Pain scale	4
Client self-report	• Tired, did not sleep well
Key changes observed by author at end of Session 3/12	• Discussion of biotensegrity greatly improved exercise execution and ability to adapt • Focused strategies for optimal use of canes
Reason behind choice of sequencing	• Improve proprioception • Pelvifemoral movement through pelvic clocks and femur-on-pelvis circles • Stimulate UE to torso activation through prone and quadruped exercises • Facilitate extensor activation for propulsion in seated and standing orientations

Session movement sequence

1. Rotational knee drops

Intent	• Support the body through using the floor in rotational movements • Sensory awareness of LE and UE contralateral movement in rotation
Gait reasoning	• Proprioception of contralateral motions of LE to torso and UE to torso • Improve hip joint glide for all phases of gait
Starting position	• Supine with knees flexed and feet flat on the floor
Movement description	• Reach right UE overhead while dropping both knees to the left and rotating the torso • Return to starting position beginning at right lateral axilla and ribs • Articulate through torso until at starting position • Repeat on other side • Complete 10 rotations, alternating sides

2. Leg slide (See Chapter 5 in Volume 1, Gentry, Knee Folds to Leg Slide)

Intent	• Facilitate hip joint glide on all planes

Chapter 8

Gait reasoning	• Couple internal rotation with extension for effective stance phase
Starting position	• Supine with knees flexed and feet on floor
Movement description	• Slide right foot along floor until knee is extended in parallel
	• With right LE extended, externally rotate LE
	• In external rotation, flex/abduct LE dragging foot back into starting position
	• Complete 8 repetitions on each side
	• Perform same movement again on each side by starting with hip joint abduction/external rotation
	• Extend LE in external rotation with foot in line with ischial tuberosity
	• Internally rotate LE to parallel with extension
	• In parallel, flex knee returning to starting position

3. Pelvic clocks with deflated ball (Black 2022; Feldenkrais 1985)

Author note
Balancing on a deflated ball creates greater demand for the torso to adapt during these leg movements, while providing immediate kinesthetic feedback. When working with individuals who have limited proprioception or sensation in general, use tools which provide this type of immediate feedback for error correction.

Editor note
Although placing the sacrum on top of a deflated ball provides the potential advantages of increasing proprioception to the posterior pelvis and elevating the pelvis relative to the thorax, it may assist in facilitating thoracolumbar fascial glide. However, consider how it contributes to increasing chaos in the vectors of lumbopelvic ground forces.

Intent	• Facilitate lumbopelvic-femoral glide that is limited due to hardware in a supported position
	• Improve proprioception of lumbopelvic-femoral glide for better execution of other exercises requiring this movement
Gait reasoning	• Improve torso orientation to midline with femoral gliding during gait
	• Increase ability to rotate torso

Set-up	• Mat
• 9 in. (23 cm) ball, one-third deflated
Starting position	• Supine with knees flexed and feet flat on floor
• Place deflated ball under pelvis
Movement description	• Rotate pelvis right and left for 20 cycles
• Anterior and posterior rotations for 10 cycles
• Articulate the pelvis in a circle following the image of a clock for 8 cycles in each direction
• Use breath to facilitate improved articulation of lumbopelvic-femoral joints
4. Modified Swan	Derivative of J. H. Pilates Swan Dive (NPCE Study Guide 2021, p. 48)
Intent	• Support torso extension in a safe range
Gait reasoning	• Increase extension activation and endurance to improve weight bearing in standing without relying on canes during gait
Starting position	• Prone on mat with pillow under pelvis
• Support head with rolled towel under forehead
• UE in flexion with elbows extended, hands on floor overhead
Movement description	• Hold starting position and exhale, sensing anterior abdominal wall drawing away from pillow
• Press hands into floor as head lifts off floor
• Extend torso in a small range activating extensors without increase in ROM due to hardware limitations
• Hold for 3–5 seconds
• Breathe naturally
• Inhale to lower down
• Complete 10 slow repetitions
5. Side plank	
Intent	• Challenging lateral movement for whole body
• UE activation for shoulder girdle continuation with torso
• Increase torso ability to be upright
Gait reasoning	• Improve one-leg stance phase with lateral activation

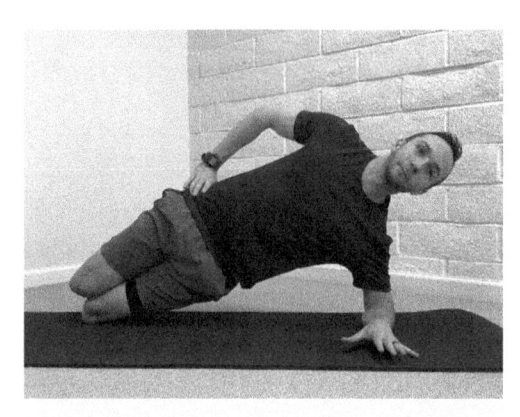

Figure 8.1

Starting position
- Sit right hemipelvis on mat
- Place right flexed elbow on mat
- Left hand on left innominate
- Knees flexed at 90 degrees stacked on top of one another
- Place roller or pillow between knees

Movement description
- Press elbow and bottom knee into floor to activate a thoracic translation away from floor
- Pelvis remains on floor
- Use left hand to traction left innominate toward heels as in "hemipelvis inferior motion" to counter the tendency to hike
- Hold for 3–5 seconds
- Sit back to starting position
- Progressed to whole torso lift after Session 6

6. Quadruped torso wave articulations

Editor note
The quadruped orientation is desirable for clients with SCI. Closed kinematic chain feedback through the hip joints and shoulder joints enhances torso control.

Intent
- Develop cranium to coccyx proprioception and articulation in sagittal plane
- Experience in generating movement from pelvis as opposed to leading with head

Gait reasoning	● Improving articulation for torso control required for gait efficiency
Starting position	● Quadruped position
Movement description	● Articulate initiating from pelvis to move sequentially like a wave into flexion ● Articulate into extension initiating with pelvis at ischial tuberosities sequentially like a wave into extension ● Complete 5 full cycles of flexion and extension
7. Kneeling Chest Expansion with band	Derivative of J. H. Pilates Chest Expansion on Trapeze Table (NPCE Study Guide 2021, p. 67)
Intent	● Activate extensors through UE resistance in kneeling
Gait reasoning	● Facilitate whole-body activation in kneeling with UE movement to improve torso adaptation strategies ● Increase loading of torso for weight bearing ● Decrease need for weight bearing through crutches during gait
Starting position	● Kneeling on mat with pillow placed under pelvis ● Sit back on pillow in hip and knee flexion ● Tie a resistance band in front at shoulder height (e.g., attached to a door at door-handle height) with two ends free to hold ● Hold the ends of the band, elbow extended

Movement description	● Extend the shoulder and pull ends of band to lateral pelvis
	● Initiate the pull from the shoulder girdle
	● Hold for 3 seconds before returning to starting position
	● Complete 10 repetitions
	● Challenge
	    ■ Perform exercise in tall kneeling
	    ■ Complete 3 sets of 5 repetitions

8. Quadruped arm reach	
Intent	● Develop coordination and control of torso with changes of base of support ● Practice UE unloading prior to LE unloading
Gait reasoning	● Proprioception of torso organization with changes in base of support ● Activate contralateral movement patterning

Chapter 8

Starting position	• Quadruped position on mat
Movement description	• In starting position, exhale and sense activation of anterior abdominal wall • Lift one hand off the floor while minimizing any weight shift • Progress to extending UE • Hold for 3 seconds and replace hand on floor • Complete 2 sets of 10 hand lifts, alternating sides

9. Quadruped extension

Intent	• Develop coordination and control of torso with changes of base of support • Practice LE unloading prior to adding combined UE and oppositional LE unloading
Gait reasoning	• Proprioception of torso organization with changes in base of support • Activate contralateral movement patterning • Activate extensors for propulsion in gait
Starting position	• Quadruped position on mat
Movement description	• In starting position, exhale and sense activation of anterior abdominal wall • Extend right LE while minimizing weight shift • Hold for 3 seconds and replace knee on floor • Complete 2 sets of 10 alternating sides

10. Seated Scooter

Intent	• Glide anterior hip joint tissues • Activate hip joint extensors • Couple extension with lumbopelvic-femoral activation
Gait reasoning	• Increase hip joint extension required for propulsion in gait
Starting position	• Sit sideways at the very front edge of a chair • Place right ischial tuberosity on edge of chair, right hip joint and knee flexion • Hold back of chair with right hand • Left ischial tuberosity off edge of chair, left hip joint extended, left knee flexed, metatarsal arch on floor • Wear socks or place towel under metatarsal arch for ease in sliding

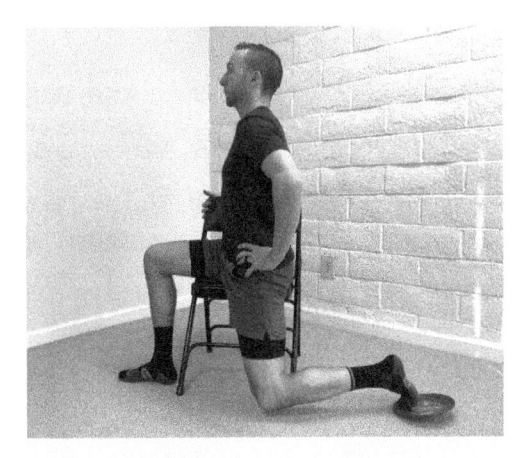

Figure 8.2

Movement description	• Find upright seated position • Reach left knee toward floor and slide left foot posteriorly • Hold for 3 seconds • Flex the hip joint by pulling the left knee anteriorly • Return to starting position • Complete 2 sets of 10 repetitions on each side

11. Standing lunge

Intent	• Increase confidence and balance in off-set stance/stride • Loading LE in standing, increasing weight bearing to minimize dependence on crutches • Activate LE during extension and flexion
Gait reasoning	• Improve extensors for propulsion • Activate extensor/flexor for leg swing
Starting position	• Stand holding onto sturdy chair with feet together • Wear socks or place towel under sliding foot for ease in sliding
Movement description	• Slide right foot posteriorly while flexing left knee into lunge position • Be mindful of stance leg tendency to internally rotate, track left knee over 2nd metatarsal • Pull right foot forward to standing in starting position • Complete 2 sets of 10 repetitions on each side

12. Standing balance

Intent	• Increase standing confidence and endurance
Gait reasoning	• Increase endurance for longer bouts of walking
Starting position	• Standing with feet parallel using crutches or any other supportive aid
Movement description	• Standing in optimal organization for 3 minutes • Take breaks as needed

Session 11/12: Studio session

Fatigue scale	3
Pain scale	1
Client self-report	• Excited about increases in control and balance during daily walks • Being diligent to take breaks during walks to reset her patterns and focus on quality
Key changes observed by author at end of Session 11/12	• Drastically increased height of bridges from Session 4 to Session 11 • Narrower stance indicative of improved midline orientation and organization of LE • General increases in self-confidence, drive, and sense of accomplishment with overall decreases in anxiety throughout the study
Reason behind choice of sequencing	• Integration of weight distribution and adaptability during stance • Efficient contralateral rotation

Session movement sequence

1. Push-Through Seated Front on Trapeze Table	Derivative of J. H. Pilates Push-Through Seated Front on Trapeze Table (NPCE Study Guide 2021, p. 63)
Intent	• Closed kinematic chain exercise to stimulate continuity of limbs to torso • Glide thoracolumbar fascia for improved shoulder ROM • Awareness of feet actively pressing into side bars • Calm and bring client's mind into session with familiar exercise

Pilates and Spinal Cord Injury: Effect on Gait

Gait reasoning	• Integrates UE and LE continuity with torso, improving standing and walking
	• Improve overall gait and comfort with use of crutches
Set-up	• 1 light spring, top-loaded on push-through bar
Starting position	• Sitting upright facing tower end with feet against vertical frame poles
	• Place hands on push-through bar overhead
	• Flex knees to maintain upright torso and optimal pelvic position
Movement description	• Pull bar down
	• As bar passes head, follow bar with crown of head
	• Articulate in flexion through torso as bar moves between side bars
	• Flex knees if necessary
	• Reverse the articulation initiating from pelvis extending to upright sitting
	• Lift bar overhead with extending elbows
	• Lean forward
	• Lean back to seated position
	• Return to starting position
	• 5 repetitions

CUES

- Stimulate flow through the torso during articulation in flexion and extension
- Press thighs into table and feet into side bars
- Allow the scapula to glide along the thorax especially when pressing the bar up

Author note

The client recognizes the integration of concepts in this "simple" exercise: control, articulation, flow, and whole-body experience.

2. Half circle saw on Trapeze Table	Derivative of J. H. Pilates Push-Through Seated Front on Trapeze Table (NPCE Study Guide 2021, p. 63) and J. H. Pilates mat exercise Saw (NPCE Study Guide 2021, p. 48)
Intent	• Segmental torso articulation
	• Improve coordination
	• Load transfer across midline of torso
	• Challenge coordination in several planes of motion

Chapter 8

Gait reasoning	• Experience variations in torso rotation, weight shifting, and subtle rotations: coupled ranges of motion experienced in gait
Set-up	• Light spring, top-loaded on push-through bar
Starting position	• Sitting upright facing tower end with feet against vertical frame poles • Place hands on the push-through bar overhead • Flex knees to maintain upright torso and optimal pelvic position
Movement description	• Left hand presses bar upward • Right hand reaches toward opposite upright pole with left torso rotation • Right UE in a sweeping motion, moves forward and passes same side vertical frame pole abducting • Right torso rotation into extension reaching for same side posterior vertical frame pole • Left UE pulls bar down during sweeping movement • Reverse the path to return to starting position • 4 sets on each side

CUE
♦ Weight shifting on ischial tuberosities: couple weight shift with thoracic lateral flexion and rotation

Editor note
When seated as in Saw, the combined motion of rotation and lateral flexion distributes the torso weight through the ischial tuberosities in varying degrees, more on one side than the other. In the thorax, right rotation is coupled with left translation that "shifts" or distributes the weight slightly more onto the left ischial tuberosity. During gait, the thoracic rotation brings the weight over the stance side for improved balance to transition to the next step. This is similar to gait patterning on the ischial tuberosities as analyzed by Serge Gracovetsky (Black 2022; Gracovetsky 1987).

3. Modified Leg Springs on Trapeze Table

Derivative of J. H. Pilates Leg Springs: Supine, Bicycle on Trapeze Table (NPCE Study Guide 2021, p. 67) and J. H. Pilates Single Leg Stretch on mat (NPCE Study Guide 2021, p. 46)

Intent	• Increase hip joint glide • Activate hip joint in all planes

Pilates and Spinal Cord Injury: Effect on Gait

Gait reasoning	• Improve femoral glide for leg swing and positioning of joint in stance phase
Set-up	• Medium long springs attached to slider bar • Velcro® thigh cuffs
Starting position	• Supine • Bilateral hip joint and knee flexion to 90 degrees • Place Velcro cuffs around mid-femurs • Hold on to vertical frame poles • Head on table

Movement description	• Full range: bilateral
	    ■ Abduction/external rotation/flexion/adduction
	    ■ Return to starting position
	    ■ Repeat 10 times
	    ■ Reverse direction
	• Unilateral
	    ■ Extend right hip joint and knee while flexing left hip joint and knee
	    ■ Change sides
	    ■ Alternate right and left 10 times
	• Progress into a larger and controlled ROM

CUES
- Observe for equal contribution between left and right femur on pelvis motion
- Track knees in center of femoral joint and over 2nd metatarsal

Author note
The difference between "Velcro thigh cuffs" versus "straps: feet in loops" facilitates improved activation of extensors. If a client has a movement pattern to extend the knee with quadriceps dominance while pulling the spring, the Velcro thigh cuffs enable activation of extensors while minimizing quadriceps dominance.

4. Pelvic clocks with deflated ball (Black 2022)

Intent	• Facilitate lumbopelvic-femoral glide that is limited due to hardware in a supported position • Improve proprioception of lumbopelvic-femoral glide for better execution of other exercises requiring this movement

Chapter 8

Gait reasoning	• Improve the torso orientation to midline with femoral gliding during gait • Increase the ability to rotate torso
Set-up	• Mat • 9 in. (23 cm) ball, one-third deflated
Starting position	• Supine with knees flexed and feet flat on floor • Place deflated ball under pelvis
Movement description	• Rotate pelvis right and left for 20 cycles • Anterior and posterior rotations for 10 cycles • Articulate the pelvis in a circle following the image of a clock for 8 cycles in each direction • Use breath to facilitate improved articulation of lumbopelvic-femoral joints

CUES
- Work to differentiate between thoracic and pelvic rotation by keeping shoulders steady on the table
- Use of tactile cueing and hands on movement pattern direction to help client feel and understand the correct movement pattern

Author note
Be aware that rotation will be limited in individuals with hardware in their lumbar vertebrae. Hemipelvis superior motion is a common compensation pattern for those who lack rotation. Support the client confirming the amount of range appropriate for them.

5. Modified Leg Springs on Trapeze Table with deflated ball under pelvis

Derivative of J. H. Pilates Leg Springs: Supine, Bicycle on Trapeze Table (NPCE Study Guide 2021, p. 67) and J. H. Pilates Single Leg Stretch on mat (NPCE Study Guide 2021, p. 46)

Intent	• Increase hip joint glide • Activate femur on pelvis in all planes with the added challenge of balancing on deflated ball
Gait reasoning	• Improve femoral glide for leg swing and positioning of joint in stance phase • Adapting to an unstable environment
Set-up	• Attach medium long springs to Velcro cuffs • 9 in. (23 cm) ball, one-third deflated

Pilates and Spinal Cord Injury: Effect on Gait

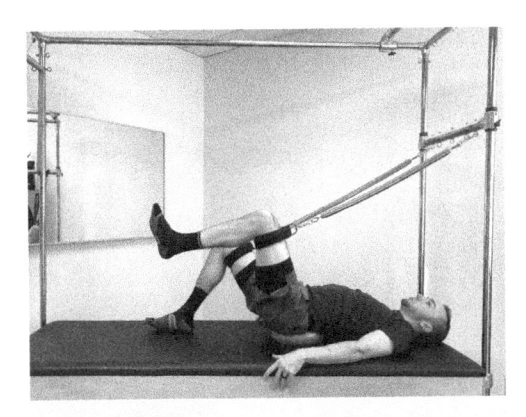

Figure 8.3

Starting position
- Supine
- Bilateral hip joint and knee flexion to 90 degrees
- Place deflated ball under pelvis
- Place Velcro cuffs around mid-femurs
- Hold on to vertical frame poles
- Head on table

Movement description
- Double Leg Stretch
  - Extend hip joints and knees
  - Slowly return to starting position
  - 10 repetitions
- Full range: bilateral
  - Abduction/external rotation/flexion/adduction
  - Return to starting position
  - Repeat 10 times
  - Reverse direction
- Unilateral
  - Extend right hip joint and knee
  - Simultaneously, flexing left hip joint and knee
  - Change sides
  - Alternate right and left 10 times

CUES
- Observe for equal contribution between left and right pelvis
- Track knees in center of femoral joint and over 2nd metatarsal
- Place fingers at sitz bones to feel activation of extensors

Chapter 8

6. Bridging with sling support

Intent
- Support and facilitate activation of extensors

Gait reasoning
- Improve ability to extend during push-off phase

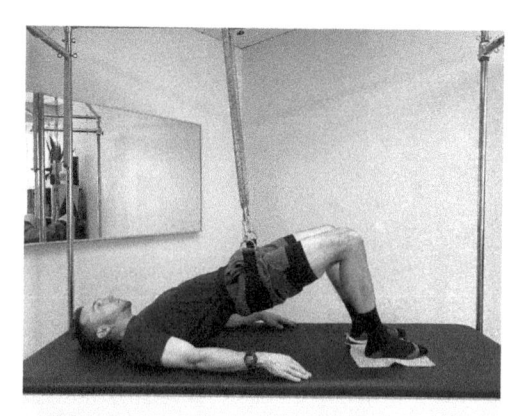

Figure 8.4

Set-up
- Non-skid rubberized mat
- 9 in. (23 cm) ball, one-third deflated
- Used in previous sessions: 2 light and/or 2 medium springs with sling suspended above client's pelvis to assist in hip joint extension

Starting position
- Supine on mat, deflated ball between knees
- Hip and knee flexion
- Feet dorsiflexed on mat
- UE by sides
- Trainer kneels at client's feet with hands on knees for support

Movement description
- Inhale to feel starting position
- Slowly exhale as feet and UE press into table
- Extend hip joints into bridge position
- Inhale at end range of bridge
- Exhale, articulate through torso to return to starting position
- 2 sets of 10 repetitions

CUE
- Allow the pelvis to be supported by the sling so that the effort is placed in the LE. The sling supports extension without over-effort of the torso extensors as a compensation for limitations of hip joint extension

Author note
Bridging can be an extremely frustrating exercise for individuals with limited sensation and movement in the LE and feet. They are unable to feel pressure through the feet, which would normally facilitate extensor activation. Assist the client by introducing a force vector with hand cueing by pressing on top of the knees, sending the force through the femur into the feet.

7. Quadruped pelvifemoral abduction

Intent
- Articulate hip joint medial glide
- Activation of posterior-lateral pelvifemoral myofascia

Gait reasoning
- Improve centration of hip joint and activation for stance balance

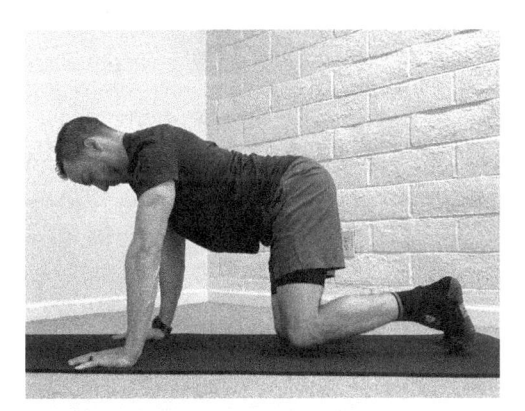

Figure 8.5

Set-up
- Optional: perform with Universal Reformer box under elbows to decrease wrist compression
- Mat

Chapter 8

Starting position	• Quadruped position with metatarsophalangeal (MTP) joints extended, metatarsal arch on mat • Option: if client is unable to meet metatarsal arch with mat, roll a mat and place under knees to bring the arch to the mat
Movement description	• Press into hands, right knee, and metatarsal arch • Abduct left femur • Minimize right lateral sway • 3 sets of 10 repetitions on each side

Editor note
Another option for quadruped orientation is including lumbopelvic-femoral rotation. Begin in quadruped pressing hands, right knee, and metatarsal arches into the mat and rotate the T/L junction, pelvis around the right femoral joint as the left LE abducts. This will facilitate lumbopelvic-femoral rotation in a closed kinematic chain orientation. Closed kinematic chain of lumbopelvic-femoral rotation is required for efficient gait.

8. Tall kneeling with sling assistance on Trapeze Table

Intent	• Springs and sling assistance allow for greater ROM in preparation for half kneeling exercises
Gait reasoning	• Functional strengthening for sit to stand
Set-up	• Hang medium long springs from horizontal frame poles with sling attached
Starting position	• Kneel holding horizontal frame poles • Place sling on posterior pelvis for sitting • Optional: place bolster behind knees to prevent excessive knee flexion
Movement description	• From tall kneeling flex and sit into sling • Extend to return to starting position • Use horizontal frame poles for assistance • 10 repetitions

CUE
♦ Press firmly into LE to extend

Author note
This set-up provides the environment for facilitating flexor and extensor coactivation which is necessary for those who tend to have flexor dominance.

9. Half kneeling balance

Intent
- Challenge balance in kneeling orientation
- Torso adaptation

Gait reasoning
- Torso adaptation to unilateral LE flexion and extension, similar to a stride step

Set-up
- Mat
- Support such as Universal Reformer box or Trapeze Table horizontal frame

Starting position
- Tall kneeling on mat holding on to support
- With assistance from trainer, move right LE anteriorly into half kneeling position

Movement description
- Press left lower limb into mat
- Trainer gently places hands on right femur cueing a sense of reaching the left knee anteriorly to facilitate a right innominate lowering to "square" the pelvis
- Hold for 1–2 minutes
- Repeat on other side

10. Side lunges on CoreAlign

Derivative of J. H. Pilates Splits on Universal Reformer (NPCE Study Guide 2021, pp. 61–62)
(See Editor note in Volume 1, Chapter 6, Session 11, exercise 4)

Intent
- Increase hip joint glide
- Activate lateral pelvifemoral myofascia
- Torso control during LE movement against resistance

Gait reasoning
- Facilitate medial glide for centration of femur and narrowing stance for midline orientation
- Awareness of torso weight distribution over stance leg

Set-up
- Stand sideways to ladder: right foot on platform and left foot on cart

Starting position
- Tall kneeling on mat holding on to support
- With assistance from trainer, move right LE anteriorly into half kneeling position

Movement description
- Right hip and knee flexion
- Simultaneously slide the cart away by pressing with left foot
- Torso weight distribution mainly over right LE
- Control cart on return
- Extend right knee to stand
- Maintain weight distribution over right LE
- 10–15 repetitions
- Repeat on other side

CUES
- Move slowly for control
- When pressing the cart out, observe how the torso's weight remains over the platform leg

11. Sagittal lunge on CoreAlign Derivative of J. H. Pilates Splits on Universal Reformer (NPCE Study Guide 2021, pp. 61–62)

Intent
- Standing environment

Gait reasoning
- Working on weight shifting for alternating LE movements and extension

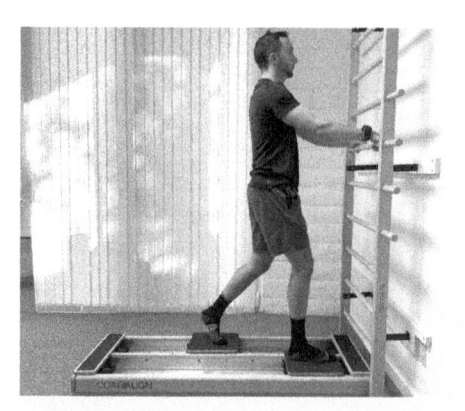

Figure 8.6

Set-up
- Bands: 1 medium and 1 light on each cart

Starting position
- Standing facing ladder, one foot on each cart

Movement description
- Bend right knee while sliding cart backward
- Control return of cart extending right knee to stand up
- 10–16 repetitions, alternating sides

CUE
- Maintain weight in the rear foot of the standing leg

The journey to Session 11

Session 4/12
Client self-report

- High fatigue and anxiety at start of session, decreased at end of session
- Fatigue scale 8
- Pain scale 3

Key changes observed

- Initial review of scapular movements informed UE motor control
- Proprioception of UE continuation to torso during foam roller balancing exercises was transposed into standing and gait integration at end of session

Reasoning behind choice of movements

- Improve balance and use of crutches through proprioception of UE, scapula to torso activation, and movement patterning

Session movement sequence
1. Trapeze Table

- Push-Through Seated Front
- Supine on roller, UE flexion/extension; extension/abduction/external rotation/adduction/internal rotation
- Unilateral Velcro cuffs on mid-femurs balancing on roller

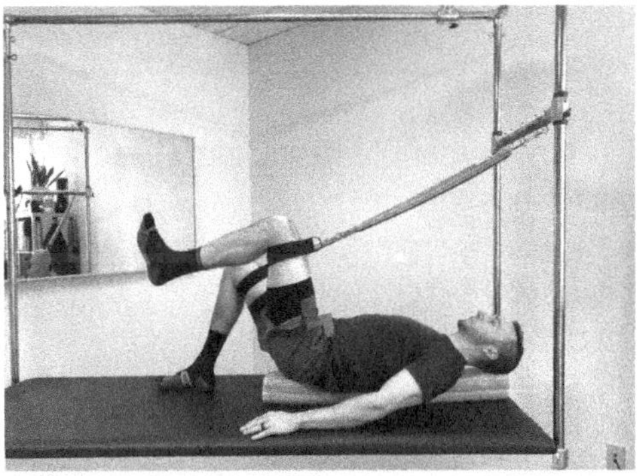

Figure 8.7

- Mermaid
- Bridging with sling

2. Mat

- Quadruped
  - Sternum drops
  - Leg extension assisted by trainer

3. Standing balance using crutches

- Standing strategy
- Standing balance: lifting 1 crutch

Session 5/12
Client self-report

- Feeling increased integration of UE to torso continuation during daily walks
- Fatigue scale 3

Chapter 8

- Pain scale 0

Key changes observed

- Continues to improve motor control of UE to torso
- More confident and balanced pelvic rotations in gait

Reasoning behind choice of movements

- Practice movement patterning of UE to torso from previous session
- Seated LE activating LE to torso to prepare for standing work
- Begin challenge in standing

Session movement sequence
1. Trapeze Table

- Push-Through Seated Front
- Arc on table
  - Sit sideways
  - Hold push-through bar
  - Laterally flex torso over arc pressing push-through bar away

2. Wunda Chair with split pedal
- Seated side leg pumps abduction

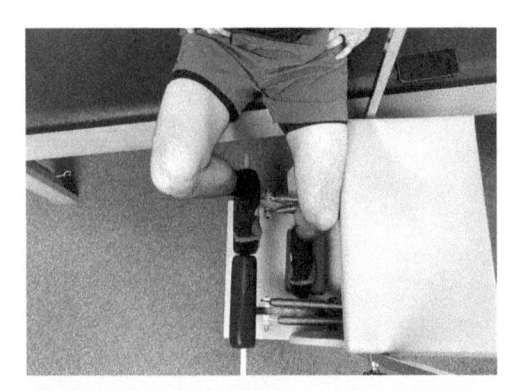

Figure 8.8

3. CoreAlign
- Ankle plantar flexion with dorsiflexion of MTP joints
- Sagittal lunge

4. Gait integration

- Focus on UE and crutch usage
- Integrating push-off

Session 6/12
Client self-report

- Increased weight distribution into LE rather than through crutches
- Fatigue scale 3
- Pain scale 4

Key changes observed

- Improved motor control in quadruped exercises
- Improved functional use of crutches
- Orientation to midline apparent

Reasoning behind choice of movements

- Build confidence in off-set stance and one-leg stance

Session movement sequence
1. Trapeze Table

- Quadruped torso wave articulations
- Supine UE flexion/extension
- Prone torso extension over arc placed on table
- Prone torso extension over arc holding light long springs, UE flexion and extension
- Prone torso extension over arc holding dowel overhead
- Plank on knees
- Side plank: lifting pelvis off mat

288

Pilates and Spinal Cord Injury: Effect on Gait

Editor note
It is common to use the Trapeze Table as a high mat. This sequence on the Trapeze Table is using the table as a high mat and at other times utilizing the springs as in supine UE flexion/extension and prone torso extension over arc with UE flexion/extension.

2. Wunda Chair with split pedal

- Seated side leg pumps
- Standing side leg pumps with 1 crutch

3. CoreAlign

- Ankle plantar flexion with dorsiflexion of MTP joints alternating with opposite hand release
- Sagittal lunge

4. Gait integration

- Shoulder continuity to torso and LE
- Integrating push-off and extension coordination

Session 7/12
Client self-report

- Shoulder soreness from workout
- Feeling sleepy, anxious, and shaky today, perhaps from heat
- Fatigue scale 7
- Pain scale 3

Key changes observed

- Client starting to understand the process of forging new movement patterns
- Tall kneeling Chest Expansion gave client confidence in extension not usually felt in supine bridging exercises
- Feet placed more narrowly throughout gait indicating orientation to midline and centration of hip joints

Reasoning behind choice of movements

- Proprioception of pressing through heels to activate extensors
- Continued development of UE to torso to LE integration, as well as off-set stance applications for gait

Session movement sequence
1. Universal Reformer with tower

- Eve's Lunge
- Footwork on heels, single leg marching
- Supine UE with straps flexion/extension
- Low kneeling Chest Expansion

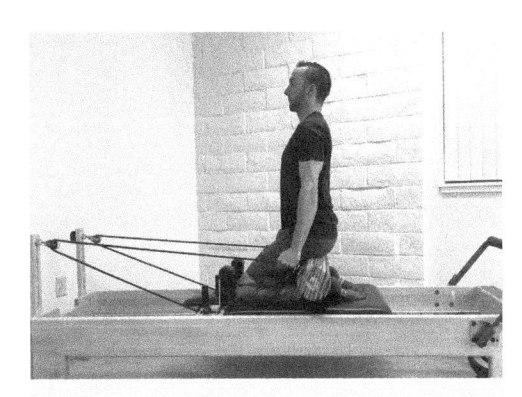

Figure 8.9

- Low to tall kneeling on carriage holding on to push-through bar
- Tall kneeling Chest Expansion

2. CoreAlign

- Ankle plantar flexion with dorsiflexion of MTP joints alternating with emphasis on weight shifting
- Sagittal lunge, alternating with opposite hand release
- Gait integration
- Walking with feet more narrowly placed (less

Chapter 8

abduction and lateral weight shift) resulting in improved rotation

Session 8/12
Client self-report

- Good energy today
- Fatigue scale 3
- Pain scale 4

Key changes observed

- Continued with narrower placement of feet throughout gait indicating orientation to midline and centration of hip joints

Reasoning behind choice of movements

- Proprioception and training of hip joint internal/external rotation in closed kinematic chain

Session movement sequence
1. Universal Reformer

- Eve's Lunge (see Chapter 5 in Volume 1, Gentry)
- Footwork using rotator discs, unilateral and bilateral

2. Seated pelvis rotation on large rotator disc

3. CoreAlign

- Lunge alternating with opposite hand release
- Standing LE rotation using rotator discs

4. Gait integration

- Working on efficient rotation in gait cycle

Session 9/12
Client self-report

- Noticed she has been needing to take more breaks during daily walks, but believes it's because she is using her legs more
- Fatigue scale 5
- Pain scale 2

Key changes observed

- Client started to play around with different walking drills on her own (i.e., walking backwards), showing confidence and willingness to explore
- Gait seems smooth with improved endurance

Reasoning behind choice of movements

- Focus on extensors to generate power for push-off in gait
- Continued progressing through established sequence

Session movement sequence
1. Add hemipelvis superior motion to Side Plank

2. Add Kneeling Chest Expansion with band exercise

3. Replace Seated Scooter with Standing Scooter/Eve's Lunge (see Chapter 5 in Volume 1, Gentry)

4. Trapeze Table

- Push-Through Seated Front
- Supine with tabletop legs/heel drops, UE flexion/extension
- Unilateral marching using spring with trainer assist
- Footwork on push-through bar, bilateral and unilateral

- Supine Leg Springs with trainer assist
    - Alternating leg marching
    - Extended knees, femoral flexion/extension, bilateral
    - Femoral abduction/external rotation/extension and adduction/internal rotation/flexion
    - Femoral extension/internal rotation/abduction/external rotation and flexion/adduction/internal rotation
- Quadruped femoral and knee extension with spring assist

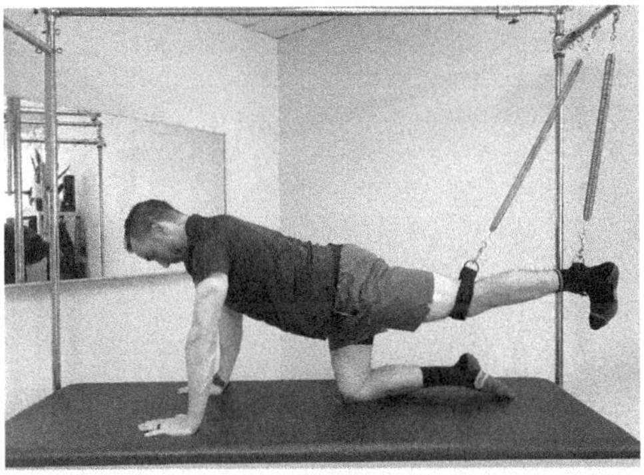

Figure 8.10

- Low and tall kneeling Chest Expansion with springs

5. Gait integration
- Focus on push-off

Editor note
Quadruped femoral and knee extension with spring assist is a sagittal plane hip and knee joint motion, with resisted flexion and controlled extension. This is gait relevant because in quadruped torso control is facilitated through the ground forces of the palms and supporting knee. Torso control in combination with unilateral limb movement prepares for limb tracking which is necessary for efficient swing phase. The spring attachment to the sliding crossbar between the vertical frame poles is crucial to the force vectors. In Figure 8.10, the Velcro thigh cuff is attached laterally to the center eye bolt. Be mindful that it places a compression force on the lateral aspect of the knee when pelvifemoral control is lacking.

Session 10/12
Client self-report

- School started this week, slightly anxious today
- Always feels stronger and confident after session
- Fatigue scale 4
- Pain scale 4

Key changes observed

- Increased ROM and control in lunges
- Improved upright posture in standing and walking
- Smoother gait rhythm

Reasoning behind choice of movements

- Challenge standing balance and endurance
- Repetition of accomplished exercises

Session movement sequence
1. Universal Reformer

- Footwork on rear foot
- Femurs in Velcro thigh cuffs
    - Hip joint flexion/extension/abduction (external rotation)/adduction (internal rotation) to midline
    - Reverse directions
- Seated on long box holding straps
    - Modified Roll-Back
    - Chest Expansion, torso leans laterally/posteriorly and laterally/anteriorly

2. CoreAlign

- Sagittal lunge
- Side lunge using ladder and 1 crutch

- Side splits using ladder and 1 crutch

3. Gait integration

- Practice patterning with orientation to midline

References

American Spinal Injury Association (ASIA) (2019) International Standards for Neurological Classification of SCI (ISNCSCI) worksheet. https://asia-spinalinjury.org/international-standards-neurological-classification-sci-isncsci-worksheet. [Accessed September 22, 2023].

Black, M. (2022) *Centered: Organizing the Body through Kinesiology, Movement Theory and Pilates Techniques.* Edinburgh: Handspring Publishing, pp. 123–125, 147–149.

Blauwet, C. and Donovan, J. (2021) Exercise after spinal cord injury. MSKTC Spinal Cord Injury Factsheets. https://msktc.org/sci/factsheets/exercise#problems. [Accessed September 22, 2023].

Bombardier, C. H. (2021) Depression and spinal cord injury. MSKTC Spinal Cord Injury Factsheets. https://msktc.org/sci/factsheets/depression. [Accessed September 22, 2023].

Christopher & Dana Reeve Foundation (2021) Autonomic dysreflexia. www.christopherreeve.org/living-with-paralysis/health/secondary-conditions/autonomic-dysreflexia. [Accessed September 22, 2023].

Feldenkrais, M. (1985 [2002]) *The Potent Self: A Study of Spontaneity and Compulsion.* Berkeley, CA: Somatic Resources/Frog Ltd., pp. 189–214.

Gracovetsky, S. (1987) *The Spinal Engine.* Springer.

NPCE Study Guide (National Pilates Certification Exam Study Guide) (2021) Miami, FL: National Pilates Certification Program, Inc.

United Spinal Association (USI) (2021) What is spinal cord injury/disorder? https://unitedspinal.org/what-is-spinal-cord-injury-disorder-scid. [Accessed September 22, 2023].

World Health Organization (WHO) (2013) Spinal cord injury. www.who.int/news-room/fact-sheets/detail/spinal-cord-injury. [Accessed September 22, 2023].

Chapter 9

Pilates and Adolescence Congenital Muscular Torticollis: Effect on Gait

Christine Egan

Congenital muscular torticollis (CMT) is a congenital locomotor system disorder characterized by unilateral shortening of the sternocleidomastoid (SCM) muscle. It presents in newborns with a reported incidence worldwide of between 0.3 percent and 1.9 percent (Minghelli and Vitorino 2022). Other studies (Stellwagen et al. 2008) indicate a ratio of 1 per 250 newborns, making it the third most common congenital orthopedic anomaly. There is a male to female predominance with a 3 to 2 ratio and it is more common to the right side (Sargent et al. 2019). CMT may be accompanied by hip joint dysplasia in 20 percent of cases (Kim et al. 2011).

When diagnosed soon after birth, CMT can be managed conservatively and rarely requires surgery. Diagnosis is made by the infant's pediatrician, using clinical and physical examination findings, and parental observation of the head having a persistent cervical lateral tilt to one side and a preference for cervical rotation to the opposite side.

The fibers of the SCM muscle originate on the sternum and run on a diagonal to insert into the mastoid process of the mandible. When the SCM muscle is shortened it causes lateral cervical flexion (head tilt) to the same side and cervical rotation of the head to the opposite side. This creates an asymmetry in two planes of movement. Persistent rotation to one side often creates a secondary diagnosis of plagiocephaly (flattening of the side of the head).

Causes of CMT include intrauterine crowding (it is common in twins), breech births, traumatic delivery or vascular phenomena, such as fibrosis from peripartum bleeds, compartment syndrome, or primary myopathy of the SCM (Amaral et al. 2019). Occasionally, there can be a fibrotic mass within the SCM muscle that dissolves over time.

The "Back to Sleep" campaign was initiated in 1994 to reduce the incidence of sudden infant death syndrome (SIDS), and the incidence of CMT has a strong correlation to the current lack of prone positioning in infants (Sargent et al. 2019). The prone position allows for normal development of the infant in gravity. Weight bearing on the face, hands, and forearms facilitated symmetrical extension of the neck and spine allowing any initial asymmetries to "self-correct." Now all babies sleep on their backs and spend most of their waking hours in supine, creating an imbalance between flexion and extension, with extension being dominant.

In most cases, CMT will resolve in two to three months with direct physical therapy treatment, parent education for handling, and therapeutic activities, including elongation of the shortened SCM muscle and facilitation of head-righting reactions, with strong focus on maintaining the head and neck in midline orientation.

The torticollis can reappear when the child may be compromised physically or they are moving toward a higher developmental skill. Occasionally, there is a generalized shortening of the whole side of the body. In the case of my subject, there was fascial shortening on the right side of her body that fostered specific body posturing that became more evident as the child's skeleton grew larger. The limited flexibility of her connective tissue did not allow for symmetrical alignment and efficient movement patterns. Surgical release of the SCM muscle was necessary to allow more freedom of movement.

Client description: 12-year-old biological female, identifies as female; Sixth Grade student

Dates of case report: Session 1: February 10, 2020; Session 12: June 3, 2020. After Sessions 1 and 2, the client fractured her clavicle. We postponed the sessions until May 5, 2020. All in-person sessions

Studio apparatus and props
Pilates equipment

- Universal Reformer modified with an adjustable footbar
- Wunda Chair

Props used with equipment

- Overball
- Small box
- Large box
- Mini Magic Circle
- Light resistance band, 4–5 ft (1.2–1.5 m)
- Soft foam roller
- Yoga block
- Mat

Home program props

- Foam roller
- Mini Magic Circle
- Light resistance band, 4–5 ft (1.2–1.5 m)
- Yoga block
- Mat

Methods and materials

Session 1/12
1. Health history interview

- DOB: 12-27-2007
- Diagnosed with right-side CMT at 5 weeks of age by her pediatrician and referred for physical therapy (PT)
- Client was seen in PT once a week until the age of 9 months when she achieved her motor milestones of sitting independently and crawling (2007–2008)
- At 7 years of age her family observed her having consistent right-side head tilt in photos (2014)
- Client was referred to a pediatric ophthalmologist to rule out any issues with her vision and was found to have normal vision (2014)
- Client was referred back to our clinic for PT where a leg-length discrepancy was observed in addition to limited range of motion (ROM) into left cervical flexion and a resting right lateral tilt of 10 degrees in standing and 15 degrees in sitting
- Palpable tightness in right SCM muscle, winging of right scapula

- Due to a rapid growth spurt, client gained 4 in. (10 cm) in height
- Client was referred to pediatric orthopedist and had surgical release of her right SCM muscle on 4-18-2015
- PT following surgery included weekly PT at clinic, home program, and 6 weeks of wearing a cervical collar 23 hours a day
- In April 2018 patient returned to clinic with complaints of pain in right pelvifemoral region
- Client began orthotic therapy that included a heel lift to accommodate her leg-length discrepancy as well as placing both subtalar joints in a neutral position (2018)
- Followed up in April 2019: client complained of arch pain, bilateral pronation, and 0.39 in. (1 cm) leg-length discrepancy, left leg being shorter. Second pair of orthotics provided
- Reevaluated in January 2020 and observed malalignment of both lower extremities (LE), with greater malalignment in the right leg, increased pronation bilaterally, and leg-length discrepancy of 0.19 in. (0.5 cm), left leg being shorter
- Mom concerned with client's gait pattern, but client not aware of anything concerning her walking and has stopped using prior pair of orthotics

2. Symptoms

- Hip pain on right
- Knee pain under patella
- Bilateral pain in feet when discontinued orthotic use

3. Movement aids

- None

Final result of case report
Client was able to walk with a wider base of support and a longer step length. She reported increased body awareness and improved strength, energy level, and coordination. I observed improved LE organization and postural symmetry overall.

Chapter 9

Session 2/12: Initial assessment

1. General observations of gait

- Walks with a narrow base of support, feet very close together
- Dorsiflexion is full bilaterally, but duration of heel strike is shorter on left than on right
- Weight lands forward of the heel and the forefoot adducts for push-off
- Knees do not fully extend during swing phase
- Stride length is short
- Reciprocal arm swing is minimal
- Torso rotation is minimal
- Right patella rotated inward
- Both femurs rotated inward, right more than left

2. Standing tests

- Full torso rotation
- Observations of inefficient side: both
  - Observed greater ROM into left rotation
  - Mid-foot movement: torso rotation right—right supination and left pronation

Session 12/12: Post-assessment

1. General observations of gait

- Walks with a slightly wider base of support
- Duration of heel strike is symmetrical
- Weight transfers across metatarsals during push-off
- Knees extend during swing phase
- Cadence increased
- Stride length is increased
- Reciprocal arm swing is about 30 degrees
- Torso rotation is improved
- Right patella rotated inward
- Both femurs rotated inward, right more than left

Editor note
Cadence has more to do with stride length, push-off, and turnover than the pace. The benefit of having a high cadence is that it reduces the impact forces that reverberate through the body when the foot hits the ground.

2. Standing tests

- Full torso rotation
- Observations of inefficient side: left
  - Observed greater ROM into right rotation
  - Mid-foot movement: torso rotation

- Mid-foot movement: torso rotation left—left supination and right pronation
- Both knees internally rotated, right more than left

◆ Hemipelvis inferior motion

● Observations of inefficient side: right
  ■ Standing alignment bilateral, internally rotated acetabular femoral joints, right more than left
  ■ Right hemipelvis inferior motion, very little pelvic translation to left
  ■ Knees move into hyperextension, right more than left

◆ Hemipelvis superior motion

● Observations of inefficient side: both
  ■ Right
    ○ Minimal adaption of torso, limited right rib translation
    ○ Lacks lumbar lateral flexion
    ○ Full ROM in ankle plantar flexion
  ■ Left
    ○ Innominate appears smoother
    ○ Limited rib translation, on left more than right
    ○ Increased ankle supination on elevated heel side

◆ Lateral pelvic shift

● Observations of inefficient side: both
  ■ Right
    ○ Left hemipelvis moves inferiorly as thorax translates left
    ○ Knee hyperextension on the weighted LE, right more than left
    ○ Right ankle supinates, left ankle pronates
  ■ Left

right—right supination and left pronation, but rear foot more stable
- Mid-foot movement: torso rotation left—left supination and right pronation, but rear foot more stable
- Ipsilateral/standing leg knee remains straight on the side she rotates toward
- Contralateral/opposite knee rotates medially

◆ Hemipelvis inferior motion

● Observations of inefficient side: right
  ■ Observed left side to move more smoothly
  ■ Rib translation and pelvic translation, more pure lateral movement with right hemipelvis inferior motion
  ■ Torso rotates to the right, rather than translates laterally, with left hemipelvis inferior motion
  ■ Resting knee position is good, not hyperextended

◆ Hip hike

● Observations of inefficient side: both
  ■ Right
    ○ Improved torso adaption of rib translation right
    ○ Improved lumbar lateral flexion
    ○ Adequate ankle plantar flexion
  ■ Left
    ○ Decreased lumbar lateral flexion
    ○ Innominate appears stiffer
    ○ Adequate ankle plantar flexion

◆ Lateral pelvic shift

● Observations of inefficient side: both
  ■ Right

Chapter 9

- ○ Right hemipelvis moves inferior as thorax translates right
- ○ Decreased control on the left
- ○ Internal rotation and relative adduction increased on the weighted LE
- ○ Right ankle pronates, left ankle supinates

- ○ Left hemipelvis moves inferiorly as thorax translates left
- ○ Knee hyperextension on the weighted LE, right more than left
- ○ Right ankle supinates, left ankle pronates
- ■ Left
  - ○ Right hemipelvis moves inferiorly as thorax translates right
  - ○ Decreased control on the left
  - ○ Internal rotation and relative adduction increased on the weighted LE
  - ○ Right ankle pronates, left ankle supinates

3. Seated tests

◆ Thoracic rotation

● Observations of inefficient side: both
  ■ Thoracic rotation limited in both directions
  ■ Right rotation is greater than left

◆ Hip joint and knee flexion

● Observations of inefficient side: both
  ■ Left femur abducts when flexed to more than 90 degrees
  ■ Both feet evert in flexion of more than 90 degrees
  ■ Slight posterior pelvic rotation with lumbar flexion during flexion bilaterally

4. Sit and stand

◆ Lateral view

● Feet pronated and everted

3. Seated tests

◆ Thoracic rotation

● Observations of inefficient side: both
  ■ Thoracic rotation limited in both directions
  ■ Right rotation is greater than left

◆ Hip joint and knee flexion

● Observations of inefficient side: both
  ■ Left femur remains in sagittal plane when flexed to more than 90 degrees
  ■ Both feet remain in contact with floor in flexion of more than 90 degrees
  ■ Pelvis and lumbar region remain in optimal position during flexion bilaterally

4. Sit and stand

◆ Lateral view

● Feet slightly pronated and everted

- Knees slightly hyperextend and then return to 2–3 degrees of flexion
- Shoulder, pelvis, knee, and ankle well aligned
- Head forward of central axis
- Leads with head and chest to assume standing

◆ Anterior view

- Head in cervical hyperextension
- Right femur adducted and internally rotated
- Knees hyperextend bilaterally
- Right ankle pronated more than left ankle
- Right foot everted more than left ankle
- Strong adduction of distal femurs on descent to bench

5. Standing balance

◆ Two-leg stance, eyes open

- 60 seconds
- Head held in slight right lateral flexion

◆ One-leg stance, eyes open

- Balance is good on both left and right
- Femur internally rotated, right more than left
- Right arm held away from body when balancing on right leg
- Slight wobble of left ankle when standing on left leg

- Knees extend and then return to 2–3 degrees of flexion
- Shoulder, pelvis, knee, and ankle well aligned
- Head on central axis
- Spinal extension smooth
- Leads with head and chest to assume standing

◆ Anterior view

- Head in slight cervical extension
- Ribs rotated slightly to the left
- Right femur adducted and internally rotated
- Knees touch/strong adduction of distal femurs on ascent and descent to bench
- Both ankles in slight pronation
- Right foot everted more than left ankle

5. Standing balance

◆ Two-leg stance, eyes open

- 60 seconds
- Head held in slight right lateral flexion

◆ One-leg stance, eyes open

- Balance is good on both left and right legs
- Femur internally rotated, right more than left
- Arm position symmetrical
- Slight wobble of left ankle when standing on left leg
- Included eyes open and eyes closed

Session 3/12: Home program

Fatigue scale	0
Pain scale	0
Client self-report	• No reports of any discomfort • Clavicle fracture healed • Excited to start program
Key changes observed by author at end of Session 3/12	• Increased ROM of hip joints in external rotation • Increased flexibility into lateral flexion bilaterally
Reason behind choice of sequencing	• Begin with gentle movement while supported • Add motor control component while performing higher level movement skills • Combine dynamic stability and mobility into exercises • Provide resistance to increase joint proprioception and body awareness

Session movement sequence

1. Warm-up on horizontal roller: Pelvic weight shift and alternating leg stretch

Intent	• Change relationship with gravity to access articulation of lumbopelvic-femoral motion • Improve proprioception of lumbopelvic-femoral motions • Stimulate adaptability of torso and LE
Gait reasoning	• Improve transverse plane motion • Activate extension to enhance step length • Increase resilience of hip joint in all planes
Starting position	• Supine on mat • Place roller horizontally under pelvis • Lift feet off mat to shift weight into hip joints • LE in adduction • Lower limbs dangling

Movement description	• Gently rock pelvis side to side • Feel the weight shift from one side of the pelvis • Repeat 5 times in each direction • Flex right hip joint and knee • Extend left hip and knee joints • Left ankle dorsiflexion, heel touching mat • Hold for a count of 10 • Repeat twice on each side
2. Articulating bridge on horizontal roller	(See Chapter 5 in Volume 1, Gentry: Spinal articulations/hip escalator)
Intent	• Hip extension with incremental articulation of the lumbar region • Symmetric pelvic movement • Activating hip abduction • Improve endurance in dynamic stabilization while in optimal LE alignment • Improve proprioception of hip joint movement
Gait reasoning	• Widen foot placement • Activate abduction bilaterally • Symmetrical weight shift into both heels
Starting position	• Lying on mat with pelvis on roller • Flex both knees • Feet on the floor, LE parallel, hip-joint-width apart • Place Mini Magic Circle with pads on the outside of mid-femurs
Movement description	• Press thighs outward into pads on Magic Circle • Press feet into the floor • Initiating from the coccyx, gently lift pelvis off roller • Visualize the coccyx like a paintbrush gently stroking up • Imagine an airplane taking off rather than a helicopter taking off (gradual rather than vertical ascent) • 5 repetitions

3. Vertical roller with Mini Magic Circle

Intent
- Improve overall proprioception
- Sense movement between head and sacrum
- Activate torso necessary for balance
- Activate dynamic stabilization of pelvis and LE
- Improve shoulder girdle proprioception
- Decrease anterior rib translation

Gait reasoning
- Improve excursion of arm swing
- Improve overall thorax and upper extremity (UE) awareness

Starting position
- Place roller on mat vertically
- Supine on mat with head and torso in contact with roller
- Place LE through Magic Circle, pads on lateral femurs
- Feet in contact with floor
- Press both feet firmly into the floor

Movement description
- Place UE on mat with palms up and elbows extended
- Move backs of hands along the mat to make "angels in the snow"
- Coordinate breathing with movement
- Inhale on superior movement
- Exhale on inferior movement
- Maintain thoracolumbar junction (TLJ) on roller while moving UE
- If TLJ lifts off roller, diminish the range of UE movement
- 10 repetitions

4. Bridge on vertical roller with Mini Magic Circle

(See Chapter 5 in Volume 1, Gentry: Spinal articulations/hip escalator)

Intent
- Activation of extension with optimal LE alignment
- Activation of lateral LE to improve hip joint positioning and glide
- Increase proprioceptive awareness of pelvic control

Gait reasoning
- Widen foot placement
- Activate posterior-lateral pelvifemoral movement bilaterally
- Symmetrical weight shift into both heels

Starting position
- Place roller on mat vertically
- Supine, with head and torso in contact with roller
- Place LE through Magic Circle, pads on lateral femurs
- Press both feet firmly into the floor

Movement description	• Maintain the resistance of the Magic Circle • Arms by sides next to roller • Press palms into the floor • Slowly bridge up, initiating from coccyx • Continue to extend the hip joints, lift pelvis up • Maintain posterior thorax on the roller • Begin lowering the bridge starting at the TLJ and articulate down to starting position • 10 repetitions
5. Ribcage Arms and shoulder drops while supine on roller	(Derivative of Grant and Gentry; see Chapter 5 in Volume 1)
Intent	• Improve overall proprioception • Sense movement between head and sacrum • Activate torso as necessary for balance • Activate dynamic stabilization of pelvis and LE • Increase shoulder girdle proprioception • Decrease anterior rib translation with UE movement
Gait reasoning	• Improve excursion of arm swing • Improve overall thoracic and UE awareness
Starting position	• Place roller on mat vertically • Supine with head and torso in contact with roller • Place LE through Mini Magic Circle, pads on lateral femurs • Press both feet firmly into the floor • Place both UE at sides, next to roller with thumbs pointing up
Movement description	• Flex UE 90 degrees with palms facing each other, elbows extended • Exhale, sustaining control at the TLJ as UE move overhead • Inhale, return to starting position • 10 repetitions • Flex UE 90 degrees with palms facing each other, elbows extended • Reach right UE toward ceiling protracting right scapula • "Drop" right UE down so the medial border of the scapula contacts the roller • Repeat for the left UE • 10 repetitions, alternating right and left

6. Swan on roller

Derivative of J. H. Pilates Swan Dive (NPCE Study Guide 2021, p. 48)

Intent
- Improve movement awareness of thoracic extension
- Coordinate movement of head, neck, and torso
- Improve dynamic stability of pelvis while activating torso into extension
- Improve shoulder girdle movement

Gait reasoning
- Improve awareness of head, neck, and torso
- Activate extensors
- Activate LE during torso extension

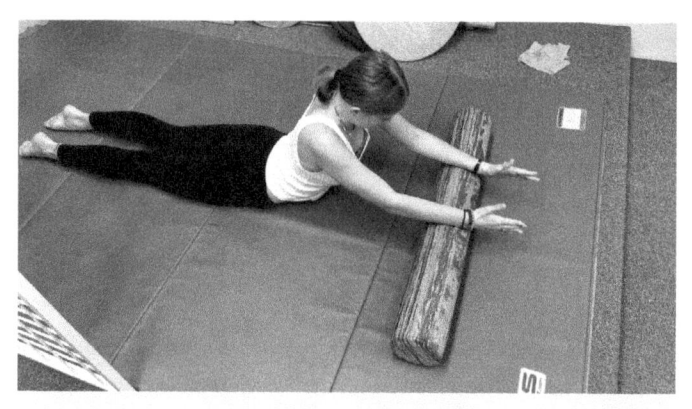

Figure 9.1

Starting position
- Prone on mat with LE extended
- Maintain centration of femoral joints throughout movement
- Place roller on the floor horizontally approximately 12 in. (30 cm) from head
- Place ulnar side of distal forearms on roller, thumbs pointed up, palms facing each other
- Head balanced in midline
- Look toward the floor

Movement description
- Bilateral elbow extension, press ulnar side of hands into roller
- Slowly glide both scapulae medially and inferiorly on thorax, moving the roller
- Extend and articulate thorax from head until weight shifts toward pelvis
- Hold for a count of 5 and slowly roll roller away
- 10 repetitions

7. Swimming	Derivative of J. H. Pilates Swimming (NPCE Study Guide 2021, p. 50)
Intent	- Facilitate proprioceptive awareness of total body integration
- Activate reciprocal UE/LE movement
- Maintain dynamic torso stability while moving extremities
- Improve activation of extension
Gait reasoning	- Enhance reciprocal UE/LE movement, contralateral movement
- Activate torso rotation

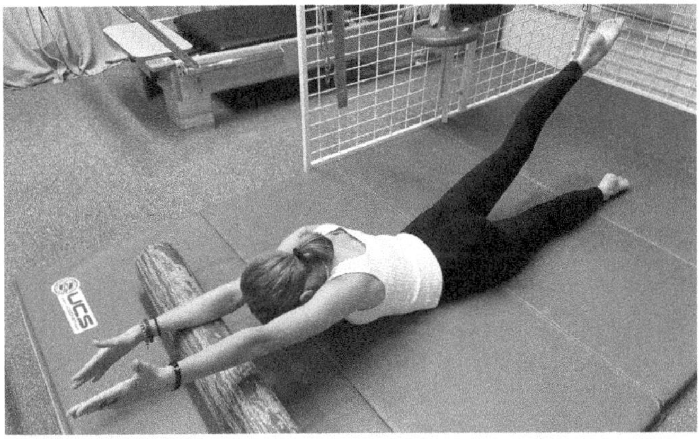

Figure 9.2

Starting position	- Prone on mat
- UE and LE fully extended
- Maintain centration of femoral joints throughout movement
- Place ulnar side of distal forearms on roller, thumbs pointed up, palms facing each other
- Head balanced in midline
- Look toward the floor
Movement description	- Flex right UE while extending left LE a few inches off the floor
- Switch sides
- Maintain extension of limbs and torso throughout movement
- Continue to alternate sides, creating a swimming motion
- 20 repetitions on each side
- Modification: maintain forearms on roller as in Swan, begin Swimming exercise moving only LE

8. Single Leg Circle

Derivative of J. H. Pilates Single Leg Circle (NPCE Study Guide 2021, p. 46)

Intent
- Experience full excursion of hip joint ROM
- Improve proprioception and differentiation of unilateral pelvifemoral movement
- Improve rotational symmetry of bilateral hip joints

Gait reasoning
- Supine position for ease of focusing on unilateral movement for leg swing
- Improve external rotation of bilateral hip joints
- Improve stride length
- Facilitate activation of dorsiflexion with knee extension

Starting position
- Supine on mat
- Hold a length of resistance band in both hands
- Place right foot in loop of band
- Flex right hip joint with knee extension to 45–60 degrees
- Left LE extended on mat

Movement description
- Create resistance to secure the band by pulling toward floor
- Move right LE in a circular motion
- Begin the circle moving toward the midline
- 10 repetitions
- Then circle away from the midline
- 10 repetitions
- Maintain the dynamic stability of the torso
- Focus on the articulation of the acetabular femoral joint

9. Heel lowers from a yoga block

Intent
- Improve glide and activation of posterior connective tissue of lower limb and ankle
- Improve graded eccentric control while ascending and descending heels off the edge of the block
- Improve joint proprioception of ankle joints and subtalar joints

Gait reasoning
- Improve ability for heel strike
- Increase stride length and cadence

Starting position
- Stand with both feet parallel about 3 in. (8 cm) apart, rear foot off the block
- Hold a chair or the wall for balance if necessary

Movement description	- Imagine you are on a diving platform and are preparing for a dive
- Plant forefoot firmly on the block with weight distributed equally through the 5 metatarsal heads of each foot
- Slowly raise calcaneus slightly while maintaining a vertical/straight position
- Hold for a count of 5
- Lower rear foot below the level of the block as much as possible while maintaining calcaneal vertical position
- Hold for a count of 10
- 10 repetitions

10. Femoral glide with Mini Magic Circle (Black 2022)

Intent	- Increase endurance of standing leg
- Improve body awareness of lateral translation of pelvis during gait
- Activate oppositional movement of thorax and pelvis
- Facilitate activation of lateral side of LE from pelvis to 5th metatarsal head
Gait reasoning	- Increase base of support
- Facilitate lateral pelvic shift over foot
- Activate standing posterior-lateral pelvifemoral movement to improve balance on stance leg
Starting position	- Stand with right side by a wall
- Place the Magic Circle just superior of the right greater trochanter and against the wall
- Weight distributed evenly between both LE
Movement description	- Keep the feet planted firmly on mat
- Press into the Magic Circle by shifting pelvis toward wall
- Observe for medial glide of left hip joint and right lateral shift of thorax
- Release pressing on circle
- 10 repetitions on each side

11. Statue of Liberty

Intent
- Increase awareness of restricted areas in coronal plane
- Improve proprioception of lateral movement
- Experience lateral heel through head through resistance

Gait reasoning
- Widen stance to improve stability
- Facilitate weight bearing through lateral aspect of both feet
- Allow for opposing forces: downward with LE and lateral flexion of torso with UE

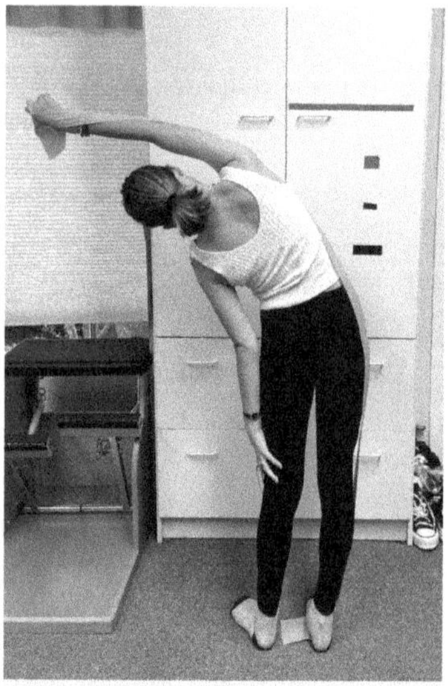

Figure 9.3

Starting position
- Standing
- Place the end of a resistance band under one heel
- Hold band in the same side hand, with palm facing forward
- Elbow extended with the band slack

Movement description
- Pull band superiorly
- Imagine creating a "racing stripe" along the side of the body
- Lean elbow into band, creating tension in band
- Continue pulling to reach toward the opposite side wall for a full torso lateral flexion
- Use a mirror to visually check remaining in coronal plane
- Avoid sagittal plane deviations
- 5 repetitions on each side

12. Mermaid	Derivative of J. H. Pilates Side Bend (NPCE Study Guide 2021, p. 50) and Mermaid on Universal Reformer (NPCE Study Guide 2021, p. 58)
Intent	• Integrate movement of head, torso, and UE • Increase proprioception of coronal plane movement • Facilitate lateral flexion of torso
Gait reasoning	• Improve symmetry of lateral flexion of torso • Improve symmetry of lateral cervical flexion • Improve torso rotation • Increase arc of UE abduction
Starting position	• Sit sideways on mat weighted more on right ischial tuberosity • Both feet to left side, both knees pointing in same direction • Place right hand on mat next to pelvis • Left UE by side • Resistance band near right pelvis
Movement description	• Abduct left UE palm facing upward • Arc left LE overhead • Rotate torso right • Rotate torso left to face forward • Adduct left UE to starting position • Perform as described above while using a resistance band placed under right pelvis • Grasp band with left hand • Reach and stretch band using an arcing motion of the arm • Gently lower the arm, allowing band to slacken • 5 repetitions on each side

Session 11/12: Studio session

Fatigue scale	0
Pain scale	0
Client self-report	• Noticing overall increased range of movement • Feels good about accomplishment during our program

Chapter 9

Key changes observed by author at end of Session 11/12	• Knee position improved • Thorax over pelvis • Gait pattern more symmetrical • Improved symmetry of pelvifemoral region, knee, and ankle
Reason behind choice of sequencing	• Begin with footwork to focus on foot position and LE alignment • Progress to LE-torso relationships • Increasing difficulty and complexity of movement

Session movement sequence

1. Footwork on Universal Reformer	Footwork (NPCE Study Guide 2021, p. 52) and Running (NPCE Study Guide 2021, p. 60)
Intent	• Activate intrinsic foot • Provide closed kinematic chain proprioceptive input from feet through torso • Reinforce proprioception of foot and ankle
Gait reasoning	• Improve gait by widening base of support • Improve symmetrical heel strike
Set-up	• Springs: 2 medium and 1 light • Footbar adjusted to allow 75 degrees hip joint flexion
Starting position	• Supine on carriage with both feet parallel • Forefoot on footbar

Movement description	• Heel raises and lowers
	  ▪ 10 repetitions
	• External rotation with metatarsals on footbar
	  ▪ Heels maintain contact under footbar
	  ▪ 10 repetitions
	• Running (2 medium springs)
	  ▪ 10 repetitions for each foot

	CUES • Tactile cueing is necessary to maintain vertical position of heels while ascending and descending • Use verbal cues to direct maintaining heels together and external rotation of both legs for the duration of the exercise

Author note
Maintaining optimal alignment of the LE was difficult because of the client's habitual posturing of her pelvifemoral region into internal rotation. The resistance provided by the springs improved her proprioceptive awareness and she could quickly self-correct foot positions.

2. Straps: feet in loops on Universal Reformer Derivative of J. H. Pilates Leg Springs: Supine on Trapeze Table (NPCE Study Guide 2021, pp. 67–68) and Single Leg Circle (NPCE Study Guide 2021, p. 46)

Intent
- Experience full excursion of hip joint ROM
- Improve proprioception and differentiation of hip joint movement
- Improve rotational symmetry bilaterally

Gait reasoning
- Supine position for ease of focusing on hip joint ROM for leg swing
- Improve external rotation
- Improve stride length
- Facilitate activation of dorsiflexion with knee extension

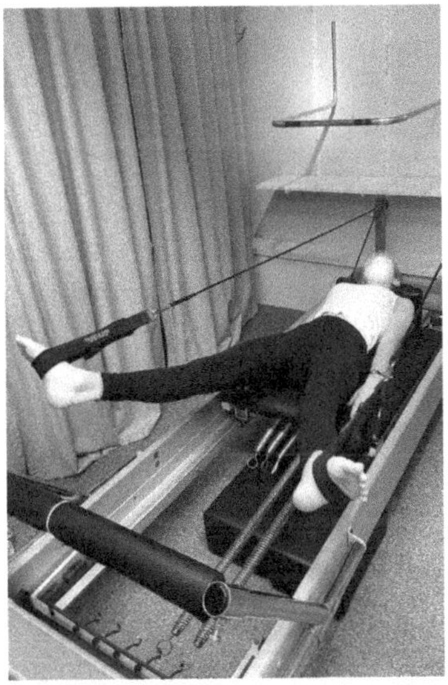

Figure 9.4

Set-up
- Springs: 1 medium and 1 very light

Chapter 9

Starting position
- Supine with feet in straps
- Hip joint flexion to 60–70 degrees and external rotation
- Knees extended
- Hands by sides, palms down

Movement description
- Pull straps into hip joint extension
- Abduct, flex, and adduct the LE to starting position
- 10 repetitions
- Reverse direction
- 10 repetitions

CUES
- Use verbal cues to maintain hands down and pressing into carriage to activate torso
- Visualize the femoral head in the acetabulum spinning
- Use tactile cues to prevent circles from getting too big
- Place hands in line with sides of Universal Reformer to demonstrate "working within the frame"

Author note
The client had good mastery over this exercise from following her home program.

3. Long Spine on Universal Reformer

Derivative of J. H. Pilates Long Spine Massage (NPCE Study Guide 2021, p. 60)
(See Chapter 5 in Volume 1, Trier)

Intent
- Provide proprioceptive input throughout the body
- Focus on eccentric, controlled movement
- Maintain symmetry of the pelvis and LE while moving in a novel way

Gait reasoning
- Torso control through sagittal plane
- Improve LE symmetry for weight distribution
- Activation of feet stimulating torso articulation

Set-up
- Springs: 1 medium and 1 light

Starting position
- Headrest down
- Supine on carriage with feet in straps
- LE extended
- Feet plantar flexed

Movement description
- Maintain resistance of both feet into straps
- Flex hip joints to the point of available range before pelvis moves
- Press into straps and lift pelvis off carriage
- Slowly articulate from pelvic base and lift torso off carriage
- LE remain extended
- Stop at the level of T8
- Reverse articulation, pressing into straps
- Control the descent
- Return to starting position
- Maintain symmetrical downward force through LE and control the torso
- 10 repetitions

CUES
- Use verbal cueing to instruct to "match the resistance" of the springs on both the ascent and descent of the torso
- Eccentric control is key to facilitate control of the torso

Author note
This exercise was a significant accomplishment by the client who had honed her ability to respond to the resistance of the equipment.

Editor note
The distribution of peripheral ground forces, with the feet in straps and the arms on the carriage, informs proximal integrity. The goal is to move with control through an active ROM to reduce hypermobility.

4. Chest Expansion on Universal Reformer

Derivative of J. H. Pilates Leg Springs: Supine on Trapeze Table (NPCE Study Guide 2021, pp. 67–68) and Single Leg Circle (NPCE Study Guide 2021, pp. 46, 57)

Intent
- Improve sagittal plane motion
- Focus on proximal organization
- Activate shoulder girdle while moving through space

Gait reasoning
- Improve organization in sagittal plane
- Increase proprioception of torso placement over pelvis

Chapter 9

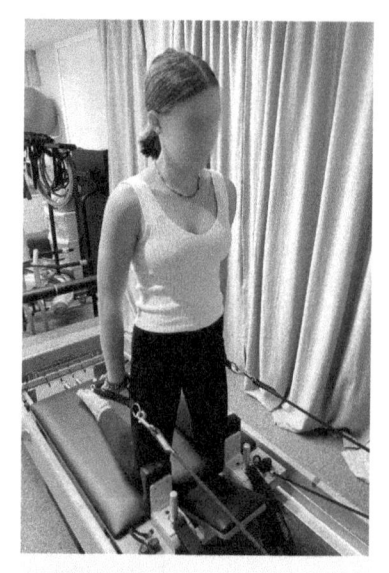

Figure 9.5

Set-up
- Springs: 1 medium and 1 very light

Starting position
- Kneeling on carriage with knees up against shoulder stops
- Shorten straps and add handles for pulling
- Ankles in plantar flexion
- Press shins into carriage to establish firm base of support with the dorsum of the foot
- Organize the torso over the knees to create a continuous midline axis

Movement description
- Pull straps, extending the UE
- Retract and depress scapulae
- Slowly flex the UE back to the starting position
- 10 repetitions

CUES
- Use tactile and verbal cues to maintain extension throughout the excursion of the movement

Author note
I often used two weighted sandbags—weighing about 10 lbs (4.5 kg) each—to give strong downward input into the shins to prevent the torso from being displaced during the movement.

5. Elephant on Universal Reformer

Derivative of J. H. Pilates Long Stretch Series: Elephant on Universal Reformer (NPCE Study Guide 2021, p. 55)

Intent
- Force generation through fully extended legs
- Improve coordination of acetabular femoral joint movement
- Strong proprioception into heels
- Total body movement

Gait reasoning
- Increase stride length
- Increase heel strike
- Improve dorsiflexion

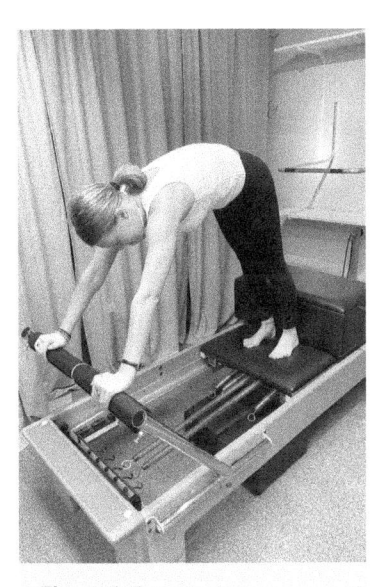

Figure 9.6

Set-up
- Medium spring
- Large box placed horizontally on carriage up against shoulder stops

Starting position
- Sitting on top of box
- Place feet hip-joint-width apart on carriage
- Find the edge where the box meets the carriage and steady or secure heels there
- Reach both arms forward and hold the bar

Chapter 9

Movement description	• Shift weight forward to distribute weight into hands • Initiate moving carriage back by activating posterior aspect of LE • Focus on energy through the heels • Press carriage back only as far as maintaining both feet firmly on the carriage • Slowly return the carriage to the starting position

CUES
- Verbal cues are necessary for maintaining contact of both heels as well as shifting weight laterally in both feet to maintain subtalar neutral position
- Emphasize moving slowly, especially on return movement to process the sensation of eccentric control of posterior aspect of LE

Author note
The client benefited from the secondary effect of improved upper body strength.

6. Mermaid on Universal Reformer   (NPCE Study Guide 2021, p. 58)

Intent	• Improve lateral flexion and thoracic rotation • Increase articulation of rib translation
Gait reasoning	• Facilitate symmetrical torso rotation and lateral flexion • Improve translation of ribcage for rotation

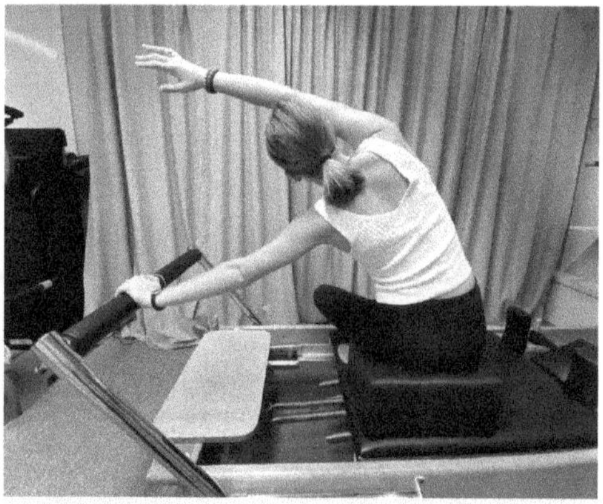

Figure 9.7

Set-up	● Light spring ● Small box
Starting position	● Sitting on small box in cross-legged position ● Right hand on bar, elbow extended ● Left arm abducted to 90 degrees
Movement description	● Right arm presses carriage away from bar ● Reach left arm in arcing motion overhead ● Rotate thorax to right ● Reach left arm toward bar ● Hold for count of 5 ● Reach left arm overhead ● Counter-rotate thorax to face forward ● Return to starting position ● 3 repetitions on each side

CUES
- Maintain ischial tuberosities on the box throughout the movement
- Make each component of the movement distinct
- Coordinate breath with movement
- Visualize a "wringing out" of the torso

Author note
The client had good carryover from her home program with two versions of this exercise while seated on the floor.

7. Eve's Lunge on Universal Reformer
(See Chapter 5 in Volume 1, Gentry, Eve's Lunge)

Intent	● Experiencing a reciprocal movement pattern ● Activate extension
Gait reasoning	● Improve organization of LE ● Increase stride length ● Reciprocal flexion and extension

Chapter 9

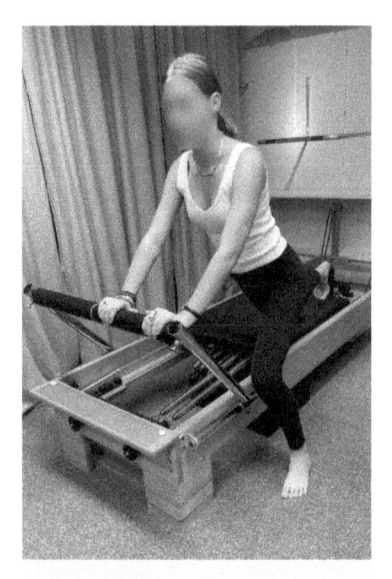

Figure 9.8

Set-up
- Springs: 1 medium and 1 very light

Starting position
- Stand on left side of Universal Reformer with left foot on floor near footbar
- Left knee centered over left ankle
- Right knee in flexion resting on carriage with foot against shoulder stops
- Hold on to footbar with both hands

Movement description
- Distribute weight laterally on left foot to maintain ankle alignment
- Press into left foot
- Extend right hip joint and knee to move carriage backward
- Return to starting position
- Pull shoulders back and down as you lift your chest gently through your arms
- Eyes are on the horizon line
- Hold for a count of 5 and slowly release
- 3 repetitions on each side

CUES
- Use tactile cues at the anterior and posterior aspects of the pelvis to teach positional awareness and draw attention to any asymmetries
- Focus on extending the hip joints rather than extending the knee
- Use tactile cues on standing knee to maintain alignment and prevent the knee from rocking in or out during the exercise

Author note
The client enjoyed the freedom of this movement.

8. Splits: Side on Universal Reformer
J. H. Pilates Splits: Side (NPCE Study Guide 2021, p. 61)

Intent
- Challenge balance while maintaining very specific organization to various joint positions
- Introduce lateral movement in coronal plane
- Create distal point of control for total body movement

Gait reasoning
- Dynamic abduction with femoral gliding
- Prevent knee hyperextension
- Improve torso organization and weight distribution in the feet

Set-up
- Medium spring
- Standing platform attached to frame of Universal Reformer

Starting position
- Standing with right foot on standing platform and left foot on carriage
- Hands on pelvis
- Eyes on the horizon line
- Externally rotate hip joints and slightly flex knees

Movement description
- Look straight ahead
- Shift weight into the lateral edges of each foot
- Gently start to move carriage away by "spreading" the feet apart
- Maintain the weight on the lateral aspects of both feet while drawing carriage in
- 10 repetitions on each side

Chapter 9

CUES
- Use tactile cues to maintain pelvic alignment in the starting position
- Use tactile cues for feet along lateral border to prevent over-pronation
- Use verbal cues to maintain slight knee flexion and to press feet down into the surface while moving carriage both away and toward standing platform

Author note
A tremendous amount of learning occurs while mastering this exercise. It is a favorite of most children who have the balance and the awareness to move through it properly.

The journey to Session 11

Session 4/12
Client self-report

- Pain scale 0
- Fatigue scale 0
- Client performed home program once since last session
- Feels more flexible
- "I have to rewire my brain" (client's response to learning new movements)

Key changes observed

- Client's awareness of feet increased
- Overall enhanced movement awareness
- Difficulty with over-effort
- Responds well to tactile cues

Reasoning behind choice of movements

- Improve body awareness
- Understand and feel the foot position with overall leg alignment
- Increase active ROM of hip joints in external rotation
- Activate laterally to improve balance
- Extension with UE movement
- Review lumbopelvic-femoral motions in bridging

Session movement sequence
1. Universal Reformer

- Footwork
    - Forefoot
    - Rear foot
    - Prehensile
    - Heel lowers

> **Author note**
> The client began with 2 medium springs and decreased resistance to 1 medium and 1 light. She required a 8–10 in. (20–25 cm) ball between the knees to prevent internal rotation and adduction of the femurs and to focus on maintaining subtalar position.

- Leg Circles
- Standing splits
- Elephant

2. Wunda Chair

- Standing Single Leg Pump
  - External rotation of acetabular femoral joint
  - 20 repetitions for each leg

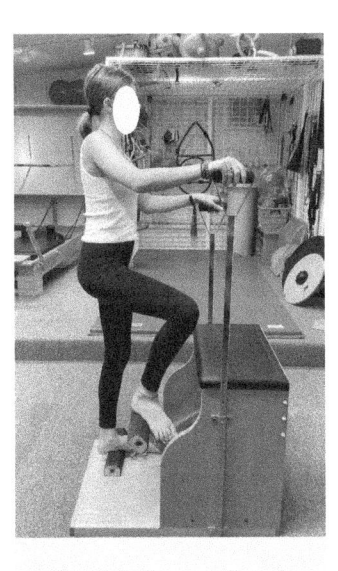

Figure 9.9

- Swan
  - 20 repetitions

Session 5/12
Client self-report

- Pain scale 0
- Fatigue scale 0
- Aware of increased focus required when performing exercises
- Enjoys Leg Circles

Key changes observed

- Client able to self-correct foot position on footbar with tactile cues and verbal prompts and throughout the session

Reasoning behind choice of movements

- Understand and feel the foot position with overall leg alignment
- Improve body awareness
- Introduce dynamic stability during LE movements

Session movement sequence

1. Universal Reformer

- Footwork
  - Forefoot
  - Rear foot
  - Prehensile
  - Heel lowers
  - Running
- Leg Circles
- Pulling Straps
- Splits: Side
- Elephant
- Eve's Lunge

2. Additional movements

- Wunda Chair
  - Seated alternating leg pumps in external rotation
  - Seated Double Leg Pump in external rotation, heels together, metatarsals on footbar

Session 6/12
Client self-report

- Pain scale 0
- Fatigue scale 2

Key changes observed

- Right knee continues to internally rotate on full extension

Chapter 9

- Improved organization and ability during Pulling Straps
- Requires verbal cues to maintain weight bearing on the lateral aspect of foot

Reasoning behind choice of movements

- Continue the focus on foot and ankle alignment and effects on overall LE function
- Activation of lateral torso
- Improve transverse plane motion

Session movement sequence
1. Universal Reformer

- Footwork: added Mini Magic Circle to improve LE alignment
- Leg Circles
- Pulling Straps
- Splits: Side
- Eve's Lunge
- Mermaid

2. Additional movement
- Reviewed Mermaid and observed limited range of motion of right thoracic rotation
- Suggest starting with left thoracic rotation in Mermaid
- Self-correction of right LE tracking required with every exercise
- Add Magic Circle Mini to increase awareness and activation of abduction and external rotation

- Wunda Chair
    - Standing side leg pump

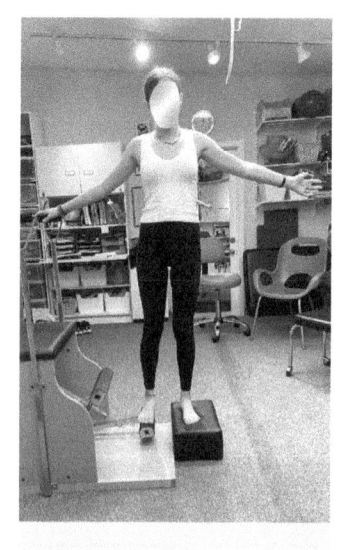

Figure 9.10

- Floor work
    - Small arc: side leg lifts, Side Kick and small circles

Session 7/12
Client self-report

- Pain scale 0
- Fatigue scale 0
- Client enjoyed balancing with one foot on a small box and the other foot on the pedal of the Wunda Chair

Key changes observed

- Observed decreased ROM in flexion with knee extended
- Upper body and UE weakness
- Feet organization improved during Footwork
- Improved ability to articulate torso

Reasoning behind choice of movements

- Understand and feel the foot position with overall leg alignment
- Improve body awareness
- Practice dynamic stability during LE movements
- Improve symmetry of torso lateral flexion and rotation

Additional movements

- Added standing LE isometric exercise: hip joint flexion, knee extension, foot on staircase
- Added supine LE isometric exercise: hip joint flexion, knee extension using Mini Magic Circle and/or resistance band on foot

1. Universal Reformer

- Footwork
- Leg Circles
- Short Spine
- Pulling Straps

2. Additional movements

- Universal Reformer
  - Eve's Lunge
  - Mermaid

Session 8/12
Client self-report

- Pain scale 0
- Fatigue scale 0

Key changes observed

- Right LE adducts and internally rotates during lunges—requires verbal and tactile cueing to improve alignment
- Improved ROM demonstrated in squats and Downward Dog

Reasoning behind choice of movements

- Understand and feel the foot position with overall leg alignment
- Improve body awareness
- Increase ROM of hip joints in external rotation
- Introduce torso articulation
- Focus on lateral movement
- Review new posterior hip joint positions and heel lowers

Session movement sequence
1. Universal Reformer

- Footwork
- Leg Circles
- Short Spine
- Pulling Straps
- Elephant

2. Additional movements

- Universal Reformer
  - Long Stretch Series: Long Stretch (Front) on knees
  - Splits: Side
- Wall
  - Side plank with knees bent

Session 9/12
Client self-report

- Pain scale 0
- Fatigue scale 4

Key changes observed

- Increased body awareness
- Improved joint proprioception in feet and ankles

323

Chapter 9

Reasoning behind choice of movements

- Integration of whole-body awareness
- Continue to increase endurance in feet and ankles to maintain optimal organization
- Upper body loading

Session movement sequence
1. Universal Reformer

- Footwork
- Short Spine
- Pulling Straps
- Mermaid

2. Additional movements

- Wunda Chair
    - Seated Double Leg Pump
    - Pull-Up/Hamstring 3

Session 10/12
Client self-report

- Pain scale 0
- Fatigue scale 2

Key changes observed

- Organized well during Long Spine
- Improved endurance overall

Reasoning behind choice of movements

- Integrate dynamic control with LE articulation
- Focus on lateral torso movement

Session movement sequence
1. Universal Reformer

- Footwork
- Short Spine
- Leg Circles
- Elephant

2. Additional movements

- Universal Reformer
    - Kneeling Side Support
- Wunda Chair
    - Seated Mermaid/Side Arm Sit
- Mat
    - Push-ups

References

Amaral, D. M., Cadilha, R. P. B. S., Rocha, J. A. G. M., Silva, A. I. G., and Parada, F. (2019) "Congenital muscular torticollis: Where are we today? A retrospective analysis at a tertiary hospital." *Porto Biomedical Journal*, 4, 3. DOI: 10.1097/j.pbj.0000000000000036.

Black, M. (2022) *Centered: Organizing the Body through Kinesiology, Movement Theory and Pilates Techniques*. 2nd Ed. Edinburgh: Handspring Publishing, pp. 89, 91.

Kim, S. N., Shin, Y. B., Kim, W., Suh, H. *et al.* (2011) "Screening for the coexistence of congenital muscular torticollis and developmental dysplasia of hip." *Annals of Rehabilitation Medicine*, 35, 4, 485–490.

Minghelli, B. and Vitorino, N. G. D. (2022) "Incidence of congenital muscular torticollis in babies from Southern Portugal: Types, age of diagnosis and risk factors." *International Journal of Environmental Research and Public Health*, 19, 15. DOI: 10.3390/ijerph19159133.

NPCE Study Guide (National Pilates Certification Exam Study Guide) (2021) Miami, FL: National Pilates Certification Program, Inc.

Sargent, B., Kaplan, S. L., Coulter, C., and Baker, C. (2019) "Congenital muscular torticollis: Bridging the gap between research and clinical practice." *Pediatrics*, 144, 2. DOI: 10.1542/peds.2019-0582.

Stellwagen, L., Hubbard, E., Chambers, C., and Jones, K. (2008) "Torticollis, facial asymmetry and plagiocephaly in normal newborns." *Archives of Disease in Childhood*, 93, 827–831.

Chapter 10

Pilates and Pregnancy-Related Diastasis Rectus Abdominis: Effect on Gait

Dawn-Marie Ickes

Diastasis rectus abdominis (DRA) is a condition where there is an abnormal widening of the abdominal midline (linea alba, LA) composed of interlacing aponeurotic expansions of the anterolateral abdominal myofascia. The excessive widening of the abdominal midline causes a bulging of the abdominal wall. The rectus fascia is intact, therefore it is not a hernia (Hall and Sanjaghsaz 2023; Jessen, Öberg, and Rosenberg 2019). DRA is often described in relation to pregnancy (Candido, Lo, and Janssen 2005; Fernandes da Mota et al. 2015) but it occurs both in post-menopausal women and in men. Between 33 and 77 percent of women experience diastasis rectus in the postpartum period more than 8 weeks after delivery (Boissonnault and Blaschak 1988; Candido et al. 2005; Mota, Pascoal, and Bo 2015). However, the condition has also been found in 38.7 percent of older parous women who underwent abdominal hysterectomy and in 52 percent of urogynecological menopausal patients. Recent studies have shown that low levels of type I and type III collagen play a key role in the development of DRA (Blotta et al. 2018).

Diastasis rectus abdominis is also found in men and is thought to be associated with increasing age, weight fluctuations, weightlifting, performing full sit-ups, congenital weakness of the abdominal muscles, chronic or intermittent abdominal distension, and activities that may induce high intra-abdominal pressure (IAP) (Nienhuijs et al. 2021).

Editor note
IAP is defined as the steady state pressure within the abdominal cavity. It results from the interaction of the abdominal wall and viscera. IAP oscillates with respiratory phase and abdominal wall resistance (Milanesi and Caregnato 2016). Breath control has been shown to influence IAP (Hagins et al. 2006).

Author note
The level of coordination beyond breathing depends on the body knowledge of the client. For some, coordinating the breath in the beginning while ensuring adequate IAP is sufficient. As the client increases their coordination and control, adding challenges to the components of diaphragmic coactivations is beneficial.

The gold standard measurement of the inter-rectus distance (IRD) is carried out via ultrasound (US) (Beamish et al. 2019). As a generalization, an IRD greater than 0.78 in. (2 cm) at the midline is considered abnormal (Michalska et al. 2018). Most experts agree that collagen changes cause lack of integrity of the associated abdominal aponeurosis. This may result in widening of the DRA.

Understanding the complex relationship of the torso's ability to respond to and transfer load is essential when working with individuals who have a DRA. The functional impacts of DRA, and changes in the biomechanical function of the LA and other structures, can guide program choices. The debate of which exercises are best for DRA continues; however, what to encourage and avoid during any exercise has recently become clearer. Case studies and experience provide guidance. The approach to program design in this population must be as unique as the client's DNA, taking into consideration objective, subjective, and theoretical knowledge to ensure the most optimal choices.

For optimal function, an appropriate load transfer requires adaptable tissue response that includes cohesion and glide between myofascial and aponeurotic layers. This model changes the paradigm of focusing on isolated training of the transversus abdominus (TrA) and pelvic diaphragm structures in the presence of DRA, pelvic girdle pain, low back pain (LBP), urinary incontinence, or pelvic organ prolapse (Michalska *et al.* 2018). The goal of movement practice is optimizing recruitment strategies of the system in its entirety during function (Lee and Hodges 2016).

Recovery is based on a combination of many psychosocial and physical factors:

- Extent of tissue integrity compromise
- Sensorimotor control training
- Capacity to support function including load transfer in full weight bearing
- Ability and openness to a change in how the body functions
- Self-recognition that one's mindset impacts outcomes

Symptoms indicating poor IAP regulation during exercise are:

- Bulge, tenting, doming, or gapping above or below the umbilicus
- Sensation of perineum pressure, internal bulging, or dragging
- Pelvic, low back, or hip area pain
- Incontinence

Manifestations in movement are:

- Instability
- Torso responds with compensatory asymmetries
- Balance dysfunction
- Postural dysfunction

Contraindications are:

- Placing the client in a position where they cannot maintain structural integrity
- Strain on the midline aponeurosis
- Exercises or movements increasing the gap
- Heavy loading until strategies are intact and well tested
- Any movement that creates leakage despite the abdominal wall being maintained

Client description: 36-year-old biological female, identifies as female; works in technology consultation

Dates of case report: Session 1: October 8, 2019; Session 12: December 30, 2019

Studio apparatus and props
Pilates equipment

- Universal Reformer
- Trapeze Table

Props used with equipment

- Long box
- Small box
- Roller
- Rotating discs
- Overball
- Resistance band
- Air cushion disc
- Mat

Home program props

- Roller
- Gliders
- 1–2 lb (0.5–1 kg) hand weights
- Mat

Methods and materials

Session 1/12
1. Health history interview

- Client has two young children, last delivery was in 2013
- Vaginal delivery, each over 10 lb (4.5 kg)
- Complains of not liking the appearance of her abdomen
- Intermittent LBP, pain scale 4 at its worst
- Experiences episodes of leakage with running, jumping, laughing, and shouting
- Has been training with husband more over the past 2 months and has noted increased left-sided tightness
- Noted an inability to pull abdominals in
- Told by MD last year there was nothing that can help bulge

2. Symptoms

- Right-sided tightness
- LBP, pain scale 4
- Excessive infrasternal angle (ISA) known as rib flare, inability to control
- Abdomen bulges with sit-ups
- Fatigue in mid-thorax, fatigue scale 3–4

3. Movement aids

- None

Final result of case report

The client had full resolution of stress urinary incontinence and eliminated LBP. She demonstrated improvement in breathing strategies and control of intra-abdominal pressure. During the phases of gait, thoracic and oppositional pelvic patterning improved and there was equal weight bearing on single stance leg. She exhibited no visible right hemipelvis inferior motion with left loading, symmetrical triplane motion of pelvis through gait cycle, and excellent dynamic control. She is able to play with young children and perform daily activities with improved awareness and strength. There is reduction in the DRA but not within the recommended range to avoid surgical repair as a consideration—it still measures more than 1.18 in. (3 cm).

Session 2/12: Initial assessment

1. General observations of gait

- Excessive right transverse plane rotation (TPR) of thorax with right loading
- Right hemipelvis inferior motion with left loading
- Left TPR of pelvis with right loading
- Shorter stance time on the right

2. Standing tests

- Full torso rotation
- Observations of inefficient side: right
  - Stands in left TPR with right foot forward
  - Minimal adaptations
  - Majority of motion at thoracolumbar junction (TLJ)

- Hemipelvis inferior motion
- Observations of inefficient side: left
  - Difficulty dropping hip, limited range
  - Poor control
  - Exaggerates left TPR with drop

- Hemipelvis superior motion
- Observations of inefficient side: right
  - Excessive left lateral shift
  - Inability to hike pelvis without pelvic torsion

- Lateral pelvic shift
- Observations of inefficient side: right

Session 12/12: Post-assessment

1. General observations of gait

- Less right TPR of thorax with right loading
- No visible hemipelvis inferior motion on right with left loading
- Balanced torso motions with all phases of gait
- Equal stance time

2. Standing tests

- Full torso rotation
- Observations of inefficient side: right
  - Distribution of motions improved, more in mid-thorax
  - Visible bilateral adaptations in rotation
  - Rotation articulates from superior torso to feet

- Hemipelvis inferior motion
- Observations of inefficient side: both
  - Improved control and more ease with hemipelvis inferior motion
  - Able to drop without TPR

- Hemipelvis superior motion
- Observations of inefficient side: right
  - Mild lateral shift
  - Smooth motion
  - Able to hike without pelvic torsion

- Lateral pelvic shift
- Observations of inefficient side: right

- Excessive left thorax shift
- Right innominate lower in starting position
- Left innominate does not lower and left lumbar lateral flexion
- Lacks adduction past midline
- Right foot from pronation to neutral, does not supinate
- Left foot pronates

3. Sit and stand

◆ Lateral view

- Left weight shift
- Center of mass (COM) anterior to phalanges
- Torso flexes to balance weight shift

◆ Anterior view

- Weight shift to left at initiation, rebalances in stance
- Poor stand to sit with TPR to left

4. Standing balance

◆ One-leg stance, eyes open

- Left leg: 25 seconds
- Right leg: 15 seconds

- Thorax shifts right with right lateral pelvic shift
- Innominates balanced in starting position
- Left innominate lowers
- Improved right hip joint adduction
- Feet adapt: right supination, left pronation

3. Sit and stand

◆ Lateral view

- Even weight bearing
- COM stays over talus
- Normal range torso to feet

◆ Anterior view

- Equal weight bearing—torso midline in sitting
- No TPR

4. Standing balance

◆ One-leg stance, eyes open

- Left leg: 60 seconds
- Right leg: 50 seconds

Chapter 10

Session 3/12: Home program

Fatigue scale	3
Pain scale	4
Client self-report	• Left and right sides feel very different, bulge not improving, seems to be worse since increasing physical activity
Key changes observed by author at end of Session 3/12	• Less prominent bulge at rest after session • Improved thorax expansion with breath
Reason behind choice of sequencing	• Establish connection and awareness maintaining the appropriate amount of IAP for optimal organ function, circulatory function and lymph balance, digestion, and a myriad of other systemic functions

Session movement sequence

1. Spine Stretch forward on wall with foam roller	Derivative of J. H. Pilates Spine Stretch (NPCE Study Guide 2021, p. 47)
Intent	• Segmental articulation • Scapulothoracic gliding • Proprioception and balanced weight bearing • Increased complexity by adding continuous movement and control in mid-range
Gait reasoning	• Decrease excessive rib translation • Improved COM and equal weight bearing through lower extremities • Sagittal plane reciprocal movement patterning
Starting position	• Sitting upright on mat leaning torso against a vertical roller on the wall • No posterior pelvic tilt in starting position • Legs shoulder-width apart, feet softly plantar flexed • Arms reaching to 90 degrees shoulder flexion
Movement description	• Inhale, sense starting position • Exhale; drawing the anterior abdominal wall toward roller, tuck the chin in gently, flex segmentally, maintaining even weight bearing through ischial tuberosities • Arms parallel to floor, head in between arms • Inhale, hold position, protract scapula, reaching forward • Use the repetition of protraction/retraction for improved scapulothoracic gliding

- Exhale; without changing the position, retract shoulders
- Inhale, extend, initiating from pelvifemoral extension
- Feel each segment on the roller
- Exhale as torso organizes upright
- Repeat 5 times

2. Supine Bent Knee Fall-Out

Intent
- Torso transverse plane movement initiating from lower extremity (LE) for reducing the ISA
- Coordinate breath with movement
- Improve pelvifemoral motion

Gait reasoning
- Integration of torso structures in all three planes to improve rotation

Starting position
- Supine on mat with feet flat, LE flexed
- Place Overball between knees for control of femoral joint centration

Author note

Posterior rotation of the lower thoracic rings in conjunction with an ISA wider than 90 degrees will cause the upper edges of the diastasis to move laterally, increasing the gap. For this client, the solution was to place a wedge pillow from the waist to the head to change the angle just enough to provide feedback for better organization of ribs.

Movement description
- Inhale, slowly lowering knees to one side with scapulae anchored to the floor with opposite hemipelvis lifting as knees move toward the floor
- Exhale, gently articulate from the torso through the feet to return to midline
- Repeat 4 times
- Hold Overball and reach toward ceiling as legs lower to one side
- Repeat 4 times
- Hold Overball and reach the ball in opposite direction to knee sway
- Repeat 4 times

Chapter 10

3. Prone extension

Intent	• Anterior torso proprioception/awareness • Mobility and activation of torso extension • Posterior leg activation coordinated with pelvic diaphragm and TrA
Gait reasoning	• Increased dynamic loading as in gait contributes to involuntary continence (consciousness of this alters the gait pattern) • Extensor recruitment to inhibit pelvic posterior rotation that limits push-off
Starting position	• Lying prone with pelvis on 0.5 in. (1.25 cm) pad for proprioception of pelvis weighted into mat • After feeling the pelvis weighted on the pad, remove pad • Palms on forehead, forehead resting on stacked hands • Place yoga block at medial malleoli
Movement description	• Inhale, feel anterior pelvis on mat • Exhale, draw abdominal wall inward • Inhale, feel breath expanding • Exhale, practice a 5-second sustained activation of pelvic diaphragm • Repeat sequence: practice 5 rapid rhythmic activations of pelvic diaphragm • Repeat 5 times alternating 5-second sustained and 5 rapid activations • Change hand position to shoulder abduction and elbow flexion, imagine Cactus Arms • Next sequence of breath cycle: exhale, extending the upper torso • Hands floating 1–2 in. (2.5–5 cm) off the floor • Hold and inhale • Exhale, shoulder flexion and elbows extending to high V • Inhale, reverse arm movement to Cactus Arms • Exhale, return to starting position • Repeat 3 times

4. Lower extremity abduction/adduction pelvic lift

Intent	• Pre-load training for torso • Coordination of breath with movement • Coordinated activation/relaxation of the abdominal wall

Gait reasoning	• Control through LE to torso activation in supine to pre-load the system
• Improve femoral joint triplanar motions for transferring loads
Starting position	• Supine on mat with knees flexed and feet in line with ischial tuberosities
• Place soft ball under sacrum for support
Movement description	• Sequentially move through the torso up to the scapula in a bridge position
• At the top of the bridge, pause
• Inhale, abduct right LE and return to center while maintaining torso control
• Exhale, pause, inhale, repeat on left side
• Exhale, articulate down to starting position
• Repeat 5 times
• Repeat, reversing inhale and exhale 5 times
• Progress using resistance band around mid-thighs
• Increase challenge by lifting heels for decreased base of support
• Progress to bilateral abduction

5. Quadruped threading

Intent	• Alignment awareness
• Whole-body system connection
• Work torso in variable positions relative to gravity
Gait reasoning	• Increase torso rotation
• Balance symmetry in sagittal plane motion

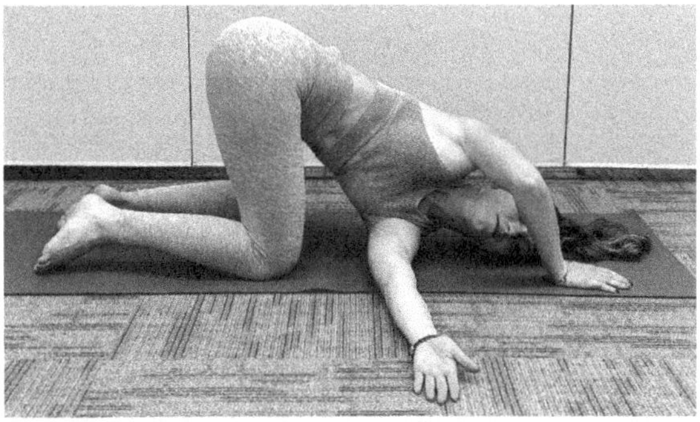

Figure 10.1

Starting position	• Kneeling in quadruped on mat • Client's optimal organization for the movement task
Movement description	• Inhale, activating upper extremity (UE) and LE by isometrically pressing laterally without changing alignment • Exhale, gently draw the abdominal wall inward • Inhale, abduct left arm • Imagine you are stretching between the top of the head and the underside of the pelvis • Exhale, rotating the torso toward the floor, threading the arm under and across the torso, rotating the torso to the level of the pelvis • Inhale, maintain position, breathing for 3 cycles • Exhale, returning to starting position • Repeat on the opposite side • Added rocking back, increasing flexion with rotation

6. Hovering

Intent	• Preparation for torso articulation and awareness of midline • Moderate challenge to anterior abdominal musculature in controlled environment • Torso dynamic midline with flexion/extension
Gait reasoning	• Proprioception of midline during all planes of motion necessary for improved efficiency • Anterior abdominal wall challenge
Starting position	• Quadruped on mat • Client's optimal organization for the movement task
Movement description	• Inhale, extend initiating from eyes looking upward, articulating into full extension of torso • Exhale, posteriorly rotate the pelvis, articulate the torso into flexion, ending by tucking in the chin/head • Repeat 3–5 times • Change position to ankle dorsiflexion, metatarsals on mat • Client's optimal organization for movement task • Isometrically press both UE and LE laterally without changing position • Exhale, lift both knees about 2 in. (5 cm) off the floor and hover, maintaining client's optimal organization • Hold for 3 seconds. Progress to 5–10 seconds

Author note

The client in the beginning was unable to maintain organization of the midline. The strategy for activating the torso to lift the knees and to ensure integrity of the anterior abdomen in midline was a small amount of torso flexion. Over time, the client improved organization and integrity of the midline without flexion and advanced to kneeling on two Overballs.

7. Quadruped with LE wall activation

Intent
- Activating torso using closed kinematic chain
- Scapular and LE coactivation and connection to torso
- To control tendency to compensate by moving into the transverse plane

Gait reasoning
- Torso loading/unloading of lower extremities
- Control in all planes necessary throughout the gait cycle
- Integration of load/force transfers of the upper and lower extremities through the torso

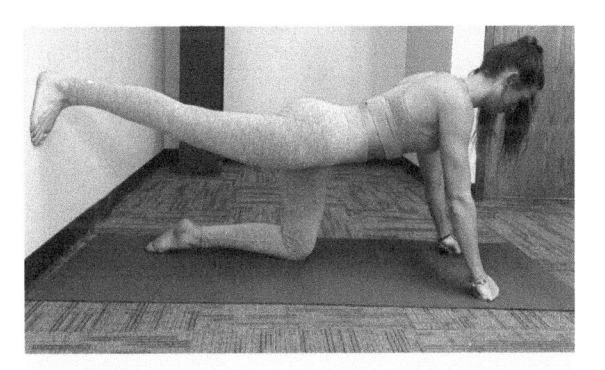

Figure 10.2

Starting position
- Position body on mat at a distance from the wall, so that foot of extended leg can touch the wall
- Quadruped
- Client's optimal organization for the movement task

Chapter 10

Movement description	• Inhale, activating the shoulders and legs by isometrically pressing laterally without changing starting position • Exhale, slide top of foot along floor, extend LE until plantar surface of foot in contact with the wall • Inhale, hiking the innominate on the weight-bearing side as foot on wall continues to press into the wall • Exhale, return to starting position, levelling pelvis as foot on wall continues to press into the wall • Repeat 3 times bilaterally, lowering leg in between each repetition

8. Squat

Intent	• Condition proper squat mechanics for carryover into activities of daily living (ADLs) • Frontal plane mobility
Gait reasoning	• Optimal distribution of ground force reactions
Starting position	• Stand with feet slightly wider than hip joints, external rotation at 7–10 degrees • Place one hand on abdomen for self-monitoring • Ground through the feet with optimal foot-ankle organization • Organize vertical orientation • UE by sides
Movement description	• Inhale, flex hip joints and knees so that the torso is at a 45-degree angle • Lift arms to 90 degrees of shoulder flexion with the descent • Exhale, keeping ischial tuberosities wide, return to standing • Reverse the breath

9. Half kneeling with hemipelvis superior/inferior motion and rotation

Intent	• Coordinate activation of torso for functional task demands with children, such as getting up/down from the floor, carrying loads, and quick movements
Gait reasoning	• Proper coordination/control of IAP with loading response

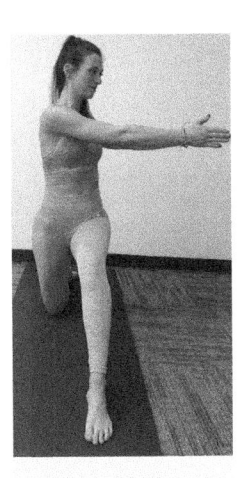

Figure 10.3

Starting position
- Half kneeling on mat in lunge position
- Even distribution of body weight between LE
- Right LE anterior
- Left LE posterior with foot plantar flexed, metatarsal arch on mat, phalanges extended
- Pelvis level without rotation, hiking, or dropping
- Torso in midline
- UE at 90 degrees flexion
- Visually check for any signs of tenting, doming, or bulging of abdominal wall
- Instruct client to self-assess abdomen and monitor any sensation of sagging, dragging, or pressure in perineum

Movement description
- Inhale, feel starting position
- Exhale, shifting weight into left leg
- Inhale, rotating torso to right, UE follow
- Exhale, returning to center
- Inhale, rotating torso to left
- Repeat 3–5 times
- Exhale, rotate torso to right, hold
- Inhale, lowering right side of pelvis toward the floor as the opposite side elevates/hikes
- Exhale, return to the level position
- Repeat 3 times focusing on the movement in the frontal plane
- Return to center, repeat with left torso rotation
- Repeat 3 times
- Progress by holding 0.5–1 lb (0.25–0.5 kg) weight at the midline at 90 degrees shoulder flexion during sequence

Chapter 10

10. Side kneeling with UE wall activation

Intent
- Proprioception of torso organization facilitates improved motor control in developing new movement strategies
- UE and LE initiating forces stimulate lateral activation

Gait reasoning
- Improve midline orientation for organizing triplanar motions necessary in gait

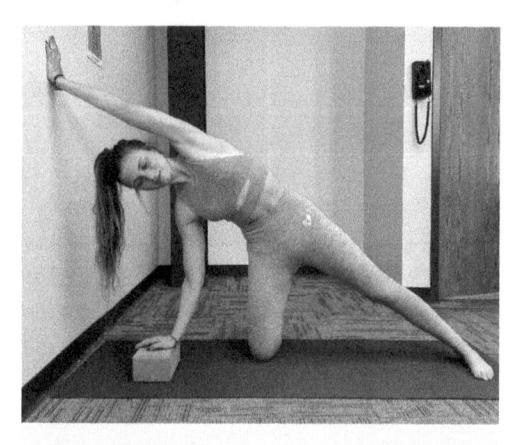

Figure 10.4

Starting position
- Place yoga block between the wall and body
- High-kneeling on mat, facing right side to wall
- Femurs parallel and abducted
- Femoral joints extended
- Left UE abducted to 90 degrees
- Right UE by side

Movement description
- Inhale, abduct left LE with knee extension and foot on floor
- Torso laterally flexes right until right hand touches yoga block
- Check torso is in a long lateral curve, minimal flexion or extension
- Exhale, left moves overhead to touch the wall
- Hold and press into the wall and yoga block while grounding right knee and left foot
- Inhale, into thorax and abdominal wall while continuing limb contact pressure

- Exhale, sliding the foot anteriorly 4–6 in. (10–12 cm)
- Inhale, return LE to mid-range position
- Exhale, sliding the foot posteriorly 4–6 in. (10–12 cm)
- Repeat 5 times
- Repeat on other side

Session 11/12: Studio session

Fatigue scale	0–1
Pain scale	2
Client self-report	• "Feeling very connected—so much more aware of my body, moving, everything I do" • Stronger—more controlled with squats, lifting, housework • "I still have bulge but I feel like I have more control over it. It doesn't pull like it used to" • "My back pain is nearly gone" • "I have not had any episodes of leakage with laughing, lifting, or chasing kids for about 3 weeks now"
Key changes observed by author at end of Session 3/12	• Improved ability of one-leg stance with increased load with and without rotation compensation • Client still unable to lean posteriorly during thigh stretch more than 10 degrees without abdominal doming • DRA distance manually and via US is stable but not less than 1.18 in. (3 cm) (goal for potential to avoid surgical repair) • Able to perform home program with increased challenge and complexity with excellent awareness

Author note

Thigh stretch is an important challenge for the DRA client. It is performed by maintaining the torso position while increasing knee flexion to lean posteriorly. It requires control through the movement relationship of the thorax and pelvis during the increase of knee flexion, that is, a well-timed approximation of the lower thoracic ring and the pelvic rim so that the xiphoid and pubis remain in continuous relationship. When leaning posteriorly, there is an increase of compression to the aponeurotic expansions of the anterolateral abdominal myofascia. This controls weight distribution during the movement.

Chapter 10

Reason behind choice of sequencing	• Increase complexity • Coordinate the timing of combined movements for dynamic input to enhance adaptability • Enhance coordination for load transfer • Challenge abdominal wall control with advanced progressions as tolerated

Session movement sequence

1. Standing Spine Stretch forward in well of Universal Reformer	Derivative of J. H. Pilates Spine Stretch (NPCE Study Guide 2021, p. 47)
Intent	• Interoception of flexors • Sequential articulation of torso • Scapulothoracic mobility • Proprioception for balance • Equal distribution of weight bearing • Increase complexity by adding continuous movement flow
Gait reasoning	• Balanced mobility in sagittal plane to help decrease shift and TPR of torso • Decrease excessive lateral rib shift • Improve COM and weight bearing

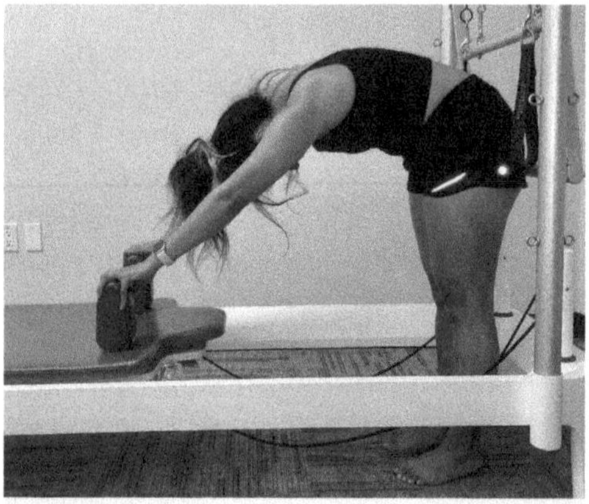

Figure 10.5

Set-up	• Springs: 1 light and 1 medium or 2 medium
Starting position	• Standing upright in well of Universal Reformer • Feet shoulder-width apart • UE reaching toward shoulder stops

Movement description	• Inhale, feel starting position
• Exhale, draw abdominal wall inward without going into flexion, tuck in the chin gently, segmentally flex the torso
• Maintain even weight through the feet front to back, side to side
• Touch the shoulder stops
• Do not shift weight posteriorly
• Inhale, protract shoulders holding the shoulder stops
• Exhale, slowly pull the shoulder stops toward the thighs, gently flexing torso and drawing abdominal wall posteriorly and superiorly
• Feel the response of torso activation
• Inhale, hold, retract shoulders
• Repeat protraction/retraction
• Reverse the sequence to move carriage toward footbar
• Exhale as articulating into extension
• Return to starting position
• Repeat 5 times
• Progression
  ▪ Add heel lift for increased challenge for decreased base of support
  ▪ Add rotation once control of abdominal wall has been established
  ▪ Place one hand on the shoulder stop, the other on the post on the same side, following same sequence
  ▪ 5 repetitions bilaterally

CUE
♦ To find a balanced starting position, shift weight on feet right to left, front to back, increasing awareness of weight distribution

Author note
Managing COM with variations in torso positions and weight shifting is a very useful way to integrate functional strategies of standing weight bearing and improve control. |

2. Standing LE activation in well of Universal Reformer

Intent	• Improve one-leg stance balance
• Extensor activation
Gait reasoning	• Improve control during stance phase in gait

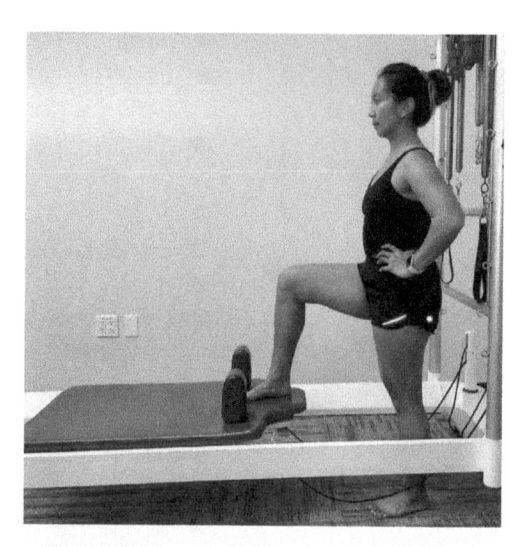

Figure 10.6

Set-up
- Light spring

Starting position
- Stand inside the well facing headrest, with feet apart slightly wider than hip joints and externally rotated 7–10 degrees
- Ground through the feet with optimal foot-ankle organization
- Reach out of the top of the head toward ceiling
- Place right foot on headrest, with less than 20 degrees knee flexion
- Standing LE extended
- Shift right stance position to left to feel balanced position

Movement description
- Inhale, sense torso uprightness
- Exhale, with heel pulling carriage toward standing leg to achieve 90 degrees knee flexion
- Inhale, return to starting position
- Monitor weight-bearing balance on standing leg
- Repeat 8–10 times
- Repeat on opposite side
- Progression
  - Add hemipelvis inferior/superior motion on standing leg at both starting position and 90 degree knee flexion
  - Add torso rotation with an inhale when knee held in flexed position
  - Hold 1–2 lb (0.5–1 kg) hand weights
  - Repeat 5 times bilaterally

CUE
- Use a dowel as feedback by holding it horizontally across pelvis during movement

3. Footwork on Universal Reformer, external rotation and abduction

Derivative of J. H. Pilates Footwork on Universal Reformer (NPCE Study Guide 2021, p. 52)

Intent
- Reverse the typical breath for activation of pelvic diaphragm
- Increase complexity of training
- Motor control of the hip joints

Gait reasoning
- Increase proprioception by stimulating foot-to-torso patterns
- Coordinate pelvic diaphragm with breath and LE movements

Author note
The pelvic diaphragm hypertonicity strategy of posterior pelvic rotation during a squat alters the pelvifemoral relationship. It decreases the ability of the femoral joint to move posteriorly and inferiorly at the bottom of the squat. It is vital to maintain the optimal pelvic position throughout the movement.

Set-up
- 3–4 medium springs
- Support torso with a wedge, prop, or pillow to bring the ISA into a normalized angle (see Author note under exercise 2, Supine Bent Knee Fall-Out, above)

Starting position
- Supine on carriage
- Heels on footbar
- Hip joints flexion, abduction, and external rotation
- Knee flexion

Movement description
- Inhale, press feet into bar, extend LE moving carriage away from footbar
- Exhale slowly, return carriage home by flexing, externally rotating, and abducting hip joints, knee flexion
- Focus on maintaining the optimal position without abdominal doming as carriage returns
- Repeat 8–10 times with a 5-second count encouraging flow
- Press carriage out 1–2 in. (2.5–5 cm) away from stoppers
- Pulse 5–10 times, moving closer to stoppers
- Focus on maintaining sustained activation of pelvic diaphragm while pulsing
- Returning carriage to starting position, add 5 rapid activations
- Reverse the breathing with entire series

Chapter 10

PELVIC DIAPHRAGM IMAGERY CUES

- Elevator endurance training: Imagine a relaxed pelvic diaphragm is the basement floor. Slowly imagine the elevator is moving up to the first floor—a light activation feeling. Hold, move the elevator slowly up to the next floor, hold, repeat to three floors, then slowly lower the elevator down floor by floor until fully relaxed. Notice the breath, be steady and calm. Practice increasing the number of floors to 10 floors. Practice holding for 3–5 seconds and build to 10 seconds to improve endurance. Relax in between repetitions for 5 seconds.
- Elevator speed training: Lift elevator as quickly as possible 10 times. Relax for 5 seconds. Repeat the speed practice 10 times, gradually building to 30 repetitions
- Imagine stopping the flow of urine, hold for 5 seconds, relax and repeat for 1 minute
- Draw a connecting line from the tailbone toward the navel without changing the pelvis position
- Begin practicing supine, then seated, followed by standing

Author note

Research shows variability of motor control during training helps change urinary incontinence, pelvic girdle pain, and LBP in individuals (Hodges *et al.* 2013). Training specificity to prevent stress urinary incontinence depends upon the adequacy of activities such as rapid activation (speed) and sustained activation (endurance).

Pelvic diaphragm exercises have a modulating effect on the autonomic nerves that supply the bladder from spinal cord segments S2–S4. It is believed this is likely the mechanism by which pelvic diaphragm conditioning improves symptoms of an overactive bladder (Purves *et al.* 2001).

4. Straps: feet in loops on Universal Reformer, flexion, abduction, external rotation

Intent
- Increase complexity of training by reversing the breath pattern
- Improve pelvifemoral relative movement
- Allow self-monitoring of IAP and control of anterior abdominal structures for increased awareness

Pilates and Pregnancy-Related Diastasis Rectus Abdominus: Effect on Gait

Gait reasoning	• Enhanced motor control during gait
Set-up	• Medium spring
Starting position	• Supine on carriage
	• Both feet in straps at mid-foot
	• Hip joint flexion, abduction, and external rotation
	• Knee flexion
	• Feet plantar flexed, with right and left phalanges touching
Movement description	• Exhale to sense starting position
	• Inhale, extend and adduct LE with control
	• Exhale, return to starting position slowly
	• On the return, slight anterior rotation of pelvis to counter a posterior rotation
	• Repeat 5 times
	• Reverse breathing, repeat 5 times
	• Progress by decreasing spring tension

CUES
- Maintain LE within the well of the Universal Reformer
- The positional mid-range is the optimal place to generate tension and promote a mechanical advantage
- Avoid anterior pelvic rotation at end of knee extension
- Avoid tendency to go into posterior pelvic tilt from 110–125 degrees hip flexion
- Teach client self-monitoring of abdominal wall

Author note
Teach the client to assess their myofascial integrity and the importance of having good integrity rather than focusing on the width of the gap. Ask questions such as: "How does it feel when you touch the space between your abdominal edges?" "Does it change when pre-activated before you move into a more challenging position?"

Teaching the client self-assessment of the abdominal wall and myofascial integrity before and after exercise is an effective way to encourage embodiment and to empower them through self-control over safety, recovery, and education.

5. Pelvic lift with rotation
Derivative of J. H. Pilates Pelvic Lift on Universal Reformer (NPCE Study Guide 2021, p. 60)

Intent
- Stimulate pelvic neuromyofascia through isometric pelvic diaphragm activation and hip joint extension, abduction, and adduction
- Resistance against gravity to assist the shortening phase of slow and fast pulse activations

Gait reasoning
- Increase the ability for stance leg through non-moving leg and swing leg with hip joint abduction/adduction movements
- Extensor activation for push-off

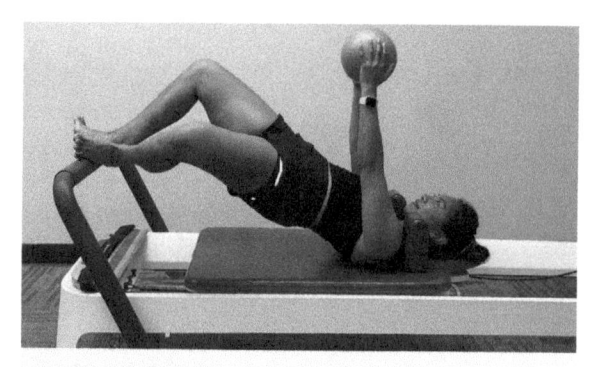

Figure 10.7

Set-up
- 2 medium springs

Starting position
- Supine on carriage with feet parallel on platform
- Hold ball in 90 degrees shoulder flexion

Movement description
- Inhale to prepare
- Exhale, bridging activating the pelvic diaphragm for 5 seconds
- Inhale, externally rotate/abduct right hip joint maintaining bridge position
- Exhale, adduct right hip to center of joint with quick activations of pelvic diaphragm for 5 seconds
- Inhale, pause
- Exhale, returning to starting position

CUES

- Start slowly with minimal number of repetitions
- Maintain pelvic position during the hip joint rotation and pelvic diaphragm activations
- Progress to placing feet on footbar
- Advance to unilateral bridge
- Replace the hip joint rotation with a unilateral bridge, ball at mid-femurs, adducting the ball while performing pelvic diaphragm pulses

6. Prone extension on Universal Reformer long box with overhead press

Intent
- Endurance for torso extension in relation to gravity
- Proprioception in sensing position on box, tactile feedback
- Activate whole body to sustain the position while challenging the UE

Gait reasoning
- Increase proprioception of torso
- Improve upright posture for effectiveness of propulsion in push-off

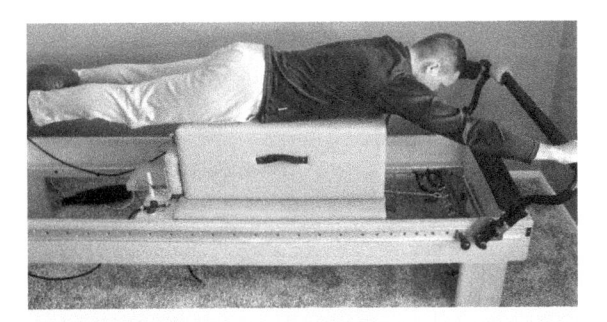

Figure 10.8

Set-up
- Long box set-up
- Springs: 1 light or 1 medium
- 8–10 in. (20–25 cm) ball between malleoli

Starting position
- Prone on long box facing footbar, mid-chest at edge of box, head aligned with torso
- Overball between the ankles
- Hold side of box
- Adding arms: move hands to footbar, gently press palms on footbar to activate UE to torso

Movement description
- Sequence
  - In prone position on box feel anterior torso, especially pelvis
  - Monitor hyperextension of TLJ promoting rib flare and sternal dumping and excessive tension of extensors
  - Exhale, gently lift anterior abdominal wall away from box while anchoring the anterior pelvis on the box
  - Inhale, lengthening through the crown of the head
  - Exhale, practice a 5-second sustained activation of pelvic diaphragm
  - Repeat 5 times
  - Repeat with 5 rapid articulations of pelvic diaphragm
- Add arms
  - Inhale, place hands on footbar
  - Elbows close to sides of torso
  - Exhale, press hands into footbar, extend elbows moving carriage away
  - Scapulae slide down the back, keeping torso unchanged on long box
  - Repeat 5 times
  - Inhale, abduct elbows with hands on footbar
  - Exhale, press hands into the footbar, extend the elbows moving carriage away
  - Repeat 5 times
- Progress to single arm with opposite arm behind back
  - Repeat 5 times
- With both hands on footbar add extension
  - Exhale, lift upper body into extension
  - Inhale, return to starting position
  - Repeat 5 times

CUES
- Keep anterior pelvis in contact with box with legs in parallel
- Activate legs by engaging the ball
- Maintain head in line with torso

Pilates and Pregnancy-Related Diastasis Rectus Abdominus: Effect on Gait

Author note
Be cautious of too much extension without anterior midline control.

7. Standing quadruped with hands on footbar of Universal Reformer	Derivative of J. H. Pilates Long Stretch Series: Elephant on Universal Reformer (NPCE Study Guide 2021, p. 55)
Intent	• Increase overall mobility and articulation • Enhance scapular glide on thorax • Standing loading of torso
Gait reasoning	• Contralateral patterning • Coordination of flexion with oppositional extension • Standing and UE weight bearing, loading the thoracodorsal fascia during femoral joint motions

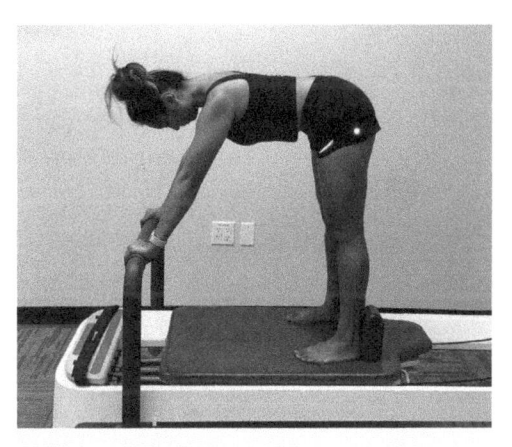

Figure 10.9

Set-up	• Springs: 1 light or 1 medium
Starting position	• Place hands on footbar, directly under shoulders with extended torso • Stand in the middle of carriage, feet under center of femoral joints • Progression: move heels back to shoulder stops (NPCE Study Guide 2021, p. 14)

Movement description
- Sequence
  - Inhale, send the heels back, initiating from the posterior pelvifemur
  - Exhale, using flexors, draw abdominal wall inward as carriage moves in while maintaining torso organization
  - Repeat 5–8 times
- Progression
  - Inhale, flex the right knee while pressing carriage back with extended left knee
  - Exhale, extend right knee, flex left as carriage moves in
  - Repeat 8–12 times alternating from side to side, keeping the movement fluid

CUES
- Sense the abdominal wall activate before moving the legs
- Keep head in line with the torso
- Maintain shoulder/upper body position during the exercise

Author note
Training with the abdominal wall in this specific relationship to gravity offers excellent feedback and proprioceptive awareness during movement.

8. Running in place on Trapeze Table

Intent
- Leg and ankle alignment awareness
- Gait patterning
- Improve coordination

Gait reasoning
- Reciprocal LE patterning with torso in mid-range

Set-up
- 1 or 2 springs, bottom-loaded
- Safety strap in place

Starting position
- Supine, with head at the open end, balls of the feet on push-through bar
- Femurs parallel
- Hip flexion in range to avoid posterior pelvic rotation, knees flexed

Movement description	• Inhale, extend both legs pressing bar up
• Exhale, left ankle dorsiflexion with extended knee as right knee flexes
• Inhale, extend right knee plantar flexing both ankles to press bar up
• Exhale, right ankle dorsiflexion with extended knee as left knee flexes
• Inhale, extend right knee plantar flexing both ankles to press bar up
• Repeat the sequence 8–10 times

CUES
- Maintain LE organization throughout each movement transition
- Improve LE control by monitoring optimal LE-ankle-forefoot organization
- Observe with knee flexion and transitions; if pelvis posteriorly rotates, cue to maintain pelvifemoral relationship without posterior rotation

Author note
Range of motion (ROM) beyond 90 degrees flexion may amplify an issue with LBP and the sacroiliac joint. It is important to maintain pelvifemoral articulation. Use a lighter load to be sure the movement is tolerated and organization is maintained before increasing the load.

9. Cat to quadruped on Trapeze Table	Derivative of J. H. Pilates Cat on Trapeze Table (NPCE Study Guide 2021, p. 63)
Intent	• Emphasis on scapular glide on thorax in variable positions
Gait reasoning	• Dynamic movement in all planes of motion
Set-up	• 1 or 2 short, medium springs, top-loaded on push-through bar
Starting position	• High kneeling with hands on push-through bar
• Knee placement is in relation to torso length, so when arms are straight the push-through bar will be lined up with the upright bars (will not pass them)
• Push-through bar at chest height with elbow flexion
• Place ankles under strap on table to add stability to resist creating activation of LE

Movement description
- Inhale, press the bar down extending elbows, keeping torso upright
- Exhale, articulate torso into flexion maintaining starting degree of knee flexion
- Inhale; as torso articulates into extension horizontal to the table push through the bar toward the upright bars
- Frame the ears with elbows, keeping head in line with torso
- Exhale, as torso articulates from flexion through extension to high kneeling starting position, initiate from pelvifemoral extension
- Inhale, pressing bar down slightly, extending upper thorax slightly, but only as far as the anterior torso structures can be maintained
- Exhale, return to starting position
- Repeat 5 times
- Stand on the outside at the tower end with the bar sprung from the high position
- Follow movement sequence
- Repeat 5 times

CUE
- Monitor activation of the abdominal wall and integrity of DRA throughout the phases of movement

Author note
Promote control to counteract compensatory strategies that could aggravate and/or increase the diastasis.

10. Cat to quadruped on Universal Reformer

Intent
- Torso control
- Activate flexors and extensors
- UE and torso activation

Gait reasoning
- Adapt to various forces
- Torso control
- Sagittal plane movement
- Arm swing

Set-up
- 1 or 2 medium springs
- 2 rotating discs placed on platform

Starting position
- Quadruped position
- Feet against shoulder stops, with metatarsals on carriage, metatarsal joints extended, heels touching shoulder stops
- Hands shoulder-width apart on rotating discs

Pilates and Pregnancy-Related Diastasis Rectus Abdominus: Effect on Gait

Movement description
- Inhale, press feet into shoulder stops extending LE 45 degrees, maintaining shoulders over hands while pushing carriage back
- Exhale, pull carriage in flexing hip joints, with abdominal wall drawn inward, maintaining shoulders over hands
- Repeat extension sequence 5 times
- Inhale, press carriage back
- Exhale; maintaining extension position press carriage further, allowing shoulder flexion
- Inhale, return shoulders over wrists
- Exhale, pull carriage flexing hip joints
- Repeat 5 times

CUE
- Maintain activation of abdominal wall throughout monitoring of the DRA

11. Seated rotation on Trapeze Table

Intent — Build variability using:
- Load
- Coordinated movement in different planes
- Position changes

Gait reasoning
- Adaptation to variable forces

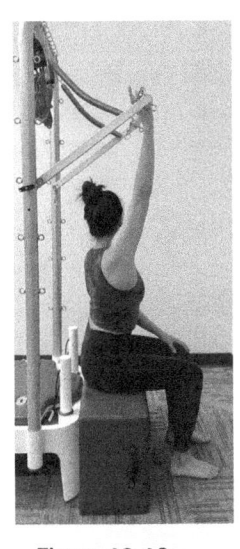

Figure 10.10

Chapter 10

Set-up	• Universal Reformer box placed on floor horizontal to table at push-through bar end
• Push-through bar on outside of table
• No spring or 1 short, light spring, top-loaded
• Air cushion disc
Starting position	• Seated on box with back to table
• Hold bar
Movement description	• Inhale, pressing bar superiorly initiating from upward scapula glide
• Exhale, pull bar inferiorly initiating from downward scapula glide
• Repeat 5–8 times
• Inhale, pressing bar superiorly initiating from upward scapula glide, rotating torso away from UE in contact with bar
• Exhale, pull bar inferiorly initiating from downward scapula glide, rotating torso toward UE in contact with bar
• Repeat 5–8 times
• Place air cushion disc on box and sit on it
• Repeat movement sequence adding hemipelvis superior/inferior motion at end of range of rotation movement
• Repeat 5 times
• Repeat movement sequence adding hemipelvis superior/inferior motion through rotation movement creating continuous movement patterning
• Repeat 5 times

CUES

- Focus on creating fluidity throughout the movement
- During hemipelvis superior/inferior motion, drive the movement from the ischial tuberosities

Author note

Smith, Coppieters, and Hodges (2007) found that women with severe incontinence had overactivation of the pelvic diaphragm and anterolateral abdominals with postural challenges, compared to continent women who showed the least amount of activation. Smith *et al.* concluded that better outcomes were produced by considering the functional interrelationship between coordinated activation patterns of the pelvic diaphragm and neuromyofascia rather than isolated engagement of the pelvic diaphragm (Woodley *et al.* 2020).

12. Push-Through Seated Front and Circle Saw on Trapeze Table

Derivative of J. H. Pilates Push-Through Seated Front on Universal Reformer (NPCE Study Guide 2021, p. 63) and mat exercise Saw (NPCE Study Guide 2021, p. 48)

Author note
It is a commonly held belief that those with DRA should avoid torso flexion to protect further separation; however, linea alba (LA) stiffness and inter-rectus distance are significant predictors of how much the LA distorts during a semi-curl-up task when women have DRA (Lee and Hodges 2016). More LA distortion is seen among those who generate less LA stiffness during the semi-curl-up. The significance of this with mild DRA is that a wider abdominal aponeurosis may not be functionally problematic if the LA is able to appropriately stiffen when a task demands load transfer across the midline of the body.

Editor note
The intention of the peripheral movement description in this exercise is cueing the hands and feet, initiating the lines of force proximally. The purpose is to direct the movement forces into the torso facilitating load transfer across the midline as required in functional gait patterning.

Intent
- Segmental torso articulation
- Improve coordination
- Load transfer across midline of torso

Gait reasoning
- Movement coupling through torso proprioception and weight-bearing awareness
- Combined flexion, lateral flexion, and rotation movements
- Variability
- Enhance global movement patterning

Set-up
- Short, light, or medium spring, top-loaded
- Bar should be at the highest setting

Starting position
- Sitting upright facing tower end with feet against the vertical frame poles
- Place hands on push-through bar overhead
- Flex knees to maintain upright torso and optimal pelvic position

Movement description
- With both hands on bar, inhale, and in one smooth movement pull bar down flexing elbows while keeping the torso tall and pushing bar toward vertical frame poles while extending the elbows
- Prepare with scapular protraction/retraction glides
- Inhale, pressing the bar forward, gliding scapulae into protraction
- Exhale, gliding scapulae into retraction
- Repeat 5 times
- Release right arm, wrap arm across anterior torso to opposite rib
- Inhale, right rotation of torso protracting left scapula as bar moves forward
- Exhale, retract left scapula, rotating through the center pulling bar in
- Continue to rotate left
- Repeat 5 times
- Repeat on the other side
- Return to starting position
- With both hands on bar, inhale, and in one smooth movement pull bar down flexing elbows while keeping the torso tall and push bar between vertical frame poles extending elbows
- Exhale, flex from the head tucking chin in toward chest, press the bar forward
- Articulate sequentially through torso flexion
- Inhale, anchor the sitz bones
- Exhale, articulate the torso from bottom to top, extending to upright, pulling bar inward
- Inhale, press bar overhead with extended elbows and shoulder flexion, lean forward increasing hip joint flexion
- Exhale, return to starting position
- Reverse breath pattern to experience a different connection with the breath
- Progress to half Circle Saw
- With the bar in up position with extended elbow and shoulder flexion, inhale, reach one hand across toward the opposite bar rotating the torso
- Exhale; in a sweeping movement reach the UE 90 degrees anterior to lateral abduction rotating the torso, then posterior toward vertical frame poles behind
- Inhale, reversing path of UE to push-through bar, return to starting position
- Repeat 3 times on each side

CUES
- Anchor the sitz bones before any movement
- Imagine the articulation sequentially from top down, bottom up
- Broaden the shoulder blades as you press the bar toward the ceiling

Author note
The protraction/retraction at the end of the ranges improves the gliding of the scapula on the thorax. The movement stimulates the shoulder girdle activations that are continuous into the torso.

13. Mermaid on Universal Reformer
Derivative of J. H. Pilates Mermaid on Universal Reformer (NPCE Study Guide 2021, p. 58)

Intent
- Improve rotation and lateral flexion
- Abdominal coordinated activation during rotation
- Mobility with balanced weight bearing in variable positions
- Lateral torso mobility through UE

Gait reasoning
- Improve torso movement limitations seen in assessment
- Breath coordination with movement
- Midline awareness: anterior to posterior, left to right, normalizing ISA

Set-up
- Medium spring

Starting position
- Sit sideways on carriage with knees bent
- Left leg positioned with shin flush against shoulder stops
- Right heel in contact with left knee creating a triangle position
- Place right hand on footbar in front of shoulder approximately 30 degrees from frontal plane

Movement description
- Inhale, press carriage away from footbar as left UE reaches overhead and laterally flex to right
- Exhale, return to starting position, reestablish sitz bones evenly weighted on carriage
- Inhale, reverse lateral flexion to left by reaching right UE toward the ceiling as right arm rests on the shoulder stop
- Repeat 3 times
- Repeat, pressing carriage out and laterally flex, hold
- Rotate torso toward floor bringing left hand to footbar, unweighting right hand to reposition toward far side of footbar

- Inhale, breathe into lateral thorax deepening flexion
- Exhale, derotate, reposition support arm in center of footbar maintaining lateral flexion
- Inhale, return to starting position
- Repeat, end range of flexion in the well, exhale, pause
- Inhale, pressing through hand, lifting upper torso into extension, broadening shoulders, opening across the chest
- Exhale, return to deep flexion facing the well, derotate, follow the return sequence to starting position
- Progress to end-range hip joint flexion position, exhale, reaching arm under side of torso in rotation while pressing away
- Inhale, returning from rotation facing the well
- Exhale, derotate out of position, bring carriage in returning to starting position

CUES
- Try gentle anterior-posterior motion of the pelvis to increase mobility and congruency with surface of carriage
- Reach in opposition of support arm and opposite LE as pressing carriage out

Author note
Rotation and counter-rotation exercises improve gait patterning through client awareness of rotational movements, oppositional rotational movements, and how the UE drives the thoracic rotation.

The journey to Session 11

Session 4/12
Client self-report

- Soreness along thorax, left more than right
- Paying more attention to posture
- Home program is hard—there is so much to think about
- Fatigue scale 3
- Pain scale 4

Key changes observed

- Ability to correct proper abdominal activation with verbal cues in standing
- Improvement in sternal positioning in standing posture with proper abdominal wall activation
- Difficulty with proprioception in supine
- Increased challenge with one-leg stance activity; however, balance on stance leg improved
- One-leg stance balance appears steadier on right

Reasoning behind choice of movements

- Balancing extensibility, left and right

- Reorient weight bearing
- Prone on the Trapeze Table to enhance proprioception of anterior torso and provide support to anterior abdominal wall
- Coordinate proper breath patterns during dynamic activities for better IAP management for decreasing stress urinary incontinence

Session movement sequence
1. Add Overball to quadruped threading for ease of rotation

2. Universal Reformer

- Standing Spine Stretch in well
- Standing LE activation in well

3. Trapeze Table

- Prone extension

4. Universal Reformer

- Footwork
    - Abduction and external rotation, knee flexion
- Cat
- Eve's Lunge (see Chapter 5 in Volume 1, Gentry)

Session 5/12
Client self-report

- "My stomach is much flatter feeling for 2–3 days after session but still has big bulge"
- "I may be experiencing less accidents with laughing/coughing"
- "Low back tightness feels like a sheet"
- Fatigue scale 3
- Pain scale 2

Key changes observed

- Beginning to self-correct without cues about 25 percent of the time
- Appears less tense in effort in standing and during gait
- Imbalanced abdominal wall strategy when supine

Reasoning behind choice of movements

- Enhance integration of torso
- Coordinate breath cycle with pelvifemoral joint movements
- Improve adaptation of forces and balance

Session movement sequence
1. Universal Reformer

- Standing Spine Stretch in well
- Standing LE activation in well
- Footwork
    - Abduction and external rotation, knee flexion
    - Reverse breathing
- Straps: feet in loops
    - External rotation/flexion with knee flexion
- Prone extension on long box
- Cat
- Elephant Flat Back

Editor note
In Flat Back the TLJ is supported by the counterbalance of the anterior rotation of the lower thoracic ring and the posterior rotation of the pelvic rim to bring the TLJ posterior. The torso is supported as a whole unit throughout the exercise. Spine articulation is minimized. The primary articulation is at the pelvifemoral joints.

2. Trapeze Table

- Running in place

3. Universal Reformer

- Eve's Lunge

Session 6/12
Client self-report

- Soreness of abdomen is better
- Continued soreness in arms
- Stomach feels less bulgy
- Fatigue scale 2
- Pain scale 2

Key changes observed

- Improved overall awareness of torso to LE relationship
- Self-correcting 50 percent of time without verbal cues
- Decreased left TPR in pelvis
- Weight bearing more balanced in standing and sitting
- Improve abdominal wall coactivation

Reasoning behind choice of movements

- Establish improved alignment, breath, and coordination
- Increase activities in lateral flexion to assist improved abdominal wall activation
- Ability to manage rotation with good control of DRA without abdominal doming
- Beginning to build in variability using:
    - Load
    - Coordinated movement in different planes and during positional changes
    - Speed

Session movement sequence
1. LE abduction/adduction pelvic lift

2. Universal Reformer

- Standing Spine Stretch in well
- Standing LE activation in well
- Footwork
    - Abduction and external rotation, knee flexion
- Straps: feet in loops
    - External rotation/flexion with knee flexion
- Prone extension on long box
- Cat: introduced discs
- Elephant Flat Back

3. Trapeze Table

- Running in place
- Push-Through Seated Front
    - Flat Back and rotation

4. Universal Reformer

- Eve's Lunge: added torso lateral flexion
- Mermaid

5. Additional movements

- Added LE abduction with quadruped UE activation for home program
- Push-Through Seated Front

Session 7/12
Client self-report

- "I do the Cat/Elephant stretch a few times every day. It helps open everything up and seems to make it easier to sit"
- Getting through home program faster, doing some stretches twice a day
- Bulge still there but seems more isolated above belly button
- Fatigue scale 2
- Pain scale 1

Key changes observed

- Better awareness of midline
- Fewer cues necessary for midline
- Increased mobility in forward-bend movements
- Decreased rib shift and lessening of excessive ISA
- Unable to wiggle ribs during abdominal connect cue—an indication of excessive stiffness in torso
- Difficulty controlling abdominal doming at end of range leg extension

Reasoning behind choice of movements

- Increase activities promoting symmetry, alignment, breath, and coordination for improved awareness of gait
- Enhance awareness through varying sensory input and feedback
- Added self-check by wiggling ribs for awareness of unconscious holding
- Limited angle of hip joint flexion in abduction/external rotation on Universal Reformer to 70 degrees to maintain pelvifemoral movement without posterior rotation

Session movement sequence
1. Universal Reformer

- Standing Spine Stretch in well
- Standing LE activation in well
- Footwork
  - Abduction and external rotation, knee flexion
  - Reverse breathing
- Straps: feet in loops
  - External rotation/flexion with knee flexion
- Pelvic lift with rotation
- Prone extension on long box with overhead press
- Cat
- Elephant Flat Back

2. Trapeze Table

- Running in place
- Push-Through Seated Front, torso axial elongation
- Cat

3. Universal Reformer

- Eve's Lunge with lateral flexion
- Mermaid

4. Additional movement

- Add hemipelvis superior/inferior motion at end of range of rotation in half kneeling in both directions
- Adduction activations to challenge lateral movements
- Increase challenge

- Cat on Universal Reformer

Session 8/12
Client self-report

- Feeling sore, but a good sore after sessions
- LBP is practically gone
- Feeling more flexible, less stiffness in back overall
- Fatigue scale 2
- Pain scale 1

Key changes observed

- Control of abdominal doming with increasingly complex movement
- Increased awareness/ability to self-correct in standing and supine
- Fewer cues necessary for midline
- Able to maintain midline in one-leg stance
- Improved pelvifemoral ROM

Chapter 10

Reasoning behind choice of movements

- Coordinate transfer of loads across torso to UE and LE
- Addition of increased challenge in variable positions relative to gravity
- Establish optimal patterns for functional movements
- Continue to increase awareness by introducing subtle shifts in movements creating challenge with familiar movements

Session movement sequence
1. Add seated Mermaid

2. Add opposite lateral flexion to kneeling UE activation

3. Universal Reformer

- Standing Spine Stretch in well
- Standing LE activation in well
- Footwork
  - Abduction and external rotation, knee flexion
  - Reverse breathing
- Straps: feet in loops
  - External rotation/flexion with knee flexion
- Pelvic lift with rotation
- Prone extension with overhead press
- Cat
- Elephant Flat Back

4. Trapeze Table

- Running in place
- Push-Through Seated Front, flexion/extension and lateral flexion
- Cat

5. Universal Reformer

- Eve's Lunge with lateral flexion
- Mermaid

6. Additional movements

- Universal Reformer
  - Reciprocal patterning in Walking Elephant

Session 9/12
Client self-report

- Almost zero accidents—when it happens it's minor
- Very little soreness now after sessions
- Bulge still there but much less "pully" and tense
- Feeling more energy and sleeping better
- Fatigue scale 0
- Pain scale 0

Key changes observed

- Able to maintain position in one-leg stance with increased load
- Managing lateral flexion with fair/good control of DRA
- Unable to lean posteriorly during thigh stretch more than 10 degrees without abdominal doming
- Managing extension/torso shift off midline with poor/fair control
- DRA distance measured manually and via US is stable but not less than 1.18 in. (3 cm) (goal for potential to avoid surgical repair)

Reasoning behind choice of movements

- Increase complexity by coordinating the timing of combined movements
- Enhance optimal movement strategies available of the correct structures at the correct time
- Coordination for dynamic load transfer through the torso
- Chose to challenge abdominal wall control with addition of thigh stretch at the end of Cat sequence to challenge motor control

Session movement sequence

1. Add hemipelvis superior motion/inferior motion at end of range rotation in half kneeling in both directions

2. Universal Reformer

- Standing Spine Stretch forward in well
- Standing LE activation in well
- Footwork
  - Abduction and external rotation, knee flexion
  - Reverse breathing
- Straps: feet in loops
  - External rotation/flexion with knee flexion
- Pelvic lift with rotation
- Prone extension on long box with overhead press
- Cat plus rotating disc arch and curl
- Elephant Flat Back and Walking Elephant

3. Trapeze Table

- Running in place
- Push-Through Seated Front
  - Flexion/extension, rotation, lateral flexion
- Seated scapular mobilization and rotation
- Cat quadruped with thigh stretch

4. Universal Reformer

- Eve's Lunge with lateral flexion
- Mermaid

5. Additional movements

- Shifting off midline into extension
- Scapular mobility work with torso control

Session 10/12
Client self-report

- LBP completely gone
- Much less stiff even before home program/stretches
- Fatigue scale 1–2 depending on activity level
- Pain scale 0
- Consultation with surgeon scheduled for next month

Key changes observed

- Excellent control of torso and midline of torso in lateral flexion and rotation
- Unable to extend past midline through torso without compensations

Reasoning behind choice of movements

- Continue with current program in preparation for potential of surgical intervention
- Continue the practice for developing confidence
- Self-assessments and corrections for daily home program

Session movement sequence

1. Reviewed squat, added band around thorax

2. Quadruped threading review for proper movement and self-awareness

3. Universal Reformer

- Standing Spine Stretch in well
- Standing LE activation in well
- Footwork
  - Abduction and external rotation, knee flexion
  - Reverse breathing
- Straps: feet in loops
  - External rotation/flexion with knee flexion
- Pelvic lift with rotation
- Prone extension on long box with overhead press
- Elephant Flat Back and Walking Elephant

4. Trapeze Table

- Running in place

Chapter 10

- Cat quadruped on table
- Seated scapula mobilization/rotation off tower end
- Push-Through Seated Front
  - Flexion/extension, rotation, lateral flexion, thigh stretch
- Thigh stretch weight shift at end of Cat sequence

5. Universal Reformer

- Eve's Lunge with lateral flexion
- Mermaid

References

Beamish, N., Green, N., Nieuwold, E., and McLean, L. (2019) "Differences in linea alba stiffness and linea alba distortion between women with and without diastasis recti abdominis: The impact of measurement site and task." *JOSPT, 49,* 9, 656–665.

Blotta, R. M., Costa, S. D. S., Trindade, E. N., Meurer, L., and Maciel-Trindade, M. R. (2018) "Collagen I and III in women with diastasis recti." *Clinics (Sao Paulo), 73.* DOI: 10.6061/clinics/2018/e319.

Boissonnault, J. S. and Blaschak, M. J. (1988) "Incidence of diastasis recti abdominis during the childbearing year." *Physical Therapy, 68,* 1082–1086.

Candido, G., Lo, T., and Janssen, P. A. (2005) "Risk factors for diastasis of the recti abdominis." *Journal of the Association of Chartered Physiotherapists in Women's Health, 97,* 49–54.

Fernandes da Mota, P. G., Pascoal, A. G., Carita, A. I., and Bø, K. (2015) "Prevalence and risk factors of diastasis recti abdominis from late pregnancy to 6 months postpartum, and relationship with lumbo-pelvic pain." *Manual Therapy, 20,* 1, 200–205.

Hagins, M., Pietrek, M., Sheikhzadeh, A., and Nordin, M. (2006) "The effects of breath control on maximum force and IAP during a maximum isometric lifting task." *Clinical Biomechanics (Bristol, Avon), 21,* 8, 775–780.

Hall, H. and Sanjaghsaz, H. (2023) Diastasis Recti Rehabilitation. [Updated 2023, Aug 8]. In: StatPearls [Internet]. Treasure Island, FL: StatPearls Publishing; 2023 Jan-. https://ncbi.nlm.nih.gov/books/NBK573063. [Accessed September 10, 2023].

Hodges, P. W., Van Dillen, L., McGill, S., Brumagne, S., Hides, J., and Moseley, L. (2013) "Integrated clinical approach to motor control interventions in low back and pelvic pain." In: P. W. Hodges, J. Cholewicki, and H. Van Dieen (Eds.) *Spinal Control: The Rehabilitation of Back Pain—State of the Art and Science.* Edinburgh: Churchill Livingstone Elsevier, p. 265.

Jessen, M. L., Öberg, S., and Rosenberg, J. (2019) "Treatment options for abdominal rectus diastasis." *Frontiers in Surgery, 6,* 65. DOI: 10.3389/fsurg.2019.00065.

Lee, D. (2022) *Diastasis Rectus Abdominus: A Clinical Guide for Those Who Are Split Down the Middle.* Canada: Learn with Diane Lee.

Lee, D. and Hodges, P. W. (2016) "Behavior of the linea alba during a curl-up task in diastasis rectus abdominis: An observational study." *JOSPT, 46,* 7, 580–589. DOI: 10.2519/jospt.2016.6536.

Mens, J. M., Vleeming, A., Snijders, C. J., Koes, B. W., and Stam, H. J. (2001) "Reliability and validity of the active straight leg raise test in posterior pelvic pain since pregnancy." *Spine (Phila Pa 1976), 26,* 10, 1167–1171.

Michalska, A., Rokita, W., Wolder, D., Pogorzelska, J., and Kaczmarczyk, K. (2018) "Diastasis recti abdominis – a review of treatment methods." *Ginekologia Polska, 89,* 2, 97–101.

Milanesi, R. and Caregnato, R. C. (2016) "Intra-abdominal pressure: An integrative review." *Einstein (Sao Paulo, Brazil), 14,* 3, 423–430.

Mota, P., Pascoal, A. G., and Bo, K. (2015) "Diastasis recti abdominis in pregnancy and postpartum period: Risk factors, functional implications and resolution." *Current Women's Health Reviews, 11,* 1, 59–67.

Nienhuijs, S. W., Berkvens, E. H. M., de Vries Reilingh, T. S., Mommers, E. H. H., Bouvy, N. D., and Wegdam, J. (2021) "The male rectus diastasis: A different concept?" *Hernia, 25,* 4, 951–956.

NPCE Study Guide (National Pilates Certification Exam Study Guide) (2021) Miami, FL: National Pilates Certification Program, Inc.

Purves, D., Augustine, G. J., Fitzpatrick, D. *et al.* (Eds.) (2001) *Neuroscience.* 2nd Ed. Sunderland, MA: Sinauer Associates. Autonomic Regulation of the Bladder. https://ncbi.nlm.nih.gov/books/NBK10886. [Accessed September 10, 2023].

Smith, M. D., Coppieters, M. W., and Hodges, P. W. (2007) "Postural response of the pelvic floor and abdominal muscles in women with and without incontinence." *Neurourology Urodynamics, 26,* 3, 377–385.

Woodley, S. J., Lawrenson, P., Boyle, R., Cody, J. D., Mørkved, S., Kernohan, A., and Hay-Smith, E. (2020) "Pelvic floor muscle training for preventing and treating urinary and faecal incontinence in antenatal and postnatal women." *Cochrane Database of Systematic Reviews, 5,* 5. DOI: 10.1002/14651858.CD007471.pub4.

Appendix

Diastasis Rectus Abdominus

Special tests

ABLR (active bent leg raise)
This test is a modification of the ASLR where the leg is lifted 2 in. (5 cm) off the bed from a supine hook-lying position (Lee 2022).

ASLR (active straight leg raise)
This is a validated clinical loading test which is used to assess pain provocation and the ability to load the pelvis through the limb and transfer load between the torso and lower extremity. It is performed in lying, and the client is instructed to lift the leg 8 in. (20 cm) off the bed (Mens *et al.* 2001). A positive response is a complete inability to lift the leg off the bed; however, this response can vary from a slight difference in heaviness to complete inability.

Auto CU (automatic curl-up)
Without any instruction about abdominal muscle contraction, the client lifts the head and neck until the tops of the scapulae have just cleared the bed (arms by sides) (Lee and Hodges 2016).

IRD (inter-rectus distance)
When using ultrasound, the measurements are in centimeters or inches based on the tool. If using the finger method, the number of fingers which fit within the separation is used.

Pelvic diaphragm muscle layering cues (during palpation)
Verbal cues were used during the assessment to elicit symmetrical coactivation of the TrA with the pelvic diaphragm.

TrA CU (curl-up with pre-activation of TrA)
The curl-up task described in Auto CU is repeated but with the instruction to activate the TrA gently prior to the curl-up (arms by sides).

Appendix

Assessment findings for Chapter 15: DRA special tests

Pre-assessment

- ◆ ASLR

- Right: 2/5, with approximation correction 4/5
- Left: 3/5, with approximation correction 4/5

- ◆ Auto CU

- Doming
- ISA—widening
- IRD
  - Fingers—4
  - US—2.31 in. (5.89 cm)

- ◆ TrA CU

- Doming
- ISA—widening
- IRD
  - Fingers—3
  - US—2.05 in. (5.23 cm)
- + Recti displacement manually—yes, above umbilicus

Post-assessment

- ◆ ASLR

- Right: 3/5, with approximation correction 4+/5
- Left: 4/5, with approximation correction 4+/5

- ◆ Auto CU

- Doming
- ISA—widening
- IRD
  - Fingers—3
  - US—1.89 in. (4.82 cm)

- ◆ TrA CU

- Doming
- ISA—widening
- IRD
  - Fingers—3
  - US—1.69 in. (4.31 cm)
- + Recti displacement manually—yes, above umbilicus

Chapter 11

Pilates and Bone Health: Effect on Gait

Rebekah Rotstein

Osteoporosis is a condition of excessive bone loss and changes in architectural structure of the bone which make it susceptible to fracture. Worldwide, 1 in 3 women and 1 in 5 men over the age of 50 will break a bone from osteoporosis (International Osteoporosis Foundation 2023). The loss of bone mass is asymptomatic and often goes undetected, but signs can include loss of height and hyperkyphosis. As of 2021 the gold standard for measurement of bone mineral density is with a DEXA (dual energy X-ray absorptiometry), a scan using low radiation. The proximal femur, spine (vertebra), and wrist (distal radius) are the most commonly fractured bones and therefore the sites of measurement in a DEXA exam.

Bone loss is natural, but excessive bone loss can lead to fragility fractures, generally defined as a fracture occurring from standing height or less. Excessive bone loss can occur as a result of changes in sex hormones, and from certain medications and specific medical conditions. Lack of exercise and poor diet, especially in youth and adolescence, can contribute to lower bone mass later in life. Osteopenia refers to bone loss that is not yet at the degree of osteoporosis but where the bones are still vulnerable to fracture.

Nutrition and exercise are promoted for bone health for their chemical and mechanical effects on bone metabolism. Exercise guidelines advise weight-bearing movement with impact and resistance training, along with balance training for fall prevention (Royal Osteoporosis Society 2019).

Thoracic flexion at end range and when loaded is contraindicated for those with osteoporosis (Giangregorio *et al.* 2015). Such positioning imposes an amount of force on the vertebra that it might not withstand and that could make it fracture. Side bending and rotation should not be combined with flexion either in this population, and seated end range rotation should be avoided.

Back extension and pelvifemoral strength should be encouraged, along with whole-body integration for improved motor control. Body-wide proprioception and coordination, in addition to standing balance, should also be practiced. Along with upright weight bearing, quadruped work should be encouraged to load the wrists. This facilitates continuous activation from the palm to the torso. Pilates offers an excellent environment in which to work on all these skills and actions. Additionally, heart rate variability with recovery through cardiovascular training and multi-component exercise programs including strength, balance, and functional training are advocated as well (Giangregorio *et al.* 2015).

Bone strength typically refers to bone density, but it is not the only aspect of bone health. A number of factors contribute to the integrity of bone structure and its ability to withstand fracture, including the size of the bone, its architecture, and metabolic turnover. Focusing just on bone density overlooks important movement skill sets (coordination, balance, mobility), which does a disservice to this population physically and emotionally.

Chapter 11

Psychological effects of osteoporosis include depression, fear, and anxiety. An important aspect of an exercise intervention for this population is to restore confidence in the patient's or client's perceived ability to move and in their self-image, both of which may be tarnished during the medical diagnosis when informed of their skeletal fragility.

The program of exercises used in this case report considered the aforementioned protocols while taking into account the needs and history of the individual client. She did not represent the stereotypical client with osteoporosis in that she was not hyperkyphotic and was not lacking extensor strength, two common characteristics of this population.

Unlike other conditions and pathologies, osteoporosis does not affect one's gait, which was the focus of this case report. In most cases with an underlying physiological effect of fear or anxiety, gait hesitancy may be expressed. In addition, the client's knee replacement, fall history, and scoliosis were relevant to the assessments and offered another lens through which to view the outcomes.

Author note

Bone requires external load forces to build and maintain its mass and structure. These forces can come from gravity, weights, bands, and springs. A bone's ability to adapt and strengthen from this is also dependent on a host of factors including age, absorption, and metabolic processes. When it comes to exercise, research has shown a correlation between back extensor strength and reduced vertebral fractures and falls (Kasukawa *et al.* 2010; Sinaki *et al.* 2002). Additionally, a movement program including Pilates mat exercises without thoracic spinal flexion has been shown to improve back extensor strength, using gravity and light weights (Kistler-Fischbacher *et al.* 2021).

Client description:	69-year-old biological female, identifies as female; real estate agent
Dates of case report:	Session 1: March 5, 2020; Session 12: May 8, 2020. Sessions 1–7 in person; Sessions 8–12 virtual due to pandemic interruption. Final session with assessment delayed 4 weeks
Note:	COVID-19 lockdown occurred halfway through this case report. The second half of the sessions utilized small props from home rather than Pilates studio equipment

Studio apparatus and props
Pilates equipment

- Universal Reformer
- Ladder Barrel
- Wunda Chair

Props used with equipment

- 1 soft foam roller, 36 in. long x 6 in. in diameter (90 cm x 15 cm)
- 5 ft (1.5 m) dowels
- 26 in. (65 cm) ball
- Mat
- Non-skid rubberized pad, 7.5 in. x 14 in. x 1/2 in. (19 cm x 36 cm x 1.3 cm)

Home program props

- 1 soft foam roller, 36 in. long x 6 in. in diameter (90 cm x 15 cm)
- Medium resistance band
- Mat

Methods and materials

Session 1/12
1. Health history interview

- Menopause at age 51 (perimenopause at age 47)
- Never before participated in a Pilates program
- Osteoporosis in spine, osteopenia in proximal femur
- Family history of osteoporosis, no personal history of medical/medication risk factors (secondary osteoporosis)
- Never taken osteoporosis medications
- Fractured left olecranon when pre-menopausal, slipping on ice
- Lost 3–4 in. (7.5–10 cm) in height but no visible hyperkyphosis
- Osteoarthritis in knees and had total right knee replacement in 2017
- Torn right meniscus in 2008, surgically repaired in 2009
- Later fell twice hurting right knee—first in 2017 just prior to arthroplasty, then again in 2018 in the same way, damaging ligaments but not prosthesis
- Occasional low back pain around left sacroiliac joint discomfort
- C4 and C5 (neck) "feel electric when pressed on" (car accident in early 30s with whiplash)

2. Symptoms

- Loss of height: 3–4 in. (7.5–10 cm), but osteoporosis asymptomatic
- Has pain around right patella, especially going up or down stairs, and lacks full knee extension
- Fearful of falling again

3. Movement aids

- None

Final result of case report

The client felt more confident in walking, less fearful of falling, and better in her mood and outlook. She no longer felt knee pain in daily activities and could climb stairs with ease. Weight transference was more evenly distributed and scoliotic patterns less exaggerated.

Chapter 11

Session 2/12: Initial assessment

1. General observations of gait

- Stance time, longer on right than left
- Right thoracic rotation and left pelvic rotation
- Left arm swing longer than right arm
- Heavy right heel strike, less heavy on left
- Limited right hip joint extension

2. Standing tests

- Full torso rotation

- Observations of inefficient side: both
  - Right side rotation follows scoliotic curve
  - Left rotation
    - Limited right thoracic translation
    - Scoliotic curve straightens
    - Elevates right shoulder
    - Limited cervical rotation
    - Limited pelvic rotation
  - Minimal bilateral pelvis on femur
  - Both directions—neither foot adapts

- Hemipelvis inferior motion

- Observations of inefficient side: left
  - Limited on left side
  - Right pelvic rotation
  - Scoliosis pattern amplified

- Hemipelvis superior motion

- Observations of inefficient side: right

Session 12/12: Post-assessment

1. General observations of gait

- Even stride lengths
- Improved thorax-pelvis orientation
- Oppositional arm swing even slightly, left more than right
- Softer heel strike
- Improved and bilateral hip joint extension and push-off

2. Standing tests

- Full torso rotation

- Observations of inefficient side: left
  - Right scoliotic curve less pronounced
  - Left rotation
    - Improved right thoracic translation but limited
    - Scoliotic curve straightens
    - Elevates right shoulder
    - Improved cervical rotation and less hesitancy
  - Improved bilateral pelvis on femur rotation
  - Feet and ankle adaptation improved but limited

- Hip drop

- Observations of inefficient side: left
  - Limited drop still on left side but more motion
  - Right pelvic rotation
  - Scoliosis pattern amplified

- Hemipelvis superior motion

- Right rotation of pelvis and thoraco-lumbar junction (TLJ)
- Right lateral flexion in thorax, but not in lumbar region
- Elevates right shoulder

◆ Lateral pelvic shift

● Observations of inefficient side: left
  - Increases existing thoracic right lateral flexion
  - No right hemipelvis inferior motion
  - Limited femoral glide on both sides
  - Left foot no supination
  - Right foot pronates

3. Seated tests

◆ Hip joint and knee flexion

● Observations of inefficient side: left
  - Pelvic left rotation
  - Leans to right
  - End range discomfort

Author note
Included dorsiflexion and knee flexion test. Left was inefficient. During ankle dorsiflexion left foot pronated. During ankle plantar flexion left ankle inverted. Included hip abduction with external rotation. Both were inefficient bilaterally. Left side compensated with pelvic rotation. Right hip joint had less range of motion (ROM).

4. Sit and stand

◆ Lateral view

● Extends back, retracts scapulae
● Reaches upper extremity (UE) to counterbalance and assist rising

---

● Observations of inefficient side: right
  - Right rotation of pelvis and TLJ
  - Left lateral flexion in thoracic region but increased in lumbar region
  - No longer elevates shoulder

◆ Lateral pelvic shift

● Observations of inefficient side: left
  - Stands with weight more evenly distributed
  - Increases existing thoracic right lateral flexion
  - No right hemiplevis inferior motion
  - Femoral glide improved but limited
  - Left foot no supination
  - Right foot pronates

3. Seated tests

◆ Hip joint and knee flexion

● Observations of inefficient side: left
  - Almost no rotation
  - Almost no leaning
  - No more discomfort

Author note
Included dorsiflexion and knee flexion test. Left was inefficient. During ankle dorsiflexion no pronation. During ankle plantar flexion left ankle inverted. Included hip abduction with external rotation. Both were inefficient bilaterally. Pelvic rotation in the direction of moving leg. Improved right ROM and no mention of pain.

4. Sit and stand

◆ Front view

● Cautious—reaches left hand to help sit back down to assist right knee

- Cautious—reaches left hand to help sit back down to assist right knee

◆ Posterior and anterior views

- Retracts scapulae to assist rising
- Knees adduct when lowering and looks down for reassurance
- Weight bears on left leg

5. Standing balance

◆ Two-leg stance, eyes open

- 60 seconds

◆ One leg stance, eyes open

- Left leg: 29 seconds
- Right leg: 33 seconds

◆ One-leg stance, eyes closed

- Left leg: 4 seconds
- Right leg: 5 seconds

◆ Two-leg stance, cervical rotation

- Left leg preferred
- Shifts ribs to left when looking right

Author note

The addition of the balance assessments below is referencing commonly used screening assessments performed in osteoporosis management. The tandem stance provides additional balance challenge through a narrow base of support, and the foam pad creates an unstable surface to test the somatosensory aspect of balance. The screening assessments referred to are: Fullerton Advanced Balance

- Good form, no longer extends back or retracts scapulae
- Rises without UE compensation
- Moves with confidence and ease, unassisted and at faster speed

◆ Posterior and anterior views

- No longer retracts scapulae
- Knees still adduct but minimal
- Equal weight distribution between legs

5. Standing balance

◆ Two-leg stance, eyes open

- 60 seconds

◆ One-leg stance, eyes open

- Left leg: 44 seconds
- Right leg: 51 seconds

◆ One-leg stance, eyes closed

- Left leg: 4 seconds
- Right leg: 7 seconds

◆ Two-leg stance, cervical rotation

- Left leg preferred
- Less rib shift when looking right

◆ One-leg stance, on foam pad, eyes open

- Left leg: 12 seconds
- Right leg: 12 seconds

◆ Two-leg stance, on foam pad, eyes closed

- 60 seconds

◆ Tandem stance, eyes closed

Scale (Fullerton Center for Successful Aging 2008; Physiopedia 2024a); Balance Error Scoring System (Physiopedia 2024b; Sports Medicine Research Laboratory 2024); The 4-Stage Balance Test (bpacnz 2024; CDC 2017; Physiopedia 2024c).

◆ One leg stance, on foam pad, eyes open

- Left leg: 2 seconds
- Right leg: 8 seconds

◆ Two-leg stance, on foam pad, eyes closed

- 6 seconds

◆ Tandem stance, eyes closed

- Left leg front: 9 seconds
- Right leg front: 5 seconds

- Left leg front: 8 seconds
  - With cues: 17 seconds
- Right leg front: 8 seconds
  - With cues: 9 seconds

Chapter 11

Session 3/12: Home program

Editor note
In order to encourage bone health one needs to be in full weight bearing and loaded. This sequence is carefully designed to safely prepare the client's organization in non-weight bearing and partial weight bearing before full weight bearing with load.

Fatigue scale	5
Pain scale	6
Client self-report	• Excited, curious
Key changes observed by author at end of Session 3/12	• More ease in movements such as squatting, lunges, and reaches • Increased thoracic rotation • Motivated for daily practice • Improved motor control and coordination
Reason behind choice of sequencing	• Address right knee pain affecting client's gait rhythm • Improve articulation of thorax to enhance excursion of ribs • Increase medial-lateral glide of pelvifemoral joint • Closed kinematic chain activation for improved standing balance • Extension to improve bone health • Weight bearing and bone loading

Session movement sequence

1. Breathing with resistance band (See Chapter 5 in Volume 1, Gentry, Bellows breathing)

Intent	• Facilitate breathing to enhance thoracic articulation, circulation, and diaphragm excursion for ease in oppositional rotation of thorax and pelvis • Use band to enhance excursion of lower thorax and provide proprioceptive feedback
Gait reasoning	• Improve motor control of thoracic and oppositional pelvic rotation patterning • Due to scoliosis, lessen potential progression of increasing asymmetrical gait pattern • Reduce stress in the body and mind

Pilates and Bone Health: Effect on Gait

Editor note
Efficient gait includes thoracic and oppositional pelvic rotation. Breathing practices facilitate rib excursion in all dimensions. Breathing allows for connective tissue gliding and increases the ability of the tissues to respond and support thoracic lateral flexion with coupled rotation. The coupled movement is necessary in torso oppositional rotation in gait.

Starting position
- Sit comfortably on floor or chair
- Wrap band at T5–T6
- Cross band anteriorly
- Elbows resting downward

Movement description
- Slowly inhale
- Feel the breath widen the band
- Slowly exhale
- Continue for 1 minute

2. Rolling on soft roller: lateral and anterior aspect of thigh

Intent
- Facilitate glide of connective tissue at anterior aspect of thigh

Gait reasoning
- Improve glide of anterior connective tissues for improved extension in push-off
- Enhance lateral femoral glide for stance phase

Editor note
Efficient gait involves coordinated motions in figure 8 patterns from the feet through to the head. Improving the capacity for movement in all planes is essential for gait patterning.

Starting position
- Propped on one forearm facing sideways with bottom thigh on roller and top foot planted
- Support torso with other hand on mat

Movement description
- Roll from proximal femur toward knee
- Lateral aspect of lower extremity (LE)
- Change orientation to anterior aspect of thigh
- Pause if a challenging area is identified, change orientation of roller to roll medially/laterally. This changes the force vector with respect to the grain of the fibers
- Breathe throughout
- If too painful, pause or stop
- Perform for 5–15 repetitions

3. Rolling on soft roller: posterior thorax

Intent
- Articulation of torso extension

Gait reasoning
- Improve accessibility of movement in all planes

Editor note
Efficient gait involves coordinated motions in figure 8 patterns from the feet through to the head. Improving the capacity for movement in all planes is essential for gait patterning.

Starting position
- Seated, hip and knee joints flexion
- Lie with back to mid-thorax on roller
- Hands cradling head

Movement description
- Press into feet and extend hips to roll along posterior thorax
- Lower pelvis at intervals to extend and articulate
- Perform for 5–15 repetitions

4. Limb reach

Intent
- UE and LE articulation from distal to proximal
- Enhance continuous activation of UE and LE to torso

Gait reasoning
- Improve LE and UE swing through increased tissue gliding and joint articulation
- Awareness of distal contact of foot and oppositional torso extension for push-off
- Stance leg continuous activation from foot to torso

Starting position
- Supine on mat
- Right hip and knee joints flexion, foot on floor
- Left LE extended, foot dorsiflexion
- Left arm overhead by ear

Movement description
- Inhale, reach left heel inferiorly and left hand superiorly, moving heel and hand away from one another
- Exhale and relax
- Repeat several times before changing sides

5. Side lying rotation

Intent
- Safe unloaded position for torso rotation
- Improve extensibility of torso, neck, and shoulders
- Improve control and proprioception of rotation

Gait reasoning	- Enhanced torso articulation
- Increase rotation for arm swing and reciprocal torso motions
Starting position	- Lying on side on mat with 90 degrees hip and knee joint flexion
- Place pillow to support head
- Touch top hand to same side shoulder
Movement description	- Exhale while rotating toward ceiling with control
- Hold for 3 breath cycles
- Slowly return to starting position
- Repeat 3 times on each side

6. Leg series with resistance band

Intent	- Experience continuity of feet through torso
- Improve ankle and hip joint articulation
- Posterior pelvifemoral continuous activation
- Practice flexion-extension pattern of knee and hip joint with ankle
Gait reasoning	- Enhanced torso articulation
- Increase rotation for arm swing and reciprocal torso motions
Starting position	- Supine on mat
- Left hip and knee joint flexion
- Right LE extended with band covering metatarsals and toes
- Holding band with elbows by sides
Movement description	- Alternate plantar flexion and dorsiflexion
- Repeat 8 times on each side
- Arcs: exhale, extend right hip joint toward floor
- Inhale, flex right hip joint
- Return to starting position
- Repeat 4 times on each side
- Circles: exhale, extend LE, abduct and flex
- Return to starting position
- Repeat 4 times, then reverse direction and repeat 4 times
- Repeat on other side
- Adduct the LE crossing midline to increase lateral femoral glide
- Hold for 2–4 breath cycles
- Abduct LE switching hands on band
- Hold for 2–4 breath cycles

7. Prone extension

Intent	• Continuous activation from LE to torso • Extension for bone health and fall prevention • Quadruped for balance, weight bearing at wrists, continuous activation
Gait reasoning	• Extensor activation for push-off • Loading progression from prone to quadruped for stance phase • Activation for knee extension
Starting position	• Lying prone on mat with hands under forehead • LE extended
Movement description	• Extend right LE • Repeat 6 times on each side • Progress to holding for 5 seconds, repeat 6 times on each side • Next progression: float head off hands and hold for 5 seconds, repeat 6 times on each side • Final progression: move UE to sides and hold for 10 seconds, repeat 6 times on each side • Change to quadruped position • Weight shift forward and back slowly 8 times • Progress to extending LE unilaterally to pelvis height and holding for 10 seconds each side

8. Side lying abduction

Derivative of J. H. Pilates Side Kick (NPCE Study Guide 2021, p. 49)

Intent	• Activation of hip joint in abduction, extension, and flexion • Control of knee extension • Torso adaptability to LE movements
Gait reasoning	• Prior to heel strike the coordination and timing of knee extensor and hip flexor • Lateral support in stance phase • Extension for push-off
Starting position	• Lie against a wall or line up against back edge of mat • Legs extended with feet stacked • Head resting on bottom arm

Pilates and Bone Health: Effect on Gait

Movement description
- Side leg lift
  - Slowly abduct LE to pelvis height and then lower
  - Repeat 4 times
- Side Kick
  - Move feet forward to front edge of mat, hip joints in 30 degrees flexion
  - Abduct LE to pelvis height
  - With control move LE anteriorly with ankle dorsiflexion for hip joint flexion
  - Swing LE posteriorly for extension
  - Repeat 6–8 times
  - Progress to double kick pulses in hip joint flexion
- Repeat on other side

9. Squats

Author note
Squatting, a closed kinematic chain exercise performed with acetabular femoral glide and not torso flexion, is significant for bone health. Squats, done well, increase a positive load to the bones, especially the hip joints.

Intent
- LE force coupling for knee issues
- LE to torso loading for bone health
- Weight-bearing bone loading
- Squatting is a functional movement

Gait reasoning
- Increase loading in standing
- Continuous activation in sagittal plane
- Balance weight distribution for midline orientation
- Pelvifemoral rhythm for flexion and extension

Starting position
- Stand with feet slightly wider than femoral joint center
- Hold a door handle with both hands, elbows bent at sides

Movement description
- Pelvifemoral flexion with knee extension
  - Torso moves anteriorly in client's optimal organization for the movement task
  - Pelvis rotating on femur
  - Repeat 4 times
- Pelvifemoral flexion with knee flexion
  - Initial movement: ankles remain in dorsiflexion
  - Lift one heel, squat
  - Squat without holding on
  - Repeat 8 times

Chapter 11

Author note
The depth of the pelvifemoral-knee flexion is determined by the ability of the ankles to dorsiflex. This protects the vulnerable regions of the torso from flexion.

10. Standing balance — Derivative of J. H. Pilates Side Kick (NPCE Study Guide 2021, p. 49)

- Intent
  - Proprioception for single stance
  - Lateral glide of supporting LE
- Gait reasoning
  - Balance for stance phase
- Starting position
  - Stand with feet in line with femoral joints
- Movement description
  - Lift one heel and close eyes for 1 minute (holding on if needed)
    - Progress to lifting foot off ground (added day 9)

11. Tension tissues of anterior thigh and pelvis in standing

- Intent
  - Alleviate sensation of tightness at anterior knee
- Gait reasoning
  - Improve hip extension for push-off
  - Assist extension by facilitating glide of anterior connective tissues
  - Activate between pubis and xiphoid for optimal pelvis and hip joint organization
- Starting position
  - Stand in front of a chair as if about to sit, and hold onto a fixed object like a wall or table
  - Flex hip and knee joints, lean forward
  - Place knee on seat of chair
  - Ankle dorsiflexion with metatarsals pushing against the chair back
  - Bring torso upright
- Movement description
  - Activate between the xiphoid and pubis for 0 degree hip joint flexion
  - Hold for 30 seconds
  - Breathing throughout
  - Repeat on other side

12. Lunge for ankle dorsiflexion

Intent
- Increase ankle dorsiflexion ROM
- Continuous activation of LE to torso in forward lunge

Gait reasoning
- Adaptability of feet to various ground surfaces
- Improve dorsiflexion for heel strike

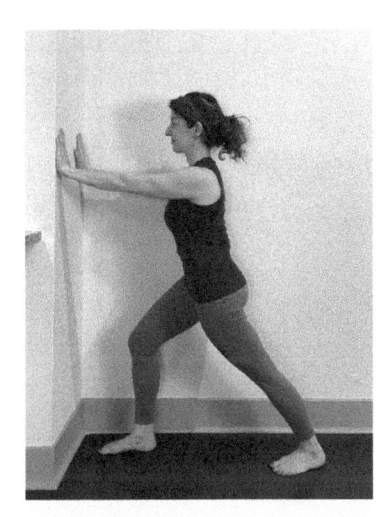

Figure 11.1

Starting position
- Standing facing wall, hands on wall
- Lunge position with posterior LE, ankle dorsiflexion

Movement description
- Hold for 30 seconds
- Repeat on other side

Chapter 11

Session 11/12: Studio session

Fatigue scale	2
Pain scale	1
Client self-report	• Feels an increase in movement strength, control, ROM, energy, and vitality
	• Notices how she's been progressing, and excited to be using her body again and feeling strong
	• "I'm going to be doing this till I'm 90! Even my husband says I'm much nicer to be around 'cause I'm no longer complaining about pain"
Key changes observed by author at end of Session 11/12	• Increased proprioception, steadier in weight bearing
	• Improved movement strategies, especially in coronal plane—no longer rotates pelvis as compensation for lateral flexion
	• Less to no pain in right knee and improved right knee extension is changing her gait strategy from pulling to pushing off
	• Holds right hip and knee joints at 90 degrees without assistance
	• Supports own body weight through UE
Reason behind choice of sequencing	• The intentions of the sequencing are to promote healthy pelvifemoral rhythm in a variety of orientations, torso extension, and balance. The sequences are designed with bone-loading principles in mind

Author note
Bone-loading principles: Bone responds to forces imposed upon it, improving the organization of the body, optimizing the ability to distribute the load, and optimizing balance.

- Additional focus for bone health is weight bearing through the wrist. Ground forces from the hand through the torso facilitate not only loading but can enhance the organization of the UE to the torso
- Client's knee pain and dysfunction that impacted her gait, daily functioning, and mental outlook was addressed
- This order was maintained once sessions switched from live in studio to virtual at home

Session movement sequence

1. Rolling on soft roller: lateral and anterior aspect of thigh

Intent
- Facilitate glide of connective tissue at anterior aspect of thigh

Gait reasoning
- Improve glide of anterior connective tissues for improved extension in push-off
- Enhance lateral femoral glide for stance phase

Editor note
Efficient gait involves coordinated motions in figure 8 patterns from the feet through to the head. Improving the capacity for movement in all planes is essential for gait patterning

Starting position
- Propped on one forearm facing sideways with bottom thigh on roller and top foot planted
- Support torso with other hand on mat

Movement description
- Roll from proximal femur toward knee
- Lateral aspect of LE
- Change orientation to anterior aspect of thigh
- Pause if a challenging area is identified, change orientation of roller to roll medially/laterally
- Breathe throughout
- If too painful, pause or stop
- Perform for 5–15 repetitions

CUES
- Roll slowly and pause when sensing a challenging area
- Roll in a transverse direction on that area, breathing throughout

Author note
Was very tender on the legs at the start but client now enjoys the experience.

2. Rolling on soft roller: posterior thorax

Intent
- Articulation of torso extension

Gait reasoning
- Improve accessibility of movement in all planes

Chapter 11

Editor note
Efficient gait involves coordinated motions in figure 8 patterns from the feet through to the head. Improving the capacity for movement in all planes is essential for gait patterning

Starting position
- Seated, hip and knee joints flexion
- Lie with back to mid-thorax on roller
- Hands cradling head

Movement description
- Press into feet and extend hips to roll along posterior thorax
- Lower pelvis at intervals to extend and articulate
- Perform for 5–15 repetitions

CUES
- Roll slowly and pause when sensing a challenging area
- Roll in a transverse direction on that area, breathing throughout

Author note
Was very tender on the legs at the start but client now enjoys the experience.

3. Eve's Lunge

Derivative of J. H. Pilates Splits: Front on Universal Reformer (NPCE Study Guide 2021, p. 62)
(See Chapter 5 in Volume 1, Gentry, Eve's Lunge)

Author note
Initially, used the Universal Reformer, but due to COVID restrictions this was substituted with a 26 in. (65 cm) ball.

Intent
- Facilitate tissue glide in anterior flexor region
- Sustained activation extensors
- Coordination of sagittal plane motion from LE to torso

Gait reasoning
- Enhance extension for push-off
- Facilitate midline organization in upright orientation

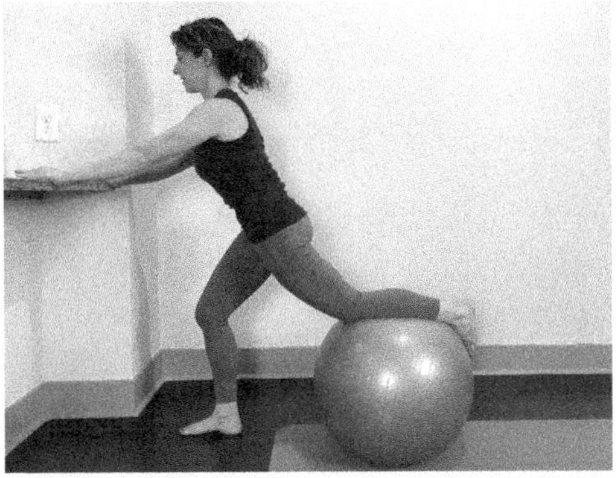

Pilates and Bone Health: Effect on Gait

Figure 11.2

Set-up	• 26 in. (65 cm) ball • Stable chair, table, or shelf to hold onto
Starting position	• Standing holding on to a stable object • Right lower limb in knee flexion and ankle dorsiflexion with dorsum of foot in contact with ball • Right hip joint in 5–15 degrees flexion • Left hip and knee joint flexion, ankle dorsiflexion
Movement description	• Exhale, roll ball posteriorly extending right LE • At the same time, increase flexion of left hip and knee joint • Inhale, sustaining organization of right hip joint extension • Exhale, return to starting position • Repeat 8 times on each side

CUES
♦ Coordinate the lowering of the standing leg with the extension of the hip joint in contact with the ball
♦ Avoid pelvic rotation when rolling posterior

4. Leg series with band   Derivative of J. H. Pilates Leg Springs Series: Bicycle, Walking, Scissors, Circles on Trapeze Table (NPCE Study Guide 2021, pp. 67–68)

Author note
Initially, Footwork and straps: feet in loops used the Universal Reformer, but due to COVID restrictions this was substituted with a resistance band

Intent	• Continuous activation from feet to torso
	• Ankle and hip joint articulation
	• Practice flexion-extension pattern of closed kinematic chain from ankle to femoral joint
Gait reasoning	• Improve proprioception through feet
	• Ankle dorsiflexion and plantar flexion for heel strike and push-off
	• Extensor activation for push-off
Set-up	• Medium resistance band
Starting position	• Supine, place band around right foot covering forefoot
	• Right hip and knee joints extended
	• Elbows by sides
	• Left foot planted, hip and knee joint flexion
Movement description	• In hip joint flexion and knee extension
	▪ Plantar flex and dorsiflex ankle
	▪ Repeat 8 times on each side
	• In knee extension
	▪ Extend and flex the hip joint
	▪ Repeat 4 times on each side
	• In hip and knee joint extension
	▪ Arc continuously from flexion to abduction/external rotation
	▪ Move LE inferiorly in abduction/external rotation
	▪ Adduction/internal rotation parallel to midline
	▪ Midline flexion to return to starting position
	▪ Repeat 4 times in one direction
	▪ Reverse direction and repeat 4 times
	• Medial-lateral femoral glides
	▪ In hip joint flexion and knee extension cross LE over midline
	▪ Hold for 2–4 breath cycles
	▪ Abduct LE
	▪ Hold for 2–4 breath cycles
	• Hip joint and knee flexion/extension
	▪ Repeat 8 times on each side
	• Hip joint flexion with knee extension and feet together
	▪ Wrap band around both feet over the midfoot, heels together
	▪ 45 degrees hip joint flexion/external rotation and knee extension (see Cues below)

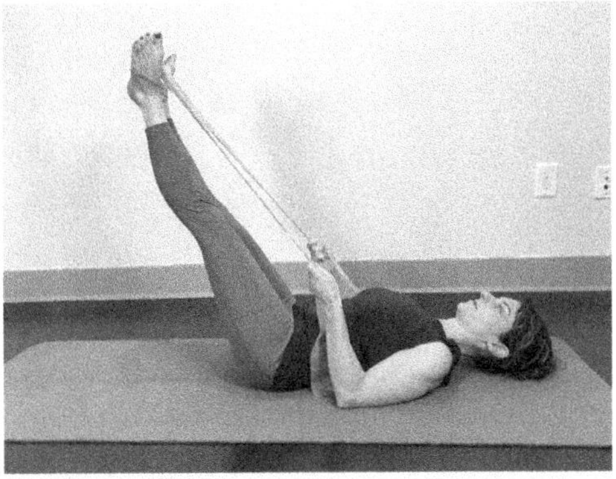

Figure 11.3

- Abduct/externally rotate hip joint with knee flexion, keeping heels together
- Return to starting position
- Repeat 8 times

CUES
- Keep elbows flexed by sides the entire time
- During hip joint flexion, especially bilateral, the degree of flexion is determined by the ROM of the hip joint relative to the lumbopelvic capacity to remain in the client's optimal organization for the movement task

5. Side lying series with roller

Author note
Initially, side lying Footwork used the Universal Reformer, but due to COVID restrictions this was substituted with a roller.

Editor note
Side lying Footwork on Universal Reformer is a closed kinematic chain exercise using the weight-bearing foot on the footbar. The closed kinematic position provides the load necessary for compression of the structures, foot through pelvis. When partial or full weight bearing is not available, sensory motor stimulation can be used as a substitute.

Intent
- Facilitate lateral flexion of lumbar region
- Continuous activation laterally from foot to torso

Chapter 11

Gait reasoning
- Improve torso adaption through lateral flexion with pelvic lift during swing-through
- Proprioception of thorax to pelvis relationship during hip hiking and lowering

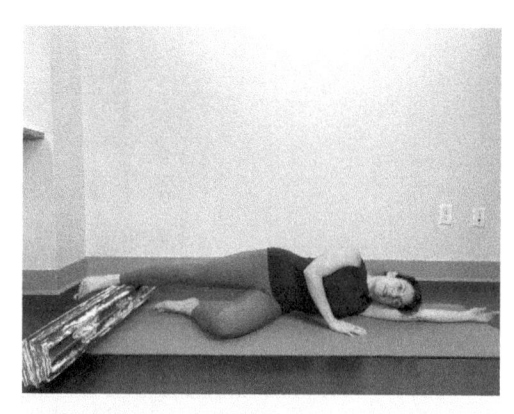

Figure 11.4

Set-up
- Roller positioned perpendicularly and distal to the body at the feet

Starting position
- Lying on side
- Mat side in hip and knee joint flexion
- Top LE extended with foot on roller

Movement description
- Slowly roll the roller away from torso, lowering top innominate
  - Lateral flexion, minimize to no rotation
  - Return to starting position
  - Repeat 8 times
- Abduct top LE to pelvis height and adduct, placing foot on roller
  - Repeat 8 times
- Remove the roller
  - Bilateral hip and knee joint flexion
  - Feet together, heels pressing together
  - Abduct and adduct top LE with heels pressing together
  - Repeat 8 times

6. **Single Leg Stretch and Double Leg Stretch** — Derivative of J. H. Pilates Overhead/Jackknife on Universal Reformer (NPCE Study Guide 2021, p. 53) and Single Leg Stretch and Double Leg Stretch (NPCE Study Guide 2021, pp. 46–47)

Author note

Initially, Overhead with arms in straps and Single Leg Stretch with hands in straps was performed on the Universal Reformer but due to COVID restrictions movement on mat was substituted. The J. H. Pilates sequence on Universal Reformer in Hundred and Overhead/Jackknife includes anterior torso activation, approximating thorax and pelvis; however, these sequences compress the vulnerable vertebrae in flexion, creating risk of fracture. The author kept the arm element of the Pilates exercise and head down. The author modified the torso and LE organization, respecting guidelines for bone health.

Intent
- Continuous activation of UE and LE to torso, stimulating flexors
- Using the mat for proprioceptive feedback of torso to address excessive rib translation

Gait reasoning
- Flexor activation for swing phase

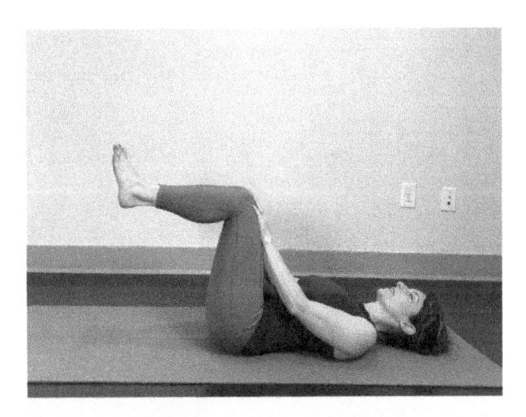

Figure 11.5

Starting position
- Supine on mat
- Hip and knee joints at 90 degrees flexion
- Hands placed on anterior inferior femur

Chapter 11

Movement description
- Preparation
  - Press hands into femurs, femurs into hands
  - Hold for 5 seconds
  - Repeat 5 times
- Single Leg Stretch
  - Exhale, extend one LE to 45 degrees hip joint flexion
  - Both hands against other flexed hip and knee
  - Repeat 4 times on each side
- Double Leg Stretch
  - UE movement only
  - Maintain hip and knee flexion to 90 degrees
  - Flex shoulders with extended elbows, UE by ears
  - Abduct UE to place hands on knees
  - Repeat arm movement 4 times

Author note
The derivatives of Single Leg Stretch and Double Leg Stretch are adapted for those with osteoporosis. The head remains on the mat to remove thoracic flexion, which can increase the risk for vertebral fracture. In this version of Single Leg Stretch, the hands press against the inferior femur during flexion instead of pulling the knee to the chest.

7. Side Bend preparation Derivative of J. H. Pilates Side Bend (NPCE Study Guide 2021, p. 50)

Author note
Initially, Side Bend preparation was performed on the Ladder Barrel, but due to COVID restrictions this was substituted with movement on mat.

Intent
- Part A: for scoliotic pattern of left rib translation in thoracic region
- Parts B and C: bone loading through upper extremities to challenge continuity of LE to torso

Gait reasoning
- Improve rib to pelvis relationship for torso rotation and arm swing

Starting position
- Side lying propped on forearm with hemipelvis on mat
- Top foot planted in front of bottom LE
- Bottom hip joint to less than 90 degrees flexion, knee flexion
- Top hand on pelvis

Pilates and Bone Health: Effect on Gait

Movement description
- A: Translate thorax toward ceiling
  - Hold for 6 seconds
- B: Press into planted foot and lift pelvis
  - Hold for 3 seconds and lower
  - Repeat 2 times
- C: Extend the elbow, planting hand on mat and stack feet

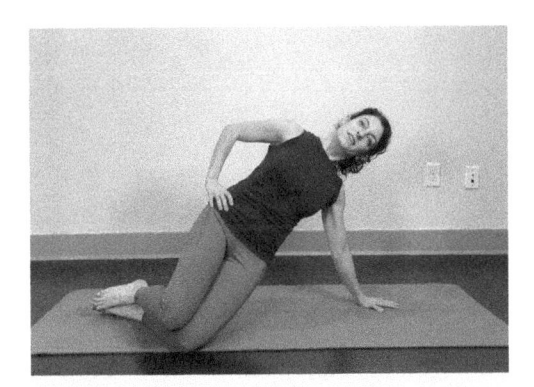

Figure 11.6

- Lift pelvis and lower
- Repeat 5 times
- Perform B and C on other side

CUES
- A: Breathe into side of the lateral ribs translating toward ceiling
- B: Press through feet and hands to elevate pelvis
- C: Press through the hand, and reach through the head

Author note
There is no instruction to perform A on second side for reason of the client's scoliotic pattern.

8. Quadruped weight shifts

Author note
Initially, Knee Stretch Series was performed on the Universal Reformer, but due to COVID restrictions this was substituted with movement on mat.

Chapter 11

Intent
- Bear weight through wrists
- Facilitate safe torso rotation
- Introduce a force vector from distal hand through torso
- Loading of femoral joints

Gait reasoning
- Lateral translation for weight shift to stance leg

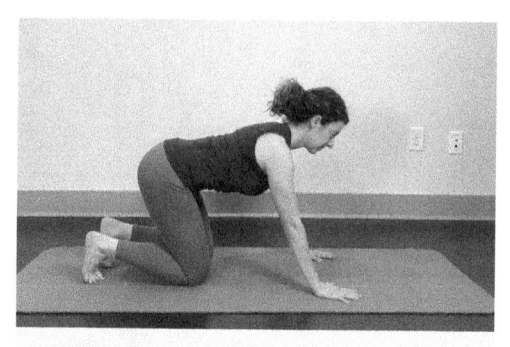

Figure 11.7

Starting position
- Quadruped in client's optimal organization for the movement task

Movement description
- Slowly flex and extend the hip joints, shifting weight
  - Repeat 8 times
- Flex one shoulder with extended elbow near ear
- Hold for 5 seconds
- Repeat 2 times
- Repeat on other side
- Place hand behind head
  - Inhale and rotate torso with slight extension away from supporting arm
  - Repeat 3 times
  - Repeat on other side

CUE
- Press into the supporting hands as if pushing the ground away using the force to assist in rotation

Author note
The addition of thoracic rotation with extension is a safe position for rotation.

9. Swan preparation — Derivative of J. H. Pilates Swan Dive (NPCE Study Guide 2021, p. 48)

Author note
Initially, Swan was performed on the Ladder Barrel, but due to COVID restrictions this was substituted with movement on mat.

Intent
- Improve articulation in extension
- Increase back extensor endurance

Gait reasoning
- Increase ability for extension improving full range of torso motions
- Increase midline orientation for thoracic rotation

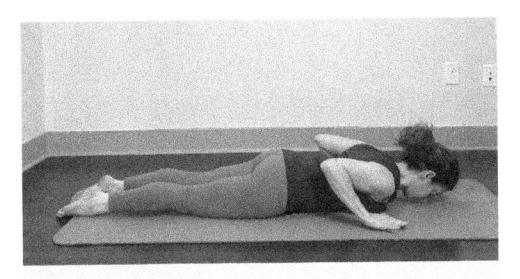

Figure 11.8

Starting position
- Prone on mat
  - Hands placed near axillas with elbows pointing posteriorly
  - LE aligned with ischial tuberosities

Movement description
- Lift hands off mat
- Lift head off mat
- Hold for 5 seconds
- Return to starting position
- Repeat 3 times
- Hold 3rd repetition
- Abduct UE to T-position
- Hold for 10 seconds

10. Splits: Side Derivative of J. H. Pilates Splits: Side on Universal Reformer (NPCE Study Guide 2021, p. 61)

Author note
Initially, Splits: Side was performed on the Universal Reformer, but due to COVID restrictions this was substituted with standing using a wall.

Chapter 11

Intent
- Standing weight bearing for bone loading
- Closed kinematic chain activation from foot to torso
- Motor control for organizing midline and balance

Gait reasoning
- Support one-leg stance
- Weight transference

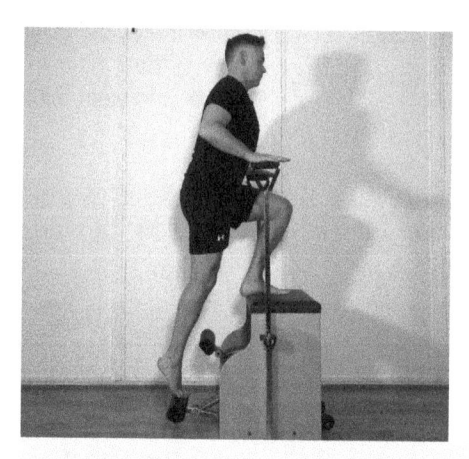

Figure 11.9

Starting position
- Stand sideways to wall with shoulder touching wall
- Shift weight to outside leg
- Abduct inside LE with knee extension
- Press foot into wall

Movement description
- Hold for 10 seconds
- Close eyes and aim to hold for 10 seconds
- Stand on a pad and aim to hold for 10 seconds, holding on to stable object if necessary

CUE
- Continuous force from standing foot as well as foot against wall

Author note
The purpose of standing on a pad is to challenge the proprioceptors with a change of surface. The client achieved standing on the pad with eyes closed for 10 seconds in the final session.

Pilates and Bone Health: Effect on Gait

11. Stepping up: front and side Derivative of J. H. Pilates Forward Lunge and Side Lunge on Wunda Chair (NPCE Study Guide 2021, p. 77)

Author note
Initially, Forward Lunge and Side Lunge were performed on the Wunda Chair, but due to COVID restrictions this was substituted with a chair.

Intent
- Activate LE in flexion and external rotation

Gait reasoning
- Transfer ground forces through LE to torso

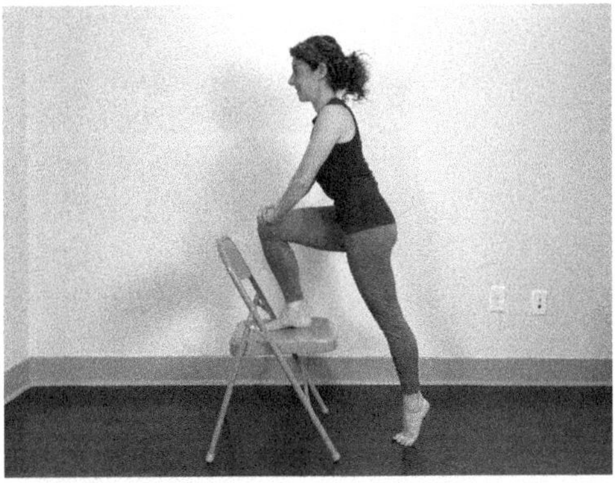

Figure 11.10

Starting position
- Standing facing a chair
- Place one foot on seat of chair with hip and knee joints flexion
- Standing LE extended

Movement description
- Press foot into seat of chair as if about to step up
- Hold for 5 seconds
- Repeat 8 times
- Facing sideways
  - Place one LE in external rotation with foot on the chair
  - Repeat pressing foot into seat as if about to step up
  - Hold for 5 seconds
  - Repeat 8 times

395

Chapter 11

12. Standing extension on chair

Author note
Initially, standing extension was performed on the Ladder Barrel, but due to COVID restrictions this was substituted with standing using a chair.

Intent	• Pelvifemoral motor control
	• Promote anterior LE to torso tissue glide
Gait reasoning	• Improve extension in push-off
Starting position	• Standing in front of a chair as if about to sit
	• Hold on to a fixed object like a wall or table
Movement description	• Flex at femoral and knee joints
	• Torso leans forward
	• Place knee on seat of chair and metatarsal arch against chair back
	• Return torso upright
	• Hold up to 30 seconds
	• Perform on other side

13. Lunge for ankle dorsiflexion

Intent	• Increase ankle dorsiflexion ROM
	• Continuous activation of LE to torso in forward lunge
Gait reasoning	• Adaptability of feet to various ground surfaces
	• Improve dorsiflexion for heel strike
Starting position	• Facing wall, hands on wall
	• Lunge position with posterior LE, ankle dorsiflexion
Movement description	• Hold for 30 seconds
	• Perform on other side

The journey to Session 11

Session 4/12
Client self-report

- Fatigue scale 3
- Pain scale 1
- Likes feeling stronger from the home program exercises and the session
- Notices increased ROM, surprised how the work affects her whole body

Key changes observed

- Developing awareness and proprioception
- Improved ability to load right LE

Reasoning behind choice of movements

- Continuous activation foot to torso
- Rib and thorax joint articulation
- Weight-bearing loading and balance

Session movement sequence

1. Reviewed details of the exercises using the band

2. Foam roller

3. Universal Reformer

- Eve's Lunge
- Footwork
- Straps: feet in loops

4. Ladder Barrel

- Side Sit-Ups preparation

5. Universal Reformer

- Splits: Side

6. Ladder Barrel

- LE extension

Session 5/12
Client self-report

- Fatigue scale 4
- Pain scale 1
- Feels she's getting stronger with more control and ROM, notices a little more energy
- Content with her progress

Key changes observed

- Client needed to hook left LE under right to lift feet to footbar and to support it in 90/90 hip and knee joints flexion
- No knee pain today during footwork
- Improved knee extension ROM

Reasoning behind choice of movements

- Lunge with ankle dorsiflexion to address lack of knee extension and connective tissue glide
- Added external rotation/abduction with knee flexion to train new pattern of pelvifemoral movement
- Continue Footwork patterning
- Continue weight bearing for loading LE and balance
- Continue thoracic articulation movements to ease scoliotic pattern

Session movement sequence
1. Prone extension

- Added 5 seconds' hold to each prone extension

2. Squats

- Added single heel lift to each squat while holding door handle

3. Foam roller

- Rolling on soft roller: lateral and anterior aspects of thigh

4. Universal Reformer

- Eve's Lunge
- Footwork
- Straps: feet in loops
- UE in straps, flexion and extension

Chapter 11

5. Ladder Barrel

- Side Sit-Ups preparation

6. Universal Reformer

- Splits: Side

7. Ladder Barrel

- Extension
- Lunge for ankle dorsiflexion

Session 6/12
Client self-report

- Fatigue scale 2
- Pain scale 1
- Turning point in enthusiasm—noticed that climbing up the stairs to the studio was easier today
- Is really enjoying the program and the homework—would be willing to do it more than twice a week

Key changes observed

- Increases Footwork spring tension
- Right knee unable to remain in line with center of hip joint, adducts while side lying with foot on footbar
- Tends to flex knee in Splits: Side to avoid medial femoral glide

Reasoning behind choice of movements

- Added side lying Footwork for foot to torso continuous activation with control in multi-dimensions
- Added Swan for activating extensors
- Continued foot to torso motor control through Footwork and straps: feet in loops

- Continued weight bearing for loading and balance
- Continued rib articulation for balance and ease of scoliotic pattern

Session movement sequence
1. Side Kick: added the double kick in hip joint flexion

2. Foam roller

- Rolling on soft roller: lateral and anterior aspect of thigh

3. Universal Reformer

- Eve's Lunge
- Footwork
- Straps: feet in loops
- Side lying Footwork
- Arms in straps: shoulder flexion/extension

4. Ladder Barrel

- Side Sit-Ups preparation
- Swan preparation

5. Universal Reformer

- Splits: Side

6. Ladder Barrel

- Extension
- Lunge with ankle dorsiflexion

Session 7/12
Client self-report

- Fatigue scale 3
- Pain scale 1
- Hasn't felt this good and without pain since before her falls (at least 2 years)

- Feels that when she is walking, she is straighter, stronger, and more confident

Key changes observed

- No longer needs left LE to assist lifting right LE or to hold in 90/90 hip and knee joints flexion
- No more knee pain or lumbopelvic pain with straps: feet in loops
- More control and fluidity in straps: feet in loops
- Performed Splits: Side hands-free and without assistance
- No longer needs assistance for standing extension on Ladder Barrel

Reasoning behind choice of movements

- Continued foot to torso motor control through Footwork and straps: feet in loops
- Continued activation of torso extensors
- Continued weight bearing to increase loading and improve balance
- Continued rib articulation for ease of scoliotic pattern

Session movement sequence

1. Add to prone: float head off hands and hold for 5 seconds, repeat 6 times

2. Add double leg balance, lifting one heel and eyes closed, up to 1 minute hold

3. Foam roller

- Rolling on soft roller: lateral and anterior aspect of thigh

4. Universal Reformer

- Eve's Lunge
- Footwork
- Straps: feet in loops
- Side lying Footwork
- UE in straps: shoulder flexion/extension

5. Ladder Barrel

- Side Sit-Ups preparation
- Swan preparation

6. Universal Reformer

- Splits: Side

7. Ladder Barrel

- Extension
- Lunge with ankle dorsiflexion

Session 8/12
Client self-report

- Fatigue scale 3
- Pain scale 1
- Feels stronger now than even last week
- Experiences sense of success: expresses satisfaction in performing the exercises because can do them better now than at the beginning

Key changes observed

- Pandemic lockdown began, so sessions became virtual and without equipment
- Eve's Lunge on ball much harder with unstable surface of ball and lack of closed kinematic chain from Universal Reformer
- Universal Reformer supine work with legs and arms prepared client well for mat work
- First time doing Single and Double Leg Stretch variations unable to fully extend knees

Reasoning behind choice of movements

- Attempting to adapt the studio program to home setting, changing sequence as little as possible

Chapter 11

- Added in quadruped and forearm propping to begin loading shoulders and wrists
- Continued to focus on foot to torso motor control
- Continued activating torso extensors
- Continued weight bearing, increasing loading and improving balance

Session movement sequence
1. Side lying thoracic rotation added

2. Prone Swan: added preparation with hands, hold for 10 seconds, repeat 6 times

3. Quadruped weight shifts added, forward and back, repeat 8 times

4. Foam roller

- Rolling on soft roller: lateral and anterior aspect of thigh

5. Physioball

- Eve's Lunge

6. Leg series with band

7. Side lying series with roller

8. Supine

- Preparation for Single and Double Leg Stretch with head down
- Single Leg Stretch with head down
- Double Leg Stretch with head down, legs only

9. Side Bend preparation

10. Prone Swan preparation

11. Quadruped

- Weight shifts

12. Standing next to wall

- Splits: Side
- Stepping up: front using chair
- Standing extension with chair
- Lunge with ankle dorsiflexion

Session 9/12
Client self-report

- Fatigue scale 1
- Pain scale 1
- Back hurt doing homework—low back spasmed in the prone head lift
- Expressed gratitude: "I feel the program is so much more than what I expected it to be, and I can't wait to continue doing this type of exercise permanently"

Key changes observed

- Improved balance in Eve's Lunge on ball and was able to lift one hand, demonstrating better motor control and balance
- Improved movement quality with more fluidity
- More confidence in balancing overall

Reasoning behind choice of movements

- Continued to focus on foot to torso motor control
- Continued activating torso extensors
- Continued weight bearing for increased loading and improved balance

Session movement sequence

1. Squat without holding on

2. Standing balance lifting the entire foot off ground with eyes open

3. Standing extension and lunge with ankle dorsiflexion added

4. Foam roller

- Rolling on soft roller: lateral and anterior aspect of thigh

5. Physioball

- Eve's Lunge

6. Leg series with band

7. Side lying series with roller

8. Supine

- Preparation for Single and Double Leg Stretch with head down
- Single Leg Stretch with head down
- Double Leg Stretch with head down, legs only

9. Side Bend preparation

10. Prone Swan preparation reviewed to improve form

11. Quadruped

- Weight shifts
- Added extension

12. Standing next to wall

- Splits: Side
- Stepping up: front using chair
- Standing extension with chair
- Lunge with ankle dorsiflexion
- Calf stretch

Session 10/12
Client self-report

- Fatigue scale 3
- Pain scale 1
- Feels more energized
- New sense of potential: "I feel up to the challenge of those things I couldn't do at first"

Key changes observed

- Increased body awareness—able to lower innominate upon cue
- No longer needs to hook ankles for support in tabletop position
- Less knee discomfort and can feel activation and even straighten knees for several Single Leg Stretch repetitions
- Improved LE control in side lying Footwork
- Could bear weight through UE into torso

Reasoning behind choice of movements

- Continued to focus on foot to torso motor control
- Continued activating torso extensors
- Continued weight bearing for increased loading and improved balance
- Continued balance and weight bearing for hand to torso loading

Session movement sequence

1. Foam roller

- Rolling on soft roller: lateral and anterior aspect of thigh

2. Physioball

- Eve's Lunge

3. Leg series with band

4. Side lying series with roller

5. Supine

- Preparation for Single and Double Leg Stretch with head down
- Single Leg Stretch with head down
- Double Leg Stretch with head down, legs only

6. Side Bend preparation

7. Prone Swan preparation

8. Quadruped

- Weight shifts

9. Standing next to wall

- Splits: Side
- Stepping up: front using chair
- Standing extension with chair
- Lunge with ankle dorsiflexion

Acknowledgements

Thank you to MOVE Studios in Denver, CO for use of its studio during this case report.

References

bpacnz (2024) The Four Stage Balance Test. https://bpac.org.nz/falls/docs/The_Four_Stage_Balance_Test.pdf. [Accessed September 19, 2023].

CDC (2017) Assessment: The 4-Stage Balance Test. www.cdc.gov/steadi/pdf/4-Stage_Balance_Test-print.pdf. [Accessed September 19, 2023].

Fullerton Center for Successful Aging (2008) Scoring Form for Fullerton Advanced Balance (FAB) Scale. https://geriatrictoolkit.missouri.edu/fab/FABScaleScoringFormwithCut-OffValues.pdf. [Accessed September 19, 2023].

Giangregorio, L. M., McGill, S., Wark, J. D., Laprade, J. *et al.* (2015) "Too Fit To Fracture: Outcomes of a Delphi consensus process on physical activity and exercise recommendations for adults with osteoporosis with or without vertebral fractures." *Osteoporosis International, 26,* 3, 891–910.

International Osteoporosis Foundation (IOF) (2023) What is Osteoporosis? www.osteoporosis.foundation/patients/about-osteoporosis. [Accessed September 19, 2023].

Kasukawa, Y., Miyakoshi, N., Hongo, M., Ishikawa, Y. *et al.* (2010) "Relationships between falls, spinal curvature, spinal mobility and back extensor strength in elderly people." *Journal of Bone and Mineral Metabolism, 28,* 1, 82–87.

Kistler-Fischbacher, M., Yong, J. S., Weeks, B. K., and Beck, B. R. (2021) "A comparison of bone-targeted exercise with and without antiresorptive bone medication to reduce indices of fracture risk in postmenopausal women with low bone mass: The MEDEX-OP randomized controlled trial." *Journal of Bone and Mineral Research, 36,* 9, 1680–1693.

NPCE Study Guide (National Pilates Certification Exam Study Guide) (2021) Miami, FL: National Pilates Certification Program, Inc.

Physiopedia (2024a) Fullerton Advanced Balance (FAB) Scale. www.physio-pedia.com/Fullerton_Advanced_Balance_(FAB)_Scale. [Accessed September 19, 2023].

Physiopedia (2024b) Balance Error Scoring System. www.physio-pedia.com/Balance_Error_Scoring_System?utm_source=physiopedia&utm_medium=search&utm_campaign=ongoing_internal. [Accessed September 19, 2023].

Physiopedia (2024c) The 4-Stage Balance Test. www.physio-pedia.com/The_4-Stage_Balance_Test. [Accessed September 19, 2023].

Royal Osteoporosis Society (2019) About exercise for osteoporosis and bone health. https://strwebstgmedia.blob.core.windows.net/media/0lhowmrk/about-exercise-fact-sheet-february-2019.pdf. [Accessed September 19, 2023].

Sinaki, M., Itoi, E., Wahner, H. W., Wollan, P. *et al.* (2002) "Stronger back muscles reduce the incidence of vertebral fractures: A prospective 10 year follow-up of postmenopausal women." *Bone, 30,* 6, 836–841.

Sports Medicine Research Laboratory (2024) Balance Error Scoring System (BESS). University of North Carolina's Sports Medicine Research Laboratory. https://atriumhealth.org/documents/carolinasrehab/bess_manual_.pdf. [Accessed September 19, 2023].

Chapter 12

Pilates and Aging Well: Effect on Gait

Kelly Kane

As Pilates professionals we can help our clients maintain and build resilience and agency by directly supporting their capacity to maintain adaptability in their neuromyofascial system in a controlled, safe, and supportive environment. Maintaining adaptability can have positive outcomes in all aspects of an individual's health and life. It is within our control to be biologically younger than our chronological age suggests based on old norms.

Typically people over 65 are at a higher risk of heart disease, diabetes, hearing and vision loss, cognitive decline, and the psychological effects associated with these declines in health than their younger counterparts (WHO 2022). The statistics vary radically based on biopsychosocial factors and should be considered in programming.

The degenerative effects of time on human physiology include inefficiency of all of the major systems of the body unless we take care of them over time. Pilates as a movement modality is uniquely able to adjust and adapt to any fitness and ability level. It supports joint health, maintains bone density, optimizes breathing, improves global movement organization, and contributes to maintaining a healthy sex life! A consistent Pilates practice can also create and maintain an adaptive and responsive nervous system. All of these are component parts of a body engaged in aging well.

An initial assessment of overall movement strategies and health history should drive your programming design, not a client's chronological age. In general, look to optimize the range of motion (ROM) of all of the joints to create adaptability and resiliency strength in the body. Note and recognize movement limitations. Slowly increase ROM, especially closed kinematic chain movements. Challenge clients with balance, coordination tasks, and progressive loading. Verbal and tactile cueing facilitates sensory perception for interoceptive and proprioceptive awareness. All aspects will have profound effects on anyone's health, especially that of older clients.

It is our job as professionals to understand health history and contraindications associated with any diagnosis ranging from osteoarthritis to joint replacement, dementia, and diabetes. But there is a new day dawning for aging well and the research supports it. Chronological age is less and less a factor of aging (Hamczyk *et al.* 2020). Support the client's capacity to adapt by administering a little healthy stress with support to facilitate change and growth. This never changes over time!

Client description:	72-year-old biological female, identifies as female; educational consultant; outdoor enthusiast; she has never engaged in strength training but does Tai Chi weekly and has for many years
Dates of case report:	Session 1: December 17, 2019; Session 12: March 11, 2020; all in-person sessions

Chapter 12

Studio apparatus and props
Pilates equipment

- Universal Reformer
- Trapeze Table
- Wunda Chair
- Ladder Barrel

Props used with equipment

- Light resistance band
- Long, full-length foam roller
- Magic Circle: light resistance
- Rotational discs: heavy resistance
- Y-loops for leg springs on Trapeze Table
- Mat

Home program props

- Light resistance band
- Soft, long foam roller
- Magic Circle
- Wall
- Light circular band
- Mat
- Small, non-skid rubberized pad, 7.5 in. x 14 in. x 1/2 in. (19 cm x 36 cm x 1.3 cm)

Methods and materials

Session 1/12
1. Health history interview

- Healthy 72-year-old female
- Educational consultant
- Active outdoor enthusiast
- Engages in outdoor activities a minimum of twice a week for cardio and mental health. Activities include road biking and hiking in the summer and cross-country skiing in the winter
- No symptoms except for some intermittent left knee pain
- She has never engaged in strength training and has never done Pilates
- She has a strong and supportive community of women friends and has been married for 15 years
- One child that was delivered vaginally with episiotomy
- Healthy balanced diet; drinks enough water generally
- Has some anxiety that she manages with breathing and meditation
- Diagnosis of osteopenia in bilateral hip joints
- Has a vaginal NuvaRing® to maintain vaginal estrogen and progesterone and reduce symptoms of vaginal atrophy and dryness

2. Symptoms
Some intermittent "achiness" on the medial knee but not present during the first session

3. Movement aids
- None

Final result of case report

Our goal was to increase overall strength and balance. Programming included fall prevention strategies aimed toward improving balance and adaptability. The client reported feeling significantly stronger and more stable during outdoor activities. There was improvement in verticality and midline orientation, longer stride length during the push phase of gait, and improved balance on the stance leg.

Session 2/12: Initial assessment

1. General observations of gait

- Gait is lively and quick

- Propulsion movement executed primarily through feet and ankles, secondarily through knees

- Left swing and heel strike phase of gait: pelvic rotation, left more than right

- Left upper extremity (UE) swings forward more than right

- Left stance phase: mild left lateral flexion in lumbar region and associated hemipelvis superior motion

- Stance phase: pelvic lateral translation bilaterally, left more than right

- Limited bilateral hip joint extension resulting in short stride length

- Adequate plantar flexion in the propulsion or push-off phase of gait

- Presents as hyperkyphotic

2. Standing tests

- Full torso rotation

- Observations of inefficient side: left
  - Left foot supinates
  - Right foot pronates
  - Cervical and lumbar rotation is limited compared to right rotation
  - Minimal sequential thoracic rotation
  - Pelvis limited in left rotation

Session 12/12: Post-assessment

1. General observations of gait

- Gait is lively and quick

- Forward propulsion executed more evenly through ankle, knee, and hip joint

- Minimal change

- UE swing evenly

- Decrease in left lateral flexion of lumbar region and hemipelvis superior motion

- Increased hip joint congruency, less translation

- Increased hip joint ROM through all phases of gait: stride is longer, accordingly pace is slower

- Increased hip joint extension and decrease in plantar flexion during push-off phase of gait

- Minimal change to hyperkyphosis, verticality improved

2. Standing tests

- Full torso rotation

- Observations of non-efficient side: left
  - Left foot supinates
  - Right foot pronates
  - Increased cervical and lumbar rotation to left
  - Minimal increase of sequential thoracic rotation to left
  - Increased pelvic rotation to left

- Limited left hip joint internal rotation with pelvic rotation to left

◆ Hemipelvis inferior motion

● Observations of inefficient side: right
  ▪ Thoracolumbar junction (TLJ) translates left with thoracic rotating right

◆ Hemipelvis superior motion

● Observations of inefficient side: both
  ▪ Left hemipelvis is already elevated
  ▪ Difference between left and right hemipelvis superior motion is minimal

◆ Lateral pelvic shift

● Observations of inefficient side: left
  ▪ Shift to left, right innominate lowers
  ▪ Thorax translates left and rotates right
  ▪ Limited left lateral glide of femoral joint, flexes right knee
  ▪ Noticed lack of femoral glide in both directions

3. Seated tests

◆ Thoracic rotation

● Observations of inefficient side: left
  ▪ Weight on left ischial tuberosity
  ▪ Non-sequential rotation to left
  ▪ Limited left rotation
  ▪ Limited right thoracic translation

◆ Hip joint and knee flexion

● Observations of inefficient side: right
  ▪ Right hip joint flexion limited by about 20 degrees as compared to left
  ▪ Right knee flexion same as left

- Increased internal rotation of left hip joint

◆ Hemipelvis inferior motion

● Observations of inefficient side: right
  ▪ Improved inferior innominate, less TLJ translation and thoracic right rotation

◆ Hemipelvis superior motion

● Observations of inefficient side: both
  ▪ Minimal change

◆ Lateral pelvic shift

● Observations of inefficient side: both
  ▪ Right innominate lowers with appropriate left thoracic translation without rotation
  ▪ Bilateral symmetry of medial and lateral glide of femur heads in both directions

3. Seated tests

◆ Thoracic rotation

● Observations of inefficient side: left
  ▪ Weight even on ischial tuberosities
  ▪ Increased sequential movement of the cervical, thoracic, and lumbar regions to left
  ▪ Increased right thoracic translation

◆ Hip joint and knee flexion

● Observations of inefficient side: right
  ▪ Right hip joint flexion improved by 10 degrees

Author note

Included dorsiflexion and knee flexion test. Right was inefficient. Right tibia externally rotates to accommodate limited dorsiflexion. Included hip abduction with external rotation. Right limited compared to left.

4. Sit and stand

◆ Lateral view

- Even weight in both legs
- Good hip glide
- Thoracic hyperkyphosis and forward head organization but overall good torso organization

◆ Anterior view

- Good midline orientation
- Mild right knee adduction on stand phase

5. Standing balance

◆ Two-leg stance, eyes open or closed

- Eyes open: 60 seconds
- Eyes closed: 60 seconds

◆ One-leg stance, eyes open or closed

- Left leg, eyes open: 60 seconds
- Right leg, eyes open: 60 seconds
- Left leg, eyes closed: 10 seconds
- Right leg, eyes closed: 12 seconds

Author note

Included dorsiflexion and knee flexion test. Right was inefficient. Less external rotation of right tibia. Improved dorsiflexion. Included hip abduction with external rotation. Right increased ROM.

4. Sit and stand

◆ Lateral view

- Improved midline orientation during movement

◆ Anterior view

- Good midline orientation
- Adduction of right knee on stand phase

5. Standing balance

◆ Two-leg stance, eyes open

- Eyes open: 60 seconds
- Eyes closed: 60 seconds

◆ One-leg stance, eyes open

- Left leg, eyes open: 60 seconds
- Right leg, eyes open: 60 seconds
- Left leg, eyes closed: 10 seconds
- Right leg, eyes closed: 17 seconds

Session 3/12: Home program

Fatigue scale	5
Pain scale	0
Client self-report	• Excited to get started. She is excited to be working on strength as opposed to her outdoor activities and cardiovascular health. She likes being seen and cared for one-on-one
Key changes observed by author at end of Session 3/12	• Challenged by verbal cues and responds better to manual cues • Feels unsuccessful when she can't easily follow verbal cues • Coordinating breath with movement is challenging • Focused on basics of breathing through her nose during movement • Holding her breath seems to be a stress response
Reason behind choice of sequencing	• Provide a home program that is replicable and easy • Increase one-leg stance balance to decrease risk of injury from falling on the ice during Vermont winters • Improve balance in one-leg stance • Facilitate integration of all aspects of physical training to support client's preferred outdoor activities • Focus on activation of extensors for balance and upright/midline orientation • Work in gravity to increase load on bones, maintaining bone density

Session movement sequence

1. Supine torso foam rolling

Intent	• Continuous articulation of torso • Gliding action to improve connective tissue resiliency • Introduce strategies of self-care and treatment
Gait reasoning	• A strategy to counter excessive hyperkyphosis and forward head organization • Improve rib articulation and respiratory capacity • Use the roller at specific points on the torso to move above and below areas lacking articulation • Increased articulation improves the ability to rotate, minimizing excessive lateral movement

Starting position	• Sitting on the ground, feet flat on mat in parallel
	• Foam roller perpendicular to torso at middle to lower ribs
	• Place hands behind head to support head and neck
	• Lie back on foam roller
Movement description	• Keeping head and neck supported, lift pelvis off mat
	• Roll the length of the torso 2–3 times
	• Place roller on one thoracic area where movement feels limited
	• Release head, neck, and shoulders posteriorly
	• Simultaneously drop the lower ribs down
	• Repeat moving up or down the thorax
	• Keep the chin slightly tucked in when extending head and neck posteriorly over foam roller

2. Articulating bridge

Intent	• Continuous articulation of torso
	• Continuous activation from feet through torso
Gait reasoning	• Reducing kyphosis, encouraging extension for midline orientation
	• Improve extension for propulsion phase of gait
Starting position	• Supine on mat, knees flexed and feet planted in parallel
	• UE overhead on mat, flexed shoulders, elbows extended
	• Hands shoulder-width distance apart or wider, palms facing each other, thumbs toward the floor
Movement description	• Exhale, ankle dorsiflexion, hip extension
	• Continuously articulate torso in flexion inferiorly to superiorly to shoulder girdle
	• Hold bridge position
	• Maintain UE overhead
	• Inhale at the top of the movement
	• Exhale, roll down, articulating torso from superior to inferior
	• Return to starting position
	• Repeat 3–5 times

3. Pelvifemoral bridge (six-part series)

Intent	• Easily replicable and scalable exercise
	• Had difficulty activating extensors in other exercises—chose this series to assist extensors

Chapter 12

Gait reasoning	• Increase extension during the push-off phase of gait • Find even force transmission through four corners of the feet to improve distribution of ground forces
Starting position	• Supine on mat, knees flexed and feet planted in parallel • Four corners of the feet press into mat • UE resting at sides, elbows extended • Scapulae are slightly adducted
Movement description	Part 1 • Elevate pelvis off mat through hip extension • Lower pelvis through hip flexion without touching pelvis to the mat • Lift pelvis through pelvifemoral extension • Repeat lift and lower 10 times • Progress to 30 repetitions Part 2 • Heels mat-width apart • Lower extremity (LE) abducted/externally rotated • Align center of knee with 2nd toe • Press into feet, extend pelvis on femur to lift pelvis • Lower down to hover pelvis above mat • Repeat lifting and lowering pelvis 10 times • Progress to 30 repetitions Part 3 • Move into bridge position • Hold • Adduct and abduct LE moving knees in toward midline and away • Repeat 10 times • Progress to 30 repetitions Part 4 • Move into bridge position • Hold • Adduct LE, knees to midline • Maintain feet in parallel • Lower pelvis down 3 in. (7.5 cm) • Lift pelvis up 3 in. (7.5 cm) • Repeat 10 times • Progress to 30 repetitions

Part 5
- Move into bridge position
- Hold
- Drop left innominate toward mat while keeping right innominate high
- Return to starting position
- Repeat on other side
- Alternate side to side
- Repeat 10 times
- Progress to 30 repetitions

Part 6
- Place Magic Circle between inner thighs above knee joint
- Move into bridge position
- Hold
- Compress the Magic Circle and release
- Repeat 10 times
- Progress to 30 repetitions

4. Prone extension

Intent
- Engage and create endurance of extensors
- Increase thoracic articulation and activation of extensors
- Train scapular retraction under minimal load

Gait reasoning
- Thorax is hyperkyphotic limiting thoracic rotation
- Activating extensors to support torso upright
- Continuous LE to torso activation

Starting position
- Prone on mat with non-skid rubberized pad placed under the forehead
- LE extended and feet plantar flexed
- Hip joints in external rotation
- UE by sides with palms facing sides

Movement description
- On exhalation retract scapulae and reach UE inferiorly
- Small extension of the torso from the head
- Reach feet away from torso and extend LE
- Monitor over-extension of cervical region
- Hold for 30 seconds
- Repeat
- Progress to 3 repetitions

5. Supported squats

Intent
- Load the torso and LE
- Improve pelvifemoral motion in flexion and extension
- Using support to ensure optimal mechanics in squat

Gait reasoning
- Increasing stride length through extensors for push-off
- Standing loading for maintaining bone density

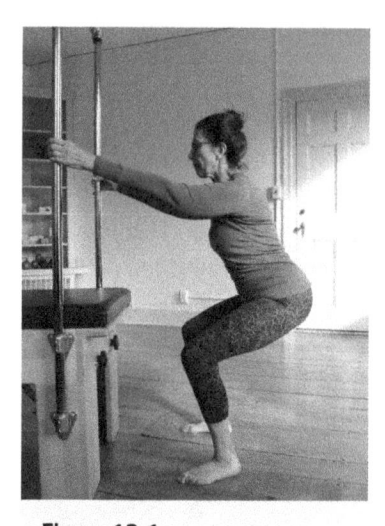

Figure 12.1

Starting position
- Stand facing kitchen sink holding onto front edge with both hands
- Feet approximately 18 in. (45 cm) away from edge
- Feet a little wider apart than shoulder-width distance, in slight external rotation
- Find equanimity in the four corners of each foot
- Gaze is forward and torso organized for the task

Movement description
- Inhale, perform hip and knee flexion as if about to sit on a chair
- Keep gaze forward, torso organized
- Keep knees over ankles
- Go slightly beyond 90 degrees of flexion
- Maintain balance in the four corners of the feet through the full squat
- Exhale to extend LE
- Return to starting position
- Repeat 25 times
- Progress to 100 repetitions

6. Elbow planks

Intent
- Integrate UE load toward maintaining bone density
- Activate torso in plank through UE continuity into torso

Gait reasoning
- Increase torso ability to be upright
- Torso and UE continuity for arm swing

Starting position
- Start in quadruped with forearms parallel on mat
- Feet dorsiflexed and metatarsals on the ground

Movement description
- Extend into plank
- Feet parallel and dorsiflexed
- Distance of xiphoid to pubis remains the same maintaining TLJ flexed
- Superior sternum and clavicles posteriorly rotated for upper thoracic extension
- Move chin toward chest and gaze slightly forward
- Hold position for 30 seconds
- Continue to breathe

7. Knee folds (See Chapter 5 in Volume 1, Gentry, Knee folds)

Intent
- Facilitate pelvifemoral flexion/extension
- Improve hip glide
- Proprioception of pelvis organization during LE movement

Gait reasoning
- Translate to standing pelvifemoral organization
- Improve ease of hip glide for leg swing
- Awareness of torso support in one-leg stance

Starting position
- Supine, knees flexed, feet planted on mat
- UE resting at sides

Movement description
- Exhale, flex right hip joint with lower limb dangling for proximal activation to 90 degrees
- Inhale in 90 degrees hip joint flexion
- Exhale, lower right LE to mat
- Repeat on left
- Alternate right to left
- Repeat 5–10 times each side
- Monitor pelvifemoral flexion/extension and avoid posterior or anterior pelvic rotation
- Progress to bilateral flexion/extension
- Repeat 10 times
- Progress to 20 repetitions

8. Pelvifemoral isometrics

Intent
- Facilitate bilateral activation of pelvifemoral joints to improve balance in standing
- Increase support for optimal medial glide of femoral head

Gait reasoning
- Facilitate lateral support during swing phase
- Increase bilateral medial glide of the hip joints during push-off

Starting position
- Supine on mat near a wall
- Place feet on wall with hip joints and knees flexed to 90 degrees
- Externally rotate and abduct right femur and place right ankle on left knee

Movement description
- Press knee toward the wall driving the hip joint into end range external rotation
- Maintain a strong and even contraction
- Hold for 30 seconds
- Progress to 60 seconds
- Repeat on other side

9. Side lying Leg Lifts (Black 2022)

Intent
- Activate femur on pelvis
- Enhance medial glide of femoral joint

Gait reasoning
- Minimize excessive movement of pelvis on femur during swing phase
- Improve congruency of hip joint for glide
- Improve balance
- Continuous activation of LE to torso

Starting position
- Lie on right side, back against a wall
- Left LE extended with heel against wall
- Right hip joint and knee flexion
- Head, thorax, and sacrum against wall
- Rest head on a support
- Pelvis stacked

Movement description
- Push back of left heel into wall and slide LE up wall
- Only abduct left LE as far as medial glide occurs and pelvis remains stacked
- Lift and lower 10 times
- Progress to 20 repetitions
- Repeat on other side

10. Shoulder extension in external rotation

Intent
- Continuous activation of UE to torso while standing
- Facilitate humeral head congruency

Gait reasoning
- Facilitate improved torso rotation and arm swing
- Improve humeral head congruency for ease in arm swing

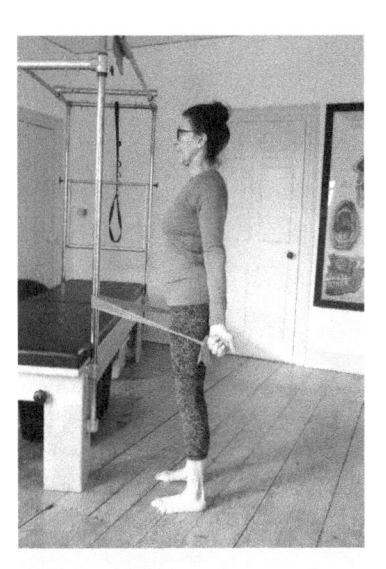

Figure 12.2

Starting position
- Anchor a light resistance band around a doorknob so that there are two even tails
- Stand facing the anchor point
- Hold the tails of the band, one in each hand
- Band a little slackened with UE by sides
- Externally rotate UE with elbows extended
- Palms facing forward

Movement description
- Exhale, retract scapulae with anteroposterior (AP) glide of humeral head for congruency
- Extend UE while maintaining scapula and humeral head positions
- Inhale, return to starting position
- Repeat 10 times
- Progress to 20 repetitions

Chapter 12

11. Standing push lunge

Intent
- Practice pushing through ball of the foot to propel body forward
- Transfer of weight (center of mass, COM) over foot
- Ground force distribution

Gait reasoning
- Coordination of extension and foot plantar flexion for push phase
- Train motor control for propulsion phase of gait

Starting position
- Stand in a short lunge in client's optimal organization for the movement task with right foot forward
- Right knee flexed, knee over ankle
- Left LE extended with left foot ankle dorsiflexion and metatarsal arch on mat
- Left knee slightly flexed
- For extra support, hold onto the edge of a kitchen sink

Movement description
- Push through the metatarsal arch to shift the body weight slightly forward by plantar flexing back foot
- Body weight moves slightly forward but not up
- Right leg maintains position
- Dorsiflex the ankle to release the left heel toward the ground
- Repeat 6–10 times on each side

12. Standing push lunge to heel lift (Black 2022)

Intent
- Transfer of weight (COM) over foot in one-leg stance
- Continuous activation from foot to torso with level changes
- Closed kinematic chain neuromuscular coordination
- Challenge balance with contralateral movement

Gait reasoning
- Improve extension patterning from LE to torso for the push-off phase of gait
- Minimize excessive lateral shifting of the pelvis during push-off phase of gait

Starting position
- Stand in short lunge facing a wall with right LE forward
- Place both hands on wall at shoulder height
- Client's optimal organization for movement task
- Right knee flexion, knee is over ankle
- Left LE extended with left foot ankle dorsiflexion and metatarsal arch on mat
- Left knee slightly flexed
- For extra support, hold onto edge of kitchen sink

Pilates and Aging Well: Effect on Gait

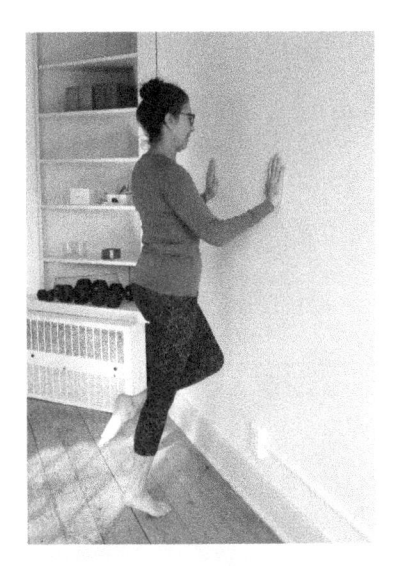

Figure 12.3

Movement description
- Push off left foot to bring the left hip joint and knee into 90 degrees flexion
- Simultaneously, plantar flex right LE with knee extension
- Return to the starting position
- Repeat 6–10 times on each side

Session 11/12: Studio session

Fatigue scale 7

Pain scale 1

Client self-report
- Client reports left medial knee pain and was treated by a physical therapist. The treatment addressed a medial torsion of tibia on femur and femoral and ankle articulation
- Discomfort abated after one treatment
- Feeling strong and energetic and more capable in all of her activities
- Noticing an increased capacity to perform daily activities with more ease and endurance
- Knee feels significantly more stable in snowshoeing and stair climbing

Chapter 12

Key changes observed by author at end of Session 3/12	• Improved one-leg stance balance • Good integration of whole-body movement with level changes • Increased confidence and neuromuscular coordination when balance and adaptability were challenged • Slight decrease of kyphosis due to overall weight distribution changes while standing
Reason behind choice of sequencing	• Increase proprioception and coordination of LE in Footwork • Cultivate coordination between movement and breath toward increasing presence, internal focus, and calm nervous system • Move from small movements to full body exercises and more complex choreography during an hour session • Progressively load during session and over time • Work in gravity to increase load for bone density • Challenge balance and adaptability toward increasing load and fall prevention

Session movement sequence

1. Footwork on Universal Reformer	Derivative of J. H. Pilates Footwork on Universal Reformer (NPCE Study Guide 2021, p. 52) and Running (NPCE Study Guide 2021, p. 60)
	
	• Footwork (five-part series)
	    ▪ Forefoot
	    ▪ Mid-foot
	    ▪ Rear foot
	    ▪ Running
	    ▪ Plantar flexion and dorsiflexion

Intent	• Facilitate breath with coordinated movement • Increase interoception and proprioception through internal focus, touch, and closed kinematic chain movement on Universal Reformer
Gait reasoning	• Focus on LE to torso patterning, coordination, and continuous activation • Establish breath and pelvifemoral movement as a concept • Increase awareness, load, and neuromuscular coordination of LE flexion and extension in all joints
Set-up	• Springs: 2 medium, 1 light, and 1 very light • Footbar in top position

Starting position	- Supine on Universal Reformer carriage
- Carriage wheels resting at stoppers
- Metatarsal arches on footbar
- UE resting at sides
- Footbar position supports 100 degrees of knee flexion
Movement description	Forefoot
- LE parallel and adducted
- Metatarsophalangeal (MTP) joints on bar
- Ankle dorsiflexion
- Heels under footbar

Mid-foot
- LE parallel and adducted
- Cuboid on bar
- Ankle dorsiflexion
- Heels under footbar
- Forefoot prehensile around footbar

Rearfoot
- Calcaneus on the bar
- Ankle fully dorsiflexed
- MTP joints neither extended nor flexed

Running
- LE parallel
- Feet hip-width-distance apart
- MTP joints on bar

Plantar flexion and dorsiflexion
- LE parallel, MTP joints on bar
- Feet hip-joint-distance apart

Forefoot, mid-foot, rear foot
- Bilateral flexion and extension
- Repeat 10 times in each position
- Small arcs of motion in 60 degrees of knee flexion
- Repeat 20 times in each position

Running
- Alternating right LE plantar flexion with knee extension and left LE dorsiflexion with knee flexion in a rhythmic pattern
- Repeat 10–20 times |

Chapter 12

Plantar flexion and dorsiflexion
- Bilateral plantar flexion and dorsiflexion with knee extension
- Repeat 10–20 times

CUES
- Exhale while extending
- Inhale while flexing
- Be attentive to maintain the rear foot through full knee extension
- Move through full ROM on both plantar flexion and dorsiflexion. Maintain weight distributed evenly through the forefoot. Imagine lifting the medial and lateral calcaneus evenly

Author note
While performing extension, a resistance band was placed behind the LE slightly higher than the knees to press against. This facilitates hip extension coordinated with knee extension. The client progresses to responding to a verbal cue to coordinate the extension without the band.

As people age, the loss of full ROM of plantar flexion and dorsiflexion occurs. Working toward full ROM of the ankle and foot is a mandate for all clients.

2. Leg Springs: Supine on Trapeze Table

Derivative of J. H. Pilates Leg Springs: Supine on Universal Reformer (NPCE Study Guide 2021, pp. 67–68)

Leg Springs Series sequence
- Flexion/abduction/external rotation/adduction/internal rotation to midline
- Legs parallel, adducted, hip and knee flexion/extension
- Hip flexion, abduction, external rotation, knee flexion, dorsiflexion with heels touching
- Hip abduction, external rotation, knee flexion, plantar flexion with toes apart

Intent
- Articulation of pelvifemoral, knee, and ankle joints through full ROM
- Closed kinematic chain from arch of foot through torso
- Train eccentric control during flexion increasing posterior glide of femoral head

Gait reasoning
- Motor control of gait pattern
- Optimizing femoral posterior glide with minimal load
- Stimulate hip joint synovium toward maintaining and improving glide

Set-up	• Medium leg springs anchored halfway up vertical bars or on crossrail
	• Feet in Y-loop straps to increase capacity to articulate foot
	• Hands holding uprights or down by sides
Starting position	• Supine on Trapeze Table
	• Feet in Y-loop double straps
	• Hip flexion, legs adducted, plantar flexion
Movement description	Flexion/abduction/external rotation/internal rotation to midline

- From starting position abduct, externally rotate legs
- Pull springs inferiorly in abduction and external rotation
- In low position, adduct legs to midline
- Strongly dorsiflex feet during flexion through midline
- Repeat 10 times
- Reverse directions and repeat 10 times

Legs parallel, adducted, hip and knee flexion/extension
- From starting position
- Flex hip joints and knees to 90 degrees
- Dorsiflex feet
- Extend knees
- Extend hip joints to 45 degrees of flexion
- Return to starting position
- Repeat 10 times

Hip flexion, abduction, external rotation, knee flexion, dorsiflexion with heels touching
- Hold starting position
- Extend and adduct LE with knee extension
- Heels together in dorsiflexion throughout movement
- Return to starting position
- Repeat 6 times

Hip abduction, external rotation, knee flexion, plantar flexion with toes apart
- From starting position abduct with knee extension
- Stay abducted
- Flex hip joints and knees and dorsiflex
- Abduct and externally rotate hip joints
- Center of knees in line with 2nd metatarsals
- Extend hip joints and knees, plantar flex foot staying abducted
- Repeat 6 times

Chapter 12

CUES
- While performing the Leg Springs Series on the Trapeze Table, observe the pelvifemoral rhythm and check that the pelvis remains in the client's optimal organization for the movement task
- Avoid anterior or posterior rotation
- Resist the springs for continuous activation of the LE through the entire series
- Movement should be fluid and connected

Author note
Be specific about foot activation. When the foot is dorsiflexed be attentive to have equanimity in the extension of the MTP, PIP, and DIP joints (see Editor note below). In plantar flexion the same holds true. Manually and verbally cue client through equal and balanced flexion in the joints of the foot and toes.

Check for even bilateral external rotation in all of the exercises of the Leg Springs Series.

Editor note
MTP refers to the metatarsophalangeal joints. PIP refers to the proximal interphalangeal joint. DIP refers to the distal interphalangeal joint. When there is even extension in each of these joints during dorsiflexion and even flexion in each of these joints when plantar flexing, it distributes the activation from the foot to the torso.

3. Pelvic Lift on Universal Reformer
J. H. Pilates Pelvic lift on Universal Reformer (NPCE Study Guide 2021, p. 60)

Intent
- Activation of extensors
- Control through LE to torso activation supine to pre-load the system

Gait reasoning
- Improve extension for push-off phase
- Improve femoral joint triplanar motions for transferring loads

Set-up
- Footbar in high or middle position
- Headrest down
- Springs: 2 medium or 1 medium and 1 light

Starting position
- Supine on Universal Reformer
- LE in parallel
- MTP joints of feet on footbar
- Heels slightly lifted

Movement description	- Exhale, pelvis lifts, hip extension without moving carriage
- Continuously articulate the torso in flexion inferiorly to superiorly to shoulder girdle
- Hold bridge position
- Push carriage halfway out to extend knees slightly
- Pull carriage back toward footbar
- Maintain LE parallel
- Repeat 6–10 times

CUES
- Maintain weight distribution through medial and lateral foot and knee
- Utilize prehensile foot to pull the carriage home
- Lift the pelvis only as high as hip joint will allow

Author note
Look for even activation from bottom of foot through the lower limb and coactivation at the pelvifemoral region.

4. Flat Back Elephant on Universal Reformer

Derivative of J. H. Pilates Long Stretch Series: Elephant (NPCE Study Guide 2021, p. 55)

Editor note
In Flat Back, the TLJ is supported by the counterbalance of anterior rotation of the lower thoracic ring and posterior rotation of the pelvic rim to bring the TLJ posterior. The torso is supported as a whole unit throughout the exercise. Spinal joint articulation is minimized. The primary articulation is at the pelvifemoral joints.

Intent	- Experience of gravity-assisted torso extension
- Work UE in closed kinematic chain
- Increase overall mobility and articulation
- Experience assisted hip flexion to activate flexors
- Address assessment finding of hyperkyphosis and associated forward head and shoulder organization
Gait reasoning	- Control LE flexion for swing through and transfer of weight
- Standing and UE weight bearing load the thoracodorsal fascia during femoral joint motions
Set-up	- Springs: 1 medium and 1 light
- Footbar in high position

Chapter 12

Starting position
- Hands on footbar shoulder-width distance apart
- Heels against shoulder stops, toes flexed
- Knees extended

Movement description
- Push carriage back with heels while maintaining shoulder and torso position
- Return carriage home
- Repeat 3–6 times

CUES
- Maintain upwardly rotated scapula, externally rotated humeri
- Allow springs to flex the LE when returning carriage
- Reach ischial tuberosities in opposition to LE flexion during return of carriage
- Maintain even distribution of weight through the feet

5. Long Stretch: Front on Universal Reformer
J. H. Pilates Long Stretch: Front on Universal Reformer (NPCE Study Guide 2021, p. 55)

Intent
- Challenging whole-body exercise for torso control through distal activation
- Facilitating loading the UE, LE, and torso in a horizontal position while moving against resistance from springs
- Closed kinematic chain exercise

Gait reasoning
- Facilitate torso organization for midline orientation to improve ability to rotate
- Ground force transmission from foot for continuous activation when foot transfers weight

Set-up
- Springs: 1 medium and 1 light

Starting position
- Hands on footbar shoulder-width distance apart
- Shoulders are over hands
- Feet on headrest, dorsiflexion with heel over ball of foot
- Body is in a plank position

Movement description
- On exhalation push the carriage away pressing from hands to torso, flexing shoulders
- Maintain position of LE and torso while performing the movement
- Inhale to return
- Repeat 3–6 times

Pilates and Aging Well: Effect on Gait

CUE
- Cue optimal organization of plank: shoulders over hands, scapula on thorax. LE actively adduct. TLJ anteriorly rotates to facilitate slight flexion throughout the movement. Sternum and clavicles in posterior rotation, with gaze slightly forward

Author note
The hip joints are fully extended to activate the continuity of LE and torso as opposed to remaining in hip flexion to hold the position.

6. Splits: Front on Universal Reformer — Derivative of J. H. Pilates Splits: Front on Universal Reformer (NPCE Study Guide 2021, p. 62)

Intent
- Eccentric load of knee extensors
- Challenge balance

Gait reasoning
- Increase range of knee extension during gait cycle
- Improve verticality and midline orientation during push-off
- Optimize LE joint positions to increase LE activation
- Facilitate pelvifemoral motion in extension unilaterally
- Activate LE in closed kinematic chain during lunge

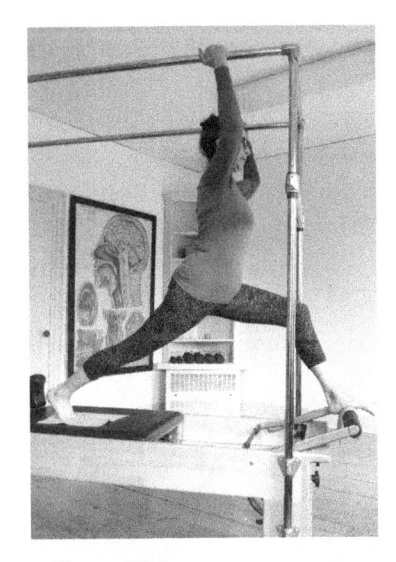

Figure 12.4

Chapter 12

Set-up	• Springs: 1 medium and 1 light • Footbar down • Standing platform attached • Hold pole for balance or overhead bars if Universal Reformer is a combination equipment
Starting position	• Standing on carriage facing footbar • Right foot on platform with knee flexed to 90 degrees • Heel of left foot on shoulder stop, knee extended • Torso upright in client's optimal organization for movement task • Pole in hand on same side as back LE
Movement description	• Keeping left knee extended, slightly extend and flex right knee, moving through a small ROM • Repeat 6–10 times • Maintain lunge position, right knee flexion • Flex and extend left knee slightly in comfortable ROM • Repeat 6–10 times

CUE
• Maintain the four corners of the foot weighted on both feet

Author note
Be confident in providing support while spotting clients in this exercise. This exercise challenges balance. Create a safe environment. For arthritic knee conditions, start slowly by holding the starting position, then progress through a minimal ROM. Increase to larger ROM when appropriate.

7. Skater on Universal Reformer	Derivative of J. H. Pilates Splits: Side on Universal Reformer (NPCE Study Guide 2021, p. 61)
Intent	• Posterior and lateral pelvifemoral activation in standing • Increase load for bone density • Medial glide of the femur head
Gait reasoning	• Increase activation in stance phase • Increase load • Improve extension for propulsion phase of gait

Pilates and Aging Well: Effect on Gait

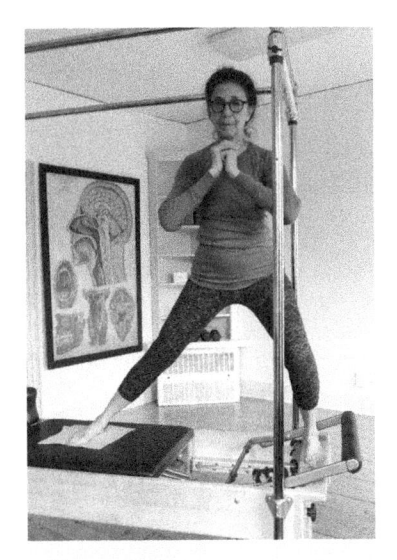

Figure 12.5

Set-up
- Medium spring
- Footbar down
- Standing platform attached

Starting position
- Stand on Universal Reformer facing the side
- Place one foot on platform and one foot on middle of carriage
- Start in a squat position
- Feet are balanced
- Knees are in alignment with 2nd toe
- Hands are clasped in front of chest and elbows are bent

Movement description
- Exhale, extend LE on carriage pushing carriage out, hold
- Maintain static hold in LE on platform
- Monitor torso organization throughout movement
- Return carriage home by flexing knee

CUE
- Look for medial glide of the femoral head on working leg

Author note
This exercise is good for increasing the load of the hip joints. The movement helps to integrate the client's home program with more complex and challenging movement that is analogous to the movement that the client engages in during winter outdoor sports.

8. Side Sit-Ups on Ladder Barrel

Derivative of J. H. Pilates Side Sit-Ups on Ladder Barrel (NPCE Study Guide 2021, p. 84)

- **Intent**
  - Strengthen core
- **Gait reasoning**
  - Improve verticality toward optimizing gait pattern
  - Engage medial line of LE continuity to torso
- **Set-up**
  - Set up the barrel appropriately for the person's height
- **Starting position**
  - Stand between ladder and barrel facing sideways with right pelvis on barrel
  - LE in front-to-back split stance with right LE to front
  - Both knees extended
  - Hands are behind head, elbows flexed
  - Torso in optimal organization for the task
- **Movement description**
  - Translate thorax to right, leaning toward barrel
  - Laterally flex torso over barrel
  - Initiate the return from the top
  - Pressing into the feet
  - Return to starting position
  - Repeat 10–20 times
  - Repeat on the other side

CUES
- Ground through the feet as the head and torso return to starting position
- Add rotation at end ranges as a progression

Author note
Watch for lateral shift of the thorax away from the barrel in the initial motion and inhibit this propensity through touch or verbal cueing.

9. Pulling Straps 1 with triceps extension on Universal Reformer

- **Intent**
  - Activate and integrate extension from all planes
  - Activate scapular retractors and posterior shoulder to counteract forward head and shoulders
  - Counteract hyperkyphosis, rounded shoulder, and forward head organization
  - Introduce an exercise to reinforce and complexify home program exercise: triceps extension exercise in external rotation performed with anchored light resistance band

Gait reasoning	• Organize torso for optimal midline orientation for improved torso rotation through increased extension
Set-up	• Medium spring • Footbar is down • Long box on Universal Reformer
Starting position	• Prone on long box, chest just off end of box • UE are extended on outside of frame holding straps • Extended torso • Feet plantar flexed
Movement description	• Exhale, pull straps to extend shoulders, bringing hands toward pelvis • Simultaneously extend torso • Return to starting position • Repeat 3–6 times • Progress to adding triceps extension

CUES
- When initiating UE extension, move the humeri in antero-posterior glide for congruency of the glenohumeral joints
- Extensors activated through action of feet through torso
- Head is organized with chin toward sternum and sternum toward chin

The journey to Session 11

Session 4/12
Client self-report

- Pain scale 0
- Fatigue scale (post-session) 7
- "Always feel good about the sessions. Feels great to be encouraged in building and demonstrating my strength physically and in my spirit"
- Client reports increased vitality, strength, and mastery of the movements

Key changes observed

- Confidence in capacity to perform exercises has increased
- Performance anxiety has decreased
- Balance has improved
- Vitality has increased

Reasoning behind choice of movements

- Repetition of choreography has been a hallmark of programming choices because of limited time of case study
- When mastery of exercises becomes apparent small incremental challenges are implemented
- UE loading to counteract forward head and shoulders and flexion of thorax assessed in gait

Session movement sequence
1. Universal Reformer

- Footwork
    - Forefoot

Chapter 12

- Mid-foot
- Rearfoot
- Running
- Plantar flexion and dorsiflexion
● Pelvic Lift
● Flat Back Elephant
● Long Stretch
● Splits: Front
● Skater
● Pulling Straps with triceps extension, 1 and 2

2. Trapeze Table

● Leg Springs Series
● Side lying Leg Springs

3. Ladder Barrel

● Side Sit-Ups

4. Additional movement

● Standing UE circle with thoracic rotation against wall

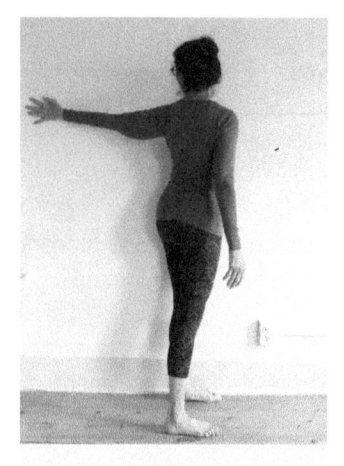

Figure 12.6

● Side lying, resistance-band-loaded thoracic rotation with internal and external rotation of UE

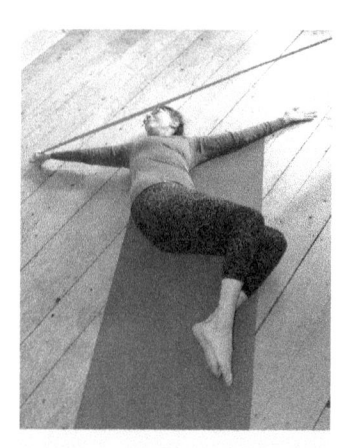

Figure 12.7

● Cervical extension and rotation/extension exercise to address forward head organization

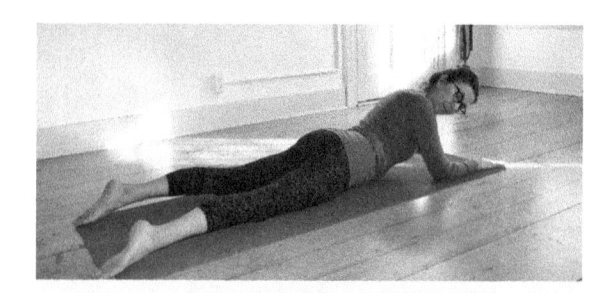

Figure 12.8

● Supine hip traction with belt against the wall

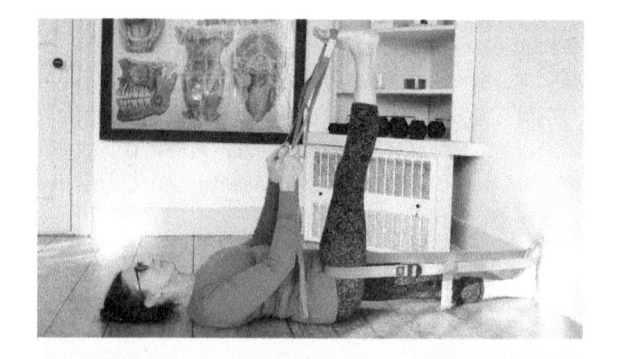

Figure 12.9

430

- Lateral torso flexion with ball against the wall

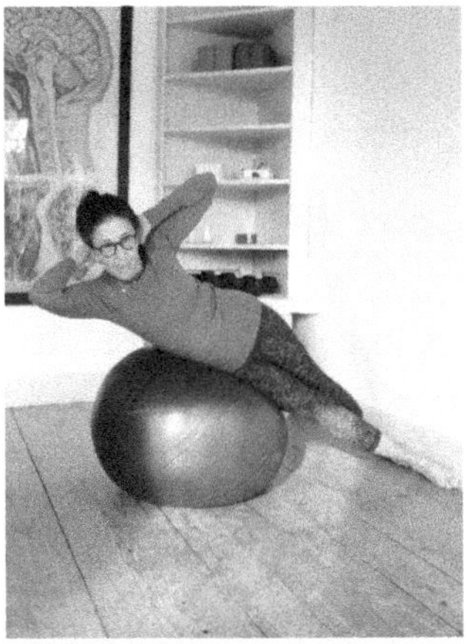

Figure 12.10

Session 5/12
Client self-report

- Pain scale 0
- Fatigue scale (post-session) 7
- "Starting to feel the effects of our work on my capacity to execute daily activities. I feel more connection in my abs"

Key changes observed

- Able to execute exercise with ease and confidence
- Neuromuscular coordination and capacity to remember exercises has improved
- Bilateral thoracic rotation has increased
- Left thoracic rotation and left shoulder horizontal extension improved as observed in standing UE circle against wall
- No report of soreness even though there are strength gains

Reasoning behind choice of movements

- Repetition toward confidence and mastery
- Working toward increasing extension activation
- Increase in bilateral thoracic rotation, which was limited in gait, especially to left
- Couple shoulder mobility with thoracic rotation toward more ease in UE during gait

Session movement sequence
1. Universal Reformer

- Footwork
  - Forefoot
  - Mid-foot
  - Rear foot
  - Running
  - Plantar flexion and dorsiflexion
- Pelvic Lift
- Flat Back Elephant
- Long Stretch
- Splits: Front, no gondola pole used but spotted for safety and security
- Skater
- Splits: Side (1 spring: very light or light)
- Pulling Straps with triceps extension, 1 and 2

2. Trapeze Table

- Leg Springs Series

3. Ladder Barrel

- Side Sit-Ups

4. Additional movements

- Standing UE circle with thoracic rotation against wall
- Side lying, resistance-band-loaded thoracic rotation with internal and external rotation of UE
- Cervical extension and rotation/extension exercise to address forward head organization

- Added rotation in flexion and extension to lateral flexion on Ladder Barrel to support increased thoracic mobility
- Seated closed kinematic chain triceps extension exercise

Session 6/12
Client self-report

- Pain scale 0
- Fatigue scale (post-session) 7
- "Am grateful for the personalized attention and program—not done a 1–1 program like this before. Feel that I am gaining knowledge of my body—the symmetries and asymmetries—in a supportive environment"

Key changes observed

- Verticality attainable in session without cueing or coaching
- Improved glide of femoral head in Skater and Splits: Front
- Mental state positive that affects client's capacity to do more repetitions
- Increasingly comfortable in level changes: from sit, to kneel, to stand on equipment

Reasoning behind choice of movements

- Added pulling UE to increase effort
- Create new challenges by standing on Trapeze Table
- Increase ability to grip

Session movement sequence

1. Foam rolling of posterior and lateral pelvis added to improve hip glide

2. Universal Reformer

- Footwork
  - Forefoot
  - Mid-foot
  - Rear foot
  - Running
  - Plantar flexion and dorsiflexion
- Pelvic Lift
- Flat Back Elephant
- Long Stretch
- Splits: Front, no gondola pole used but spotted for safety and security
- Skater
- Splits: Side (spring: 1 very light or light)
- Pulling Straps with triceps extension, 1 and 2

3. Trapeze Table

- Leg Springs Series
- Squats standing on Trapeze Table grasping top bars
- UE Hang

4. Ladder Barrel

- Side Sit-Ups

5. Additional movements

- Side lying supine, resistance-band-loaded thoracic rotation with internal and external rotation of UE
- Cervical extension and rotation/extension exercise to address forward head organization
  - Lie in supine position to increase posterior glide of femoral heads
  - Positioned near wall, legs are flat on floor, feet flat on wall
  - Extend one LE toward ceiling, place yoga strap around the ball of dorsiflexed foot
  - Practitioner places another yoga strap around superior aspect of femur and applies gentle traction caudad

Session 7/12
Client self-report

- Pain scale 0
- Fatigue scale (post-session) 7
- "I continue to feel more capable and stronger. I feel great after our sessions. Consistency feels important"

Key changes observed

- Consistently self-reports gains with each session
- Observable improvement is evident due to client's strong vitality and fitness level prior to the start of this project
- Improved verticality in gait and gaze is forward
- Client has more thoracic rotation bilaterally in gait, right side is still preferred

Reasoning behind choice of movements

- Repetition of exercises introduced in previous sessions towards client mastery

Session movement sequence
1. Squats: advancing squats from 50 a day holding on to sink to unsupported squats

- Client will start with 15 unsupported squats and add 15 every day until she gets to 60 unsupported

2. Universal Reformer

- Footwork
    - Forefoot
    - Mid-foot
    - Rear foot
    - Running
    - Plantar flexion and dorsiflexion
- Pelvic Lift
- Flat Back Elephant
- Long Stretch
- Splits: Front, no gondola pole used but spotted for safety and security
- Skater
- Splits: Side (spring: 1 very light or light)
- Pulling Straps with triceps extension, 1 and 2

3. Trapeze Table

- Leg Springs Series
- Squats standing on table grasping top bars
- UE Hang

4. Ladder Barrel

- Side Sit-Ups

5. Additional movements

- Supine, resistance-band-loaded thoracic rotation; added internal and external rotation of UE
- Cervical extension and rotation/extension exercise to address forward head organization
- Added rotation in flexion and extension to Side Sit-Ups on Ladder Barrel
- Supine with a yoga belt around superior aspect of femur to increase posterior glide of femoral heads

Session 8/12
Client self-report

- Pain scale 0
- Fatigue scale (post-session) 7
- "Sessions are feeling more challenging. It feels good"

Key changes observed

- It appears changes are being maintained and increased
- Mental state is consistently positive—curious and willing to work hard

Chapter 12

- Increased thoracic rotation but needs to be consistently reinforced through movement additions
- Mental state seems to adversely affect uprightness; after sessions client's mood is lighter and less anxious

Reasoning behind choice of movements

- Consistency and increased load in exercises and movements that are familiar
- Second and third sets of exercises were added to established program, specifically: Long Stretch, Splits: Front, Skater, Splits: Side, Pulling Straps with triceps extension, squats standing on Trapeze Table, UE Hang on Trapeze Table

Session movement sequence

1. Added circular resistance band to bridging series

2. Increased plank hold to two 1 minute timings

3. Universal Reformer

- Footwork
    - Forefoot
    - Mid-foot
    - Rear foot
    - Running
    - Plantar flexion and dorsiflexion
- Pelvic Lift
- Flat Back Elephant
- Long Stretch
- Splits: Front, no gondola pole used but spotted for safety and security
- Skater
- Splits: Side (spring: 1 very light or light)
- Pulling Straps with triceps extension, 1 and 2

4. Trapeze Table

- Leg Springs Series
- Squats standing on table grasping top bars
- UE Hang

5. Ladder Barrel

- Side Sit-Ups

6. Additional movements

- Supine, resistance-band-loaded thoracic rotation; added internal and external rotation of UE
- Cervical extension and rotation/extension exercise during prone movements to address forward head orientation
- Added rotation in flexion and extension to Side Sit-Ups on Ladder Barrel to support increased thoracic articulation

Session 9/12
Client self-report

- Pain scale 3
- Fatigue scale (post-session) 6
- "Getting into the groove of doing the home exercises well and effectively. Have been doing them all along; now feel they are more integrated"

Key changes observed

- Client arrived feeling pain in left medial knee—an apparent medial rotation of tibia on femur—referred her to the physical therapist (PT)
- Client's commitment to the home program has affected her agency in movement, her balance, and kinesthesia
- Successfully integrated movement strategies that reinforce the specific cueing based on her structure

Reasoning behind choice of movements

- Minimized the LE loading specifically by replacing standing on Universal Reformer with supine and side lying positions on Universal Reformer and Trapeze Table
- Focused on torso movement in all planes
- Eccentric load of LE
- Due to client report, decreased or ceased movement irritating knee; home program continues without pain or discomfort

Session movement sequence

1. Supported squats

- Reduced repetitions to 30 or, if pain, no squats

2. Universal Reformer

- Footwork
    - Forefoot
    - Mid-foot
    - Rear foot
    - Running
    - Plantar flexion and dorsiflexion
- Pelvic Lift
- Flat Back Elephant
- Long Stretch

3. Trapeze Table

- Leg Springs Series
- UE Hang
- Teaser with push-through bar
- Side lying Leg Springs
    - Leg Lifts
    - Abduction/flexion/extension/adduction

4. Ladder Barrel

- Side Sit-Ups

5. Wunda Chair

- Supine unilateral LE extension

6. Additional movements

- Eccentric knee flexion with resistance band
    - Supine in hook lying position
    - Place resistance band over plantar surface of MTP joints and phalanges
    - Foot plantar flexed
    - Take tails of resistance band and anchor them under the same side of pelvis
    - Keeping knees level, extend resistance-band-loaded knee and slowly descend
    - Repeat 8–10 times

Session 10/12
Client self-report

- Pain scale 0
- Fatigue scale (post-session) 6
- "Learning about my knee issues—grateful for the opportunity to see the connection between the knee pain and other functional/structural issues. Another piece to address and work on. With the opportunity to see a PT in conjunction with my session with Kelly I feel very good about addressing the hip, knee, ankle issues! Great sessions with both and I appreciate their communication with one another"

Key changes observed

- Presented pain free after the last session in conjunction with session with PT
- Returned to established program with minimal modification
- Demonstrated a primary principle of aging well: capacity to adapt and heal quickly

Chapter 12

Reasoning behind choice of movements

- Assess and correct through manual and verbal cueing, fibular mobility in plantar flexion and dorsiflexion during Footwork
- Ensure proper subtalar joint mobility in plantar flexion and dorsiflexion during Footwork
- Activate LE in all planes

Session movement sequence
1. Eccentric knee flexion with resistance band

2. Universal Reformer

- Footwork
  - Forefoot
  - Mid-foot
  - Rear foot
  - Running
  - Plantar flexion and dorsiflexion
- Pelvic Lift
- Flat Back Elephant
- Long Stretch

3. Trapeze Table

- Leg Springs Series
- Squats standing on table grasping top bars
- UE Hang
- Teaser with push-through bar
- Side lying Leg Springs
  - Leg Lifts
  - Abduction/flexion/extension/adduction
- Squats standing on Trapeze Table grasping top bars

4. Ladder Barrel

- Side Sit-Ups

5. Wunda Chair

- Supine unilateral LE extension

6. Additional movement

- Bridge with Magic Circle
  - Adduct and abduct legs
  - Repeat 10 times

References

Black, M. (2022) *Centered: Organizing the Body through Kinesiology, Movement Theory and Pilates Techniques*. Edinburgh: Handspring Publishing, pp. 87–88.

Hamczyk, M. R., Nevado, R. M., Barettino, A., Fuster, V., and Andrés, V. (2020) "Biological versus chronological aging: JACC Focus Seminar." *Journal of the American College of Cardiology, 75,* 8, 919–930.

NPCE Study Guide (National Pilates Certification Exam Study Guide) (2021) Miami, FL: National Pilates Certification Program, Inc.

WHO (World Health Organization) (2020) Ageing and health. October 1, 2020. www.who.int/news-room/fact-sheets/detail/ageing-and-health. [Accessed September 21, 2023].

Chapter 13

Pilates and Arrhythmogenic Right Ventricular Cardiomyopathy/Dysplasia: Effect on Gait

Jo Strutt

Arrhythmogenic right ventricular cardiomyopathy/dysplasia (ARVC/D)—a form of heart disease that usually appears in adulthood—is a disorder of the myocardium, the muscular wall of the heart. The myocardium breaks down over time, increasing the risk of an abnormal heartbeat (arrhythmia) and sudden death.

ARVC/D may not cause any symptoms in the early stages. Affected individuals may still be at risk of sudden death, especially during strenuous exercise. Common symptoms include a sensation of fluttering or pounding in the chest (palpitations), light-headedness, and fainting (syncope). Over time, ARVC/D can cause shortness of breath and abnormal swelling in the legs or abdomen. If the myocardium becomes severely damaged it can lead to heart failure (HF).

> ...the Pilates method may be a beneficial adjunctive treatment that enhances functional capacity in patients with HF... (Guimarães *et al.* 2012)

Diagnosis is based on meeting a set of specific criteria:

- Electrocardiogram (ECG) abnormalities
- Arrhythmias
- Structural abnormalities/tissue characteristics
- Family history
- Genetics

In a normal heart, the cells of the heart muscle are held together by proteins. In people with ARVC/D, these proteins have not developed properly and cannot keep the heart muscle cells together when under stress—such as when the heart is beating faster or working harder than normal, for example during exercise. The detached, damaged, dead heart muscle cells become fibrous. Fatty deposits build up in an attempt to repair the damage and cause scarring. As a result, the walls of the ventricle become thin and stretched, which means the heart cannot pump effectively.

Changes to the heart muscle cells mean the normal passage of electrical impulses through the heart are interrupted or altered and can cause life-threatening arrhythmias and, in some cases, sudden cardiac death.

Treatments
1. Beta blocker medication

2. Catheter ablation
An endocardial ablation treats the muscle in the inside surface of the heart via catheters sent through veins in the legs. The arrhythmic area is located and destroyed.

As many ARVC/D arrhythmias come from the outside of the heart an epicardial ablation procedure is where the catheter goes under the breastbone and into the sac around the heart.

3. Implantable cardioverter defibrillator (ICD)

An ICD is a small, thin, battery-powered device implanted just under the skin in the chest region and is designed to deliver a shock to restore normal cardiac rhythm.

Daily light exercise is safe for most people with ARVC/D.

> ...gait is a marker for overall health. (Dommershuijsen *et al.* 2019)

Other considerations

- In utero, the heart starts as a tube, spirals into shape, and beats from week 5
- The vagus nerve (10th cranial nerve) and cardiac accelerator nerves at T4–T5 moderate the heart (for additional information on the vagus nerve see Chapter 11, Volume 1)
- Heart attachments to sternum/pleura linings, hyoid, sternoclavicular joint
- The heart is located superiorly to and on top of the diaphragm in its pericardial sac; fluid fascial glide between the lungs
- The heart spins blood to the lungs for gaseous exchange throughout the body
- Front/back heart chakra, front/back solar plexus chakra, emotional physiological influences

Client description: 53-year-old biological female, identifies as female; aesthetician and mother

Dates of case report: Session 1: January 8, 2020; Session 12: February 13, 2020

Studio apparatus and props
Pilates equipment

- Trapeze Table
- Universal Reformer with clinical adaption
- Jump board
- Wunda Chair with split pedal
- Ladder Barrel

Props used with equipment

- 10 (25 cm) Overball
- Weighted ball
- Resistance band, heavy, 5 ft (170 cm)
- Mat

Home program props

- Roller
- 10 in. (25 cm) Overball
- Spikey balls
- Resistance band, heavy, 5 ft (170 cm)
- 26 in. (65 cm) ball
- 2 lb (1 kg) hand weights
- Chair
- Weighted prop (ball or sandbag)
- Mat

Methods and materials

Session 1/12
1. Health history interview

- Three children—all vaginal deliveries, left fallopian tube removed
- May 2007: ARVC/D diagnosed aged 40—an avid cardio exerciser, client discovered heart rate at 200 bpm on treadmill at gym. She was prescribed beta blocker medication (180 mg) with annual cardiology appointment checks
- December 2018: shingles
- April 2019: ventricular tachycardia ablation endoscopy
- April 2019: diagnosed coeliac
- May 2019: ICD fitted
- August 2019: epicardial and endocardial ablation
- December 2019: beta blocker medication reduced to 80 mg
- January–March 2020: DEXA (bone density) scan postponed due to COVID

2. Symptoms

- Constant right-sided lateral hip pain 8/10 (trochanteric bursitis)
- Low back pain 8/10
- Thoracic kyphosis
- Left-sided upper neck pain
- Headaches
- ICD slipped under left armpit immediately after operation, heart rate increases when raising left arm. Discomfort on left humeral adduction and sleeping
- Perimenopausal/menopausal: flushes, heat, mood swings, palpitations/anxiety
- Experiences kinesiophobia

3. Movement aids

- No movement aids
- Heart aid—ICD—implanted just under skin in chest region, designed to deliver a shock to restore normal cardiac rhythm if rate is over 150 bpm

---

Final result of case report

Client shows a reduction of forward head posture and overall improved sagittal plane organization. Decreased pain. Improved gait patterning overall. Improved reciprocal motion of thorax and pelvis. Increased stride length and pace. Even arm swing coordinated with strides. Feet articulate well from heel strike to push-off. Integrated smooth movements, walks with confidence.

Chapter 13

Session 2/12: Initial assessment

1. General observations of gait

- Eye gaze down, forward head position
- Limited thoracic rotation, excessive kyphosis
- Right hemipelvis superior motion on right step
- Uncoordinated reciprocal rotation of pelvis and thorax
- Reduced hip extension, short strides
- Right foot pronates
- Left foot flattens
- Left knee hyperextends, tibial torsion foot swivel on propulsion

2. Standing tests

- Full torso rotation
- Observations of inefficient sides: both
  - Right
    - Pelvic rotation to right at start
    - Limited thoracic articulation
    - Tibia and feet do not adapt
  - Left
    - Rotation occurs at thoracolumbar junction (TLJ)
    - Limited thoracic articulation
    - Tibia and feet do not adapt
- Hemipelvis inferior motion
- Observations of inefficient sides: both
  - Left
    - Hemipelvis, no lowering
    - Thorax translates left and flexes
  - Right
    - Hemipelvis, no lowering

Session 12/12: Post-assessment

1. General observations of gait

- Eye gaze lifted, less forward head
- Improved torso rotation, decreased kyphosis
- Smoother transference of weight and dissipation of ground forces
- Improved reciprocal motions of pelvis and thorax
- Increased hip extension, longer stride
- Reduced talus medial collapse, less pronation in both feet
- Reduced tibial torsion and ball of foot swivel on propulsion

2. Standing tests

- Full torso rotation
- Observations of inefficient side: right
  - Right
    - Pelvis orientated facing forward
    - Right limited thoracic rotation
    - Pelvis initiates rotation
    - Tibia and feet do not adapt
  - Left
    - Improved thorax articulation
    - Improved tibia and feet adaptation
- Hemipelvis inferior motion
- Observations of inefficient side: left
  - Hemipelvis, no lowering
  - Whole torso rotates right
- Hemipelvis superior motion
- Observations of inefficient side: right

440

- - - Pelvis rotates right with increased left hip flexion and adduction
  - Torso follows rotation
- ◆ Hemipelvis superior motion
- ● Observations of inefficient side: left
  - ■ Left hemipelvis unable to elevate
  - ■ Thorax translates right
  - ■ Mild supination on heel raise
- ◆ Lateral pelvic shift
- ● Observations of inefficient sides: both
  - ■ Right
    - Increased left foot pronation
  - ■ Left
    - Hemipelvis moves anteriorly
    - Thorax rotates right
    - Transfers weight to lateral left foot decreasing pronation, unable to supinate
    - Right foot pronates

3. Seated tests

- ◆ Thoracic rotation
- ● Observations of inefficient sides: both
  - ■ Right
    - Thorax increased flexion
    - Posteriorly rotated pelvis
    - Head forward
    - No segmental rotation through thorax
  - ■ Left
    - Rotates from TLJ
- ◆ Hip joint and knee flexion
- ● Observations of inefficient side: both
  - ■ Begins seated posteriorly on ischial tuberosities
  - ■ Increases torso flexion

- - ■ Pelvis rotates right with weight shift onto left leg
  - ■ Mild supination on heel raise
- ◆ Lateral pelvic shift
- ● Observations of inefficient sides: both
  - ■ Right
    - Thorax laterally flexes left
  - ■ Left
    - Hemipelvis rotates left
    - Femur internally rotates and adducts
    - Left foot pronates

3. Seated tests

- ◆ Thoracic rotation
- ● Observations of inefficient side: right
  - ■ Improved thorax relative to pelvis orientation
  - ■ Improved segmental articulation of thorax, left more efficient than right
- ◆ Hip joint and knee flexion
- ● Observations of inefficient side: right
  - ■ Reduced pelvic posterior rotation
  - ■ Maintains sagittal curvatures

Author note

Included dorsiflexion and knee flexion test. Left was inefficient. Reduction of left hemipelvis posterior rotation. Maintains anterior-posterior curves. Included hip abduction with external rotation. Left was inefficient. Maintains anterior-posterior curves, no lateral flexion.

Chapter 13

> **Author note**
> Included dorsiflexion and knee flexion test. Left was inefficient. Left hemiplevis posteriorly rotated. Included hip abduction with external rotation. Left was inefficient. To achieve the task, the torso laterally flexed left.

4. Sit and stand

- Lateral view
  - Right lateral view
    - Shoulder elevates to sit
    - Torso flexes to sit
    - Right pelvic rotation on standing
    - Forefoot extends
  - Left lateral view
    - Shoulder elevates to sit
    - Pelvis anteriorly rotates to sit and stand
    - Forefoot extends
- Anterior view

- Femurs adduct as weight transfers to standing, more on right than left
- Pelvis rotates right on knee extension
- Right knee hyperextension
- Forefoot extension on sit
- Cervical region hyperextends

5. Standing balance

- Two-leg stance, eyes open
- 60 seconds
- One-leg stance, eyes open

- Right leg: 60 seconds
- Left leg: 45 seconds
- Unable to balance with eyes closed on either leg

4. Sit and stand

- Lateral view
  - Right and left
    - Anterior-posterior curves better organized
    - Reduced forward head
    - Improved hip flexion to sit and hip extension to sit
- Anterior view

- Midline orientation maintained
- Femurs adduct less with weight transferred centrally
- Reduced pelvic rotation on knee extension
- Reduced right knee hyperextension
- Increased range of motion (ROM) of hip flexion, no forefoot extension
- No cervical hyperextension

5. Standing balance

- Two-leg stance, eyes open
- 60 seconds
- One-leg stance, eyes open

- Right leg: 60 seconds
- Left leg: 60 seconds

- One-leg stance, eyes closed

- Right leg: 10–15 seconds
- Left leg: 10–15 seconds

Session 3/12: Home program

Fatigue scale	8
Pain scale	8
Client self-report	• Client feels perpetually twisted with constant pain in right hip (8/10), low back pain (8/10), right-sided low level neck pain (1/10), and right and left shoulder pain. She is aware of kyphosis and forward head
Key changes observed by author at end of Session 3/12	• Improved anterior-posterior curves, reduced thoracic flexion • Reduced to 4/10 pain in low back and hips, 0/10 pain in shoulders • Became aware of the challenge to use breath with movement
Reason behind choice of sequencing	• Increase awareness of lower extremity (LE) organization in sitting, standing, and transitions • Improve foot loading with hip extension • Contralateral upper extremity (UE) and LE patterning • Breath work for thoracic articulation

Session movement sequence

1. Standing left hip joint extension and seated right hip joint external rotation/flexion

Editor note
These exercises are only performed on one side and in sequence. Left hip extension is followed by seated right hip joint external rotation/flexion. The author's intention is to use the oppositional hip joint placement with specific and mid-range movement. This stimulates a gliding motion of the hip joint in different planes to facilitate the minimizing of right pelvic rotation orientation.

Intent	• Self-care for pelvic organization prior to beginning home program • Minimize right pelvic rotation orientation
Gait reasoning	• Improve foot to torso adaptability to ground forces • Femoral joint centration for improved force transmission

Chapter 13

Starting position
1. Standing left hip joint extension
- Standing with back to chair
- Place left dorsal foot on chair, knee flexed in alignment with hip joint
- Right standing LE knee extended

2. Seated right hip joint external rotation/flexion
- Sitting on chair, knees extended in front

Movement description
1. Standing left hip joint extension
- Flex and extend right standing knee 10 times

2. Seated right hip joint external rotation/flexion
- Cross right ankle over left ankle maintaining evenly weighted ischial tuberosities
- Trace right ankle up left LE to above knee
- Flex left knee, foot flat on floor
- Right hand under right knee
- Left hand on right ankle
- Extend torso leaning forward increasing hip joint flexion
- Once each side for 10 breath cycles

2. Roller: Thoracic extension

Intent
- Facilitate thoracic articulation
- Focus breath to sense sternal movement
- Use lung and heart imagery with torso articulation
- Eye gaze to enhance flexion/extension
- Feet pushing and pulling for dynamic whole-body motion

Gait reasoning
- Improve verticality by activating posterior torso concentrically and anterior torso eccentrically
- Improve segmental anterior-posterior articulation through foot loading
- Establish midline orientation before rotation

Starting position
- Seated on mat, knees flexed, feet on mat
- Place roller horizontally behind torso
- Lie back to mid-thorax onto roller
- Fingers interlinked and pulling apart, cradling skull
- Elbows in peripheral vision

Movement description
- Inhale, extend torso over roller
- Exhale, flex torso
- Maintain head to cervical organization, no chin lifting or lowering
- 8–10 repetitions

CUES
- Imagery: drape upper lungs over roller allowing heart and sternum to lift on inhale
- Initiate exhale with sinking of heart between lungs into middle of back between shoulder blades

3. Roller: Bridge with plantar flexion and dorsiflexion

Intent
- Activate feet to torso for hip extension as gravity assists extension
- Increase plantar flexion maintaining knee flexion and hip extension for propulsion phase
- Increase dorsiflexion for heel strike
- Self-massage posterior torso

Gait reasoning
- Activate extensors
- Improve plantar flexion for push-off
- Improve dorsiflexion for stance

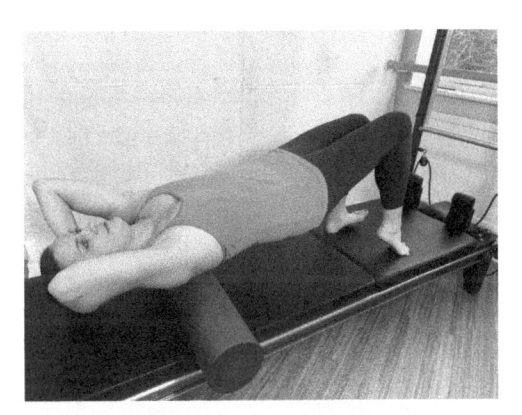

Figure 13.1

Starting position	- Seated on mat, knees flexed, feet on mat
- Roller placed horizontally behind torso
- Lying with mid-thorax on roller
- Fingers interlinked and pulling apart, cradling skull
- Elbows in peripheral vision
Movement description	- Inhale
- Exhale, extend hip joints into bridge
- Maintain neck alignment—no chin lifting or lowering
- Transfer weight through feet, plantar flexion and dorsiflexion
- Roll roller superiorly and inferiorly along posterior torso
- 8–10 times
- Inhale on plantar flexion
- Exhale on dorsiflexion

4. Coordination of hip joints with balls

Intent	- Increase hip joint articulation in all planes
- Centralize glenohumeral joints
- Homologous, homolateral, and contralateral patterning at glenohumeral and hip joints
Gait reasoning	- Coordination of contralateral patterning at glenohumeral and hip joints
- Integrate crossing midline in three-dimensional movement

Author note

Homologous refers to the symmetrical movement through midline orientation of both UE and both LE. Homolateral refers to the first asymmetrical patterns establishing sidedness and lateral orientation. Focusing on the connection of both UE and both LE (homologous), before alternating right arm, right leg with left arm, left leg (homolateral) aids the integration of opposite contralateral right arm and left leg, fine tuning the three-dimensional helical movement pattern found in gait (Bainbridge Cohen 2018).

Starting position	- Supine, spikey balls under pelvis at the posterior hip joints
- Hip joints and knees flexed beyond 90 degrees flexion
- Lower limb hanging
- Hands holding knees, fingertips facing medially, humerus in relaxed external rotation

Movement description	• Flex elbows increasing hip joint flexion
• Extend elbows increasing hip joint extension
• Repeat 5 times
• Move from hip joint flexion to extension, to abduction/flexion
• Reverse
• Repeat 5 times
• Flex right elbow and extend elbow, alternating hip joint flexion and extension
• Repeat 5 times
• Add alternating abduction/flexion/extension in figure 8 pattern
5. Roller: Four movements	• Lateral thoracic flexion
• Rotating thorax
• UE with thoracic rotation
• Diagonals
Intent	• Segmental lateral translation of torso
• Move UE through all planes to stimulate connective tissue glide
• Sensing spiral movement patterns of UE and torso

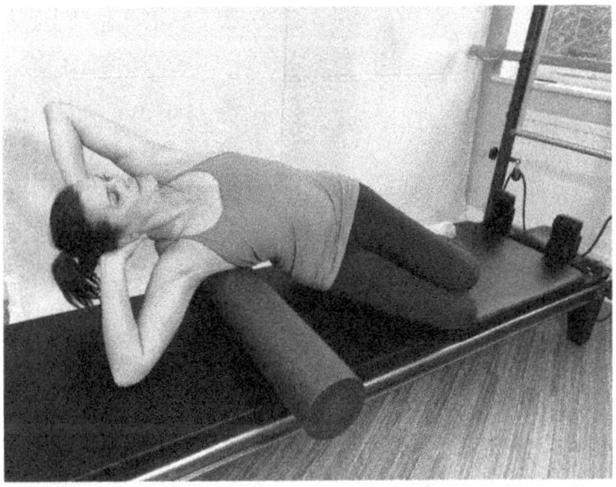

Figure 13.2

Author note

Use imagery of spirals of the arterial/venous, lymphatic systems flow throughout the torso. Coordinate the breath with the flow sensations. Interoception of the breath may cause an overwhelm of strong emotions.

Chapter 13

Editor note
Interoception is one of two neural pathways of the primary sense of proprioception. It is processed in the insular cortex of the brain. Interoception is a sense of the physiological world, including sensations from viscera, muscular effort, tickling, and sensual touch (Schleip and Jaeger 2012).

Gait reasoning	• Increase proprioception of thoracic movement using imagery of helical motions of heart, lungs, and organs above diaphragm
• Feel thorax and glenohumeral joint to improve arm swing
• Improve relative counter-rotations of pelvis and thorax
Starting position	• Sitting on mat on right lateral hemipelvis
• Hip joints and knees flexion, feet together
• Hands interlinked behind head, elbows in peripheral vision
• Roller perpendicular to torso at the level of the heart
Movement description	• Inhale, right lateral thoracic flexion over roller moving roller toward pelvis
• Exhale, push roller away, left lateral flexion
• Repeat 6–8 times
• Inhale, left thoracic rotation
• Exhale, right thoracic rotation
• Repeat 6–8 times
• Slide left LE extending knee, foot dorsiflexed, heel in line with ischial tuberosity
• Reach left hand to touch superior scapula
• Maintain left hand on scapula
• Inhale, left elbow moves inferiorly toward left hemipelvis, anteriorly to superiorly
• Exhale, left elbow moves posteriorly into extension, inferiorly toward left hemipelvis
• Repeat 6–8 times
• End with UE extended overhead and LE moving in opposition
• Change sides
• Progress to extending elbow during movement unless ICD does not allow

6. Roller: Contralateral UE and LE

Intent	• Challenge torso with moving limbs on unstable surface
• Train proprioception through sensory feedback of floor and roller
• Motor control of contralateral patterning

Pilates and Arrhythmogenic Right Ventricular Cardiomyopathy/Dysplasia: Effect on Gait

Gait reasoning	• Integrate contralateral arm and leg patterning coordinating with torso
Starting position	• Supine on mat longitudinally on roller with three points of contact: back of head, mid-thorax, and pelvis • Feet in full contact with floor, LE parallel • Pressing feet into ground • UE with palms up on mat pressing into ground

Movement description	• Alternate hip joint flexion and extension, knee remains flexed
	• Exhale, press stationary foot to initiate lift of opposite hip joint
	• Repeat 6–8 times
	• Bilateral hip joints flexion and extension
	• Press hands into ground
	• Repeat 6–8 times
	• Single Leg Stretch: LE movement
	    ■ Right hip joint and knee flexion
	    ■ Left hip joint and knee extension
	• Repeat 6–8 times
	• Scissors
	    ■ Extended knees
	    ■ Alternating hip joint flexion and extension
	• Repeat 6–8 times

7. Two progressions with resistance band and chair

Intent	• Alleviate client-reported cervical discomfort • Improve cervical and shoulder articulation • UE integration into torso via thoracolumbar fasciae
Gait reasoning	• The UE are integral to rotation of thorax • Integrate contralateral patterning

Starting position	• Standing exercise
	    ■ Stand on resistance band
	    ■ LE parallel, hip-joint-width apart
	    ■ Hold ends of bands in each hand
	• Progression to seated exercise
	    ■ Seated on chair, resistance band over top of door, knees holding door steady, hands holding ends of bands with 5th finger grip

Chapter 13

Movement description
- Standing exercise
  - Stand on resistance band: humeral internal and external rotations followed by elevation and depression
  - Circle internal humeral rotation scapula protraction, elevation then external rotation, scapula retraction and depression
  - Repeat 8–10 times
- Progression to seated exercise
  - Seated: hold ends of bands, humeral flexion and elbow extension
  - Inhale, elevate scapula in humeral flexion
  - Exhale, pull band in order of scapula depression, externally rotating humerus, flex elbow
  - Inhale, pause
  - Exhale, allow band to recoil, UE follow elevating to starting position without scapula elevation
  - Repeat 8–10 times

8. Bridges on ball

Intent
- Challenge LE organization with non-weight bearing on an unstable surface
- Challenge coordination of torso alternating weight bearing on single leg

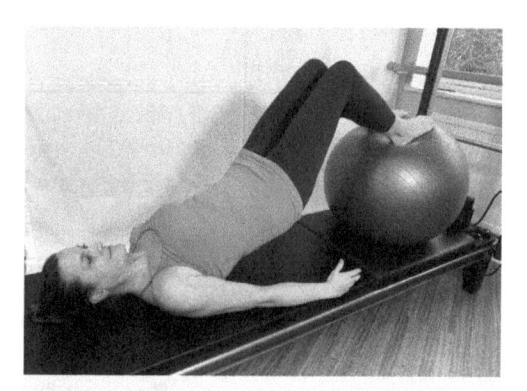

Figure 13.3

Pilates and Arrhythmogenic Right Ventricular Cardiomyopathy/Dysplasia: Effect on Gait

Gait reasoning	• Activate eccentric torso extensors and concentric torso flexors • Challenge transference of weight of LE maintaining optimal LE organization • Improve bilateral LE to unilateral LE with developmental patterning • Activate torso extensors with rotation
Starting position	• Supine on mat • UE externally rotated, palms up at 30 degrees abduction • LE extended, parallel feet on ball • Unilateral hip joint and knee 90 degrees flexion

Movement description	• Inhale, flex hip joints and knees to pull ball in
	• Exhale, press LE into ball, push ball away with hip and knee extension
	• Repeat 8–10 times
	• Repeat unilaterally with each LE 8–10 times
	• Return to starting position bilaterally
	• Bridge series progression
	    ■ Articulate torso into bridge pulling ball in
	    ■ Articulate torso down, push ball away
	    ■ Hold bridge push/pull ball with LE bilaterally
	    ■ Return to starting position
	    ■ Unilateral: hold bridge, alternate LE in marching pattern
	    ■ Hold bridge, unilateral LE push/pull ball, extending hip joint and knee

9. Breathing with weighted prop, supine and prone

Intent	• Sensations of breathing • Interoception—sensory feedback using imagery of the lungs, heart, liver, kidneys, windpipe, esophagus, and thymus movement with breath • Stimulate parasympathetic state
Gait reasoning	• Increase interoception by exploring underlying organ support during walking • Thoracic extension and rotation

Chapter 13

Starting position	- Supine
	    - Hip joints and knees flexion
	    - Feet parallel
	    - UE by sides
	    - Support forward head
	    - Place weighted prop (ball or sandbag) on heart area
	- Prone
	    - One hand on top of the other
	    - Forehead resting on back of hands
	    - LE extended and parallel
	    - Partner places weighted prop on posterior heart area

Movement description	- Breathe slowly, allow prop to follow the breath - Add eye tracking arcs and side-to-side patterns

Author note
It is important to feel the sensation of the breath moving the ball rather than the torso.

10. Prone extension on roller progressions (3 sequences)

Intent	- Activate upper thorax reducing thoracic flexion - UE articulation with resistance - Improve glenoid humeral joint congruency while flexing elbows - Stimulate sequential extension and flexion from UE
Gait reasoning	- Rebalance torso extension/flexion to reorganize glenoid humeral joint congruency for arm swing - Improve vertical orientation for improved multi-planar movement

Starting position	- Prone extension on roller 1
	    - One hand on top of the other
	    - Forehead resting on back of hands
	    - LE extended and parallel
	- Prone extension on roller 2
	    - Forearms on mat with elbows flexed
	    - Thorax extended
	    - LE extended and parallel
	- Prone extension on roller 3
	    - Forearms on horizonal roller
	    - Head on mat

Movement description	● Prone extension on roller 1
■ Elevate and depress scapula
■ Scapula set on thorax with forearms on mat, hands on top of one another, internally rotated glenoid humeral joints
■ Extend thorax sequentially: head, throat, posterior roll of clavicles
■ Pause, inhale, sensing heart extending further
■ Exhale, imagine the heart sinking and moving forward
■ Sequentially lower to starting position
■ Repeat sequential extension
■ Hold thoracic extension
● Prone extension on roller 2
■ Externally rotate glenoid humeral joints, moving elbows toward the lateral torso
■ Hands move laterally
■ Extend torso and elbows to Swan position
■ Sequentially lower torso to starting position
● Prone extension on roller 3
■ Place hands on top of roller in shoulder flexion
■ Sequentially extend the torso with extended elbows pulling and rolling roller toward body
■ Sequentially lower the torso with extended elbows pushing and rolling roller away
■ Hold torso extension
■ Inhale, flex elbows
■ Exhale, extend elbows

11. Quadruped hover, plank, and Mountain Climber

Intent	● Increase UE and LE loading
● Integrate torso and shoulder girdle activations
● Balance challenge
Gait reasoning	● Increase awareness of UE and LE relationships to torso
● Improve midline organization
Starting position	● Quadruped on forearms
● Ankles dorsiflexed with metatarsals extended on mat
● Progress to extended elbows

Chapter 13

Movement description
- Inhale into posterior thorax
- Exhale, soften sternum, hover both knees off mat
- Hover and lower 6 times
- Hold hover for 3–4 breaths
- Hover, extend right hip joint with metatarsals on mat
- In hover position, quickly alternate extension and flexion of hip joint with metatarsals on mat
- Imagine climbing a mountain
- Maintain torso organization throughout movement
- Progress to unilateral hip joint and knee extension with foot off floor

12. Standing plantar flexion and dorsiflexion series

Intent
- Challenge ankle articulations in vertical orientation in gravity
- Foot loading to stimulate LE activation
- Find standing balance in homologous pattern and contralateral pattern

Gait reasoning
- Forefoot, mid-foot, and rear foot pliability required for sequential LE tracking integration
- Deceleration adaptability of LE transmission of ground forces through the body
- Integrate LE sagittal plane with contralateral arm swing
- Efficient use of ground forces

Author note
The pumping quality of the movement from the foot and ankle has been recognized as a secondary heart pump for encouraging venous return (McLeod and Pierce 2013).

Starting position
- Standing with feet parallel, hip distance apart
- Progress to standing on bottom step

Movement description
- Hip joint and knee flexion with ankle dorsiflexion
- Hold knee flexion and plantar flex
- Extend hip joint and knees in plantar flexion
- Lower mid-foot and rear foot to dorsiflexion
- Repeat 6 times
- Return to standing position
- Raise rear foot and plantar flex

- Hold plantar flexion, flex hip and knee joints
- Lower mid-foot and rear foot to dorsiflexion, extend hip and knee joints
- Repeat 6 times
- Add alternating dorsiflexion and plantar flexion moving through mid-foot, talus, and metatarsals
- Repeat 6 times

Session 11/12: Studio session

Fatigue scale	2
Pain scale	0
Client self-report	• No pain • Cervical discomfort with no headache • More confident in movement awareness during exercises and walking • Feeling more coordinated and balanced
Key changes observed by author at end of Session 11/12	• Increased confidence, movement competency, and mind-body connection • Keen to exercise more • Breathing integration gained torso support • Improved midline organization
Reason behind choice of sequencing	• Improve thorax and pelvis reciprocal rotation with LE integration • Specifically focus on inefficient rotation and motor control

Session movement sequence

1. Eve's Lunge on Universal Reformer (left side only)	(See Chapter 5 in Volume 1, Gentry Eve's Lunge)
Intent	• Alter preference for right pelvic rotation
Gait reasoning	• Altering preference for right pelvic rotation improves right-to-left pelvis movement in transverse plane • Increase stride maximizing extensors with push-off

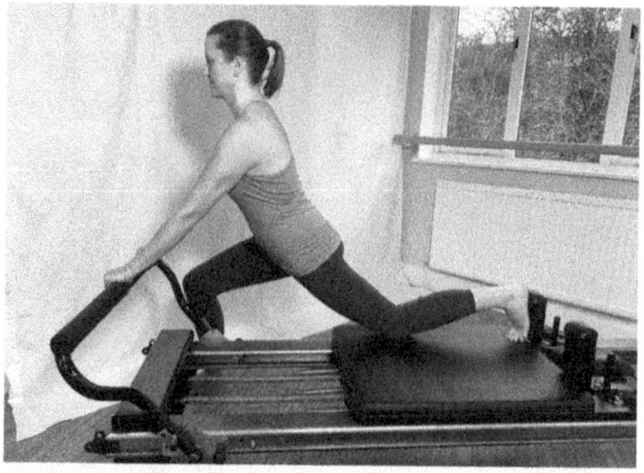

Chapter 13

Figure 13.4

Set-up	• Springs: 1 medium and 1 light
Starting position	• Left knee on carriage, metatarsal extension with phalanges on carriage, calcaneus against shoulder stop
	• Standing, right hip and knee flexion
	• Foot next to frame of Universal Reformer
	• Hands on footbar
	• Progress to hands interlinked behind head
Movement description	• Exhale, press carriage away with left knee on carriage extending left hip joint
	• Increase right knee and hip flexion
	• Inhale, return carriage to starting position
	• Repeat 4–6 times
	• Progress to pressing carriage away with left hip extension with knee extension and right hip flexion with knee extension
	• Left hip extension with knee flexion and right hip flexion with knee flexion moving carriage to stops
	• Repeat 4–6 times

CUES

- Imagine the ASIS of pelvis with headlights, shine them up the wall in front of you
- Be observant of torso hyperextension tendencies
- To prevent right hemipelvis elevation, reach right ischial tuberosity toward left medial malleolus
- Push into hands on footbar, feeling inferior angle of scapula rotate toward axilla

Pilates and Arrhythmogenic Right Ventricular Cardiomyopathy/Dysplasia: Effect on Gait

Author note
In previous sessions the client used the Ladder Barrel, Wunda Chair, or passive positions to achieve desired outcome to reduce inefficient rotation. This closed kinematic chain version of the movement proved most effective to find the organization of the pelvis in the sagittal plane.

2. Ladder Barrel (right side only)

Intent
- Follow Eve's Lunge on Universal Reformer, left side only
- Focus on right hip joint area in abduction and external rotation to oppose the tendency for right pelvic rotational orientation

Gait reasoning
- Sagittal plane orientation of the pelvis for improved thorax and pelvic counter-rotation
- Increase stride length and maximize extensor for toe push-off

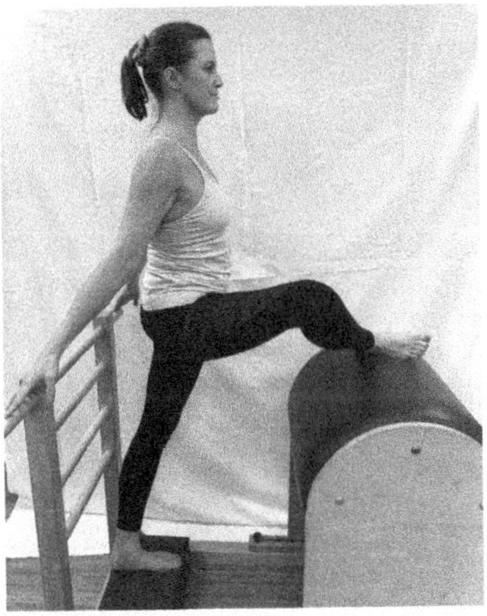

Figure 13.5

Starting position
- Stand with back to ladder, hold top rung, palms facing anteriorly, elbows supinated, glenoid humeral joint externally rotated, feet together in parallel
- Place right lateral border of right foot with ankle dorsiflexion on center of arc of Ladder Barrel
- Hip joint flexion/external rotation/abduction
- Knee flexion
- Midline organized

Movement description
- Maintain right foot position, without ankle supination, with contact of lateral malleolus into arc of Ladder Barrel
- Lean forward, increasing hip joint flexion
- Breathe in and out 6–10 times
- Inhale, flex left hip joint and knee
- Exhale, extend left hip joint and knee
- Repeat 6–10 times

CUES
- Activate extensors through hands pressing laterally on the rung
- Increase left foot loading by pressing into floor
- Imagine reversing your heart, lifting the thymus while leaning toward the Ladder Barrel to encourage thoracic and UE extension
- Right ischial tuberosity moves inferiorly without shifting pelvis left to counter right hemipelvis superior motion

3. Single leg bridge (standing on left foot only) on mat and Universal Reformer

Intent
- Activate left hip extensors
- Activate right hip flexors

Gait reasoning
- Pre-activation of the neuromyofascial system for single LE stance in a different orientation in gravity prior to standing
- Reciprocal activation of LE

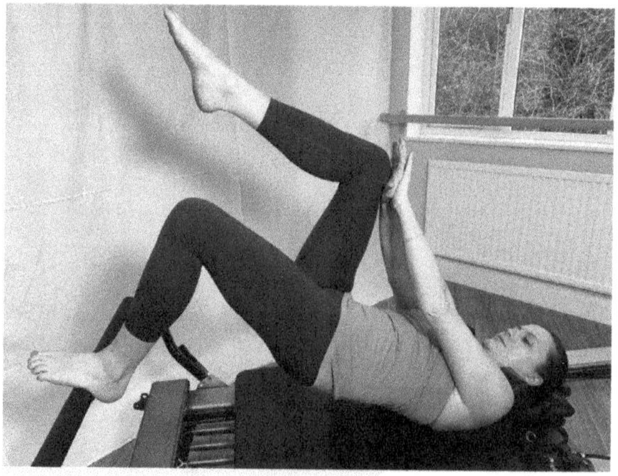

Figure 13.6 Single leg bridge

Set-up	- Attach all springs for no carriage movement
- Progress to 1 medium spring or 1 medium and 1 light
Starting position	- Supine on carriage, headrest down
- Left foot cuboid on footbar, right hip and knee flexion to 90 degrees
- Place both hands on right anterior femur
- Press hands into femur and femur into hands
Movement description	- Exhale, pre-activate hands and press into femur without disturbing orientation of pelvis
- Pause, inhale
- Exhale, extend left hip joint into unilateral stance bridge while maintaining midline organization
- Inhale, return to starting position
- Repeat until confident
- Once confident, change springs to 2 medium or 1 medium and 1 light, then progress to 1 medium
- Move into unilateral bridge
- Hold
- Extend the left knee, moving the carriage away while hands continue to press on right femur
- Avoid changing the pelvic orientation in any plane
- 4–10 repetitions

CUES

- Press hands into femur and femur into hands, sensing the coactivation prior to moving
- Press down with left foot on footbar increasing foot load without changing midline orientation
- Maintain left hip centration and left foot cuboid contact on footbar for LE organization

Author note

In preparation, teach a mat version with left foot on a small box to build confidence. The cuboid placement of the foot on the footbar minimizes mid-foot pronation or supination. Advance the movement by changing the left foot to forefoot to challenge the mid-foot and rear foot.

4. Supine upper arms and leg slides on Trapeze Table

(See Chapter 5 in Volume 1, Gentry: leg slides; Grant: upper arms)

Intent
- Improve shoulder girdle glide on thorax with glenoid humeral joint congruency
- Explore all planes of movement for stimulating connective tissue resiliency of scar adhesions
- Improve segmental movement with eye gaze directed movement

Gait reasoning
- Gain confidence
- Improve interoception of breathing and breath movements
- Train contralateral patterning of UE/LE through thoracolumbar fasciae and ground surface

Set-up
- Push-through bar, top-loaded
- Springs: 1 medium and 1 light

Starting position
- Supine, holding bar with overhand grip
- Glenoid humeral flexion, 90 degrees elbow extension
- Hip and knee flexion
- Feet parallel, hip distance apart
- For rotation, one hand in overhand grip (lower limb pronated) in center of bar
- For gliding, one hand in underhand grip (lower limb supinated) in center of bar

Movement description
- Inhale with elbows extended, protract scapulae, internally rotate humerus, medial hand grip
- Exhale, externally rotate humerus, retract scapulae, lateral hand grip
- Hold bar with right hand, lower limb pronated
- Exhale, look left
- Left thoracic rotation
- Inhale to return to midline
- Repeat on other side
- Repeat with unilateral hand, lower limb supinated
- Hold bar with both hands
- Protract, retract scapulae
- Pull the bar down, flexing elbows
- Push bar through vertical side poles
- Shoulder flexion and elbow extension, scapulae upward rotation
- Pull the bar reversing the articulation of hand to shoulder
- Return the bar to starting position
- Once coordinated with breathing, add alternate and double leg slides

CUES
- Imagine the thorax folding around the heart with the medial hand grip
- Imagine softening the heart with the lateral hand grip
- On exhale, sink heart between shoulder blades from inner collar bones
- As the bar moves overhead, allow collar bones to reverse spin like a key in a lock

CUES FOR ROTATION
- Sense the left lung lift off the table and the right lung yield into the table
- Move with the quality of a pump, flossing neural/vascular/lymph throughout the rotations
- Focus on the side leaning into the table rather than the side moving off the table to reduce the initiation of rotation at the TLJ

Author note
Time was spent naming and demonstrating the bones of the shoulder complex using Netter's *Atlas of Human Anatomy*. It is helpful to visualize the complexity of structures in this region. Experiencing the nerves, lymph, arterial and venous supply, vagus nerve, phrenic nerve, heart and lungs, and pleural linings helped with verbal cueing. Use a tactile cue by gently placing a hand on the client's elbow to introduce a force vector into the glenoid acetabular joint. This facilitates an increase of proprioception of joint congruency. It reduces the anterior humeral head orientation and increases capsule stimulation.

5. Push-Through Seated Front and Circle Saw on Trapeze Table

Derivative of J. H. Pilates Push-Through Seated Front on Trapeze Table (NPCE Study Guide 2021, p. 63) and J. H. Pilates Saw on mat (NPCE Study Guide 2021, p. 48)

Intent
- Transfer new interoception of heart into seated, vertical orientation in gravity
- Weight bearing on ischial tuberosities with spring-assisted shoulder flexion with hip joint flexion
- Facilitating anterior-posterior glide of hip joint
- Stimulate thoracic extension coupled with rotation

Chapter 13

Gait reasoning	• Stimulate rotation from opposite foot loading on vertical side bar and UE
	• Using eye gaze to facilitate transverse plane movement
	• Oppositional thoracic and pelvic movement
Set-up	• Medium spring, top-loaded
Starting position	• Sitting facing push-through bar
	• Feet dorsiflexed, plantar surface touching vertical side poles
	• Hip flexion
	• Knee flexion
	• Hands in overhand grip on push-through bar
	• Thumbs together
	• Elbows flexed without tensioning the spring
Movement description	• Increase hip flexion, pressing bar upward
	• Shoulder flexion and elbow extension
	• Return to starting position
	• Extend hip joints, moving torso posteriorly
	• Shoulder and elbow extend
	• Hold
	• Hold push-through bar with right hand
	• Abduct left UE with left thoracic rotation
	• Press into left foot on vertical side pole to stimulate right pelvic rotation
	• Return to starting position
	• Repeat 3 times
	• Repeat rotation one more time
	• Hold
	• Eye gaze to left hand, follow the hand throughout the movement
	• Left UE in external rotation/flexion coordinated with thoracic extension
	• Arcing movement overhead and toward right vertical side pole with torso in right lateral flexion
	• Press bar upward
	• Thoracic right rotation, left hand holds right vertical side pole
	• Return to starting position
	• Repeat sequence on other side

Author note

Before the exercise, we explored images of the salt or pepper grinder, lids on jam jars, and that oppositional rotational/helical patterning, discussing the need for midline orientation in sagittal plane to decrease thoracic flexion.

CUES
- Notice weight distribution on ischial tuberosities
- During left thoracic rotation weight increases on right ischial tuberosity
- Maintain contact with left ischial tuberosity
- Use imagery to the heart looking to the direction of the rotation
- Direct the eye gaze to the heart and hand and imagine them as one
- When the heart reaches its end of movement, continue eye gaze and hand stimulating segmental rotation from lower thoracic to cervical region
- Follow the UE movement with the eye gaze and heart
- In Saw, imagine wringing the heart in a spiral
- Cue the oppositional rotation of thorax and pelvis during the rotation

6. Long Stretch and Down Stretch on Universal Reformer

Derivative of J. H. Pilates Long Stretch and Down Stretch on Universal Reformer (NPCE Study Guide 2021, p. 55)

Intent
- Head, cervical region, and shoulder organization relative to torso
- Activation from feet and hands stimulating torso verticality

Gait reasoning
- Increase proprioception of transfer of ground forces from feet to crown of head
- Weight bearing on hands with feet actively pressing on shoulder stops creating a closed kinematic chain action for whole-body activation

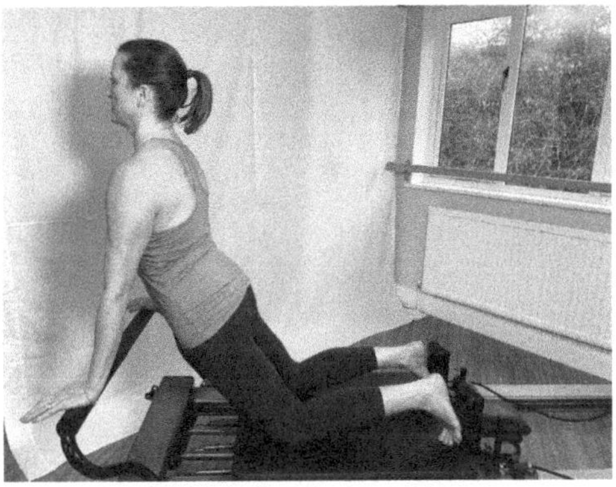

Figure 13.7

Set-up	• Springs: 1 medium and 1 light
Starting position	• Hands shoulder-width apart on footbar • Kneeling on carriage, metatarsals extended and placed on carriage • Heels against shoulder stops • Hands and feet press to activate torso toward extension
Movement description	• Posteriorly rotate pelvis to ensure limitation of pelvic anterior tilt • Exhale, feet press on shoulder stops • Extend the knees pushing carriage away • Inhale, flex knees, place on carriage returning carriage in • Extend torso into J. H. Pilates Down Stretch starting position • Repeat 6–8 times

CUES

- To assist in proprioception of torso organization, place a roller posteriorly with posterior head, heart, and torso in contact with the roller
- When bringing the carriage in, imagine the torso extending around a gym ball behind torso
- Feel the skin of the mons pubis pulling up toward the umbilicus to behind the heart and posterior head
- Press hands into footbar as carriage moves out
- Pull hands as carriage moves in

Author note

Due to the potential for osteopenia and postural reflex of flexion, this exercise focused on extension. Initially, thoracic extension was difficult. The client progressed from quadruped with hands on the Universal Reformer frame, focusing on quadruped position with knees hovering off the carriage, advancing to pressing carriage away and in. Thoracic extension was introduced slowly, changing to hands on footbar.

7. Leg Springs Supine on Trapeze Table with arm springs long-spring crossover series	Derivative of J. H. Pilates Leg Springs Supine: Bicycle, Walking, Scissors, Circles, and Magician (NPCE Study Guide 2021, pp. 67–68) Derivative of J. H. Pilates Arm Springs: Circles Supine (NPCE Study Guide 2021, p. 69)
Intent	• Improving femur on pelvis movement • Torso adaptability to LE movement • Activate the LE in all planes
Gait reasoning	• Ensure conscious awareness of torso support with UE and LE movement • Breathing stimulating movement • Improve proprioception of contralateral UE and LE patterning

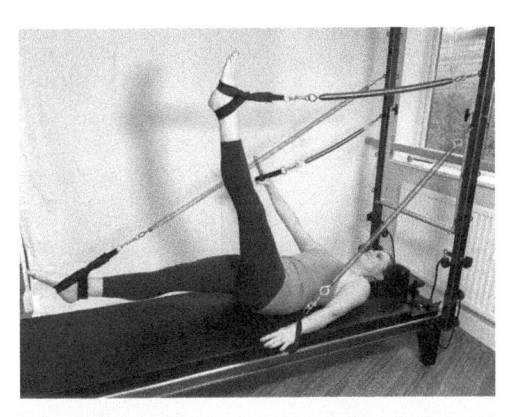

Figure 13.8

Set-up	• 2 light long springs at the top eyelets • Progressing to 2 medium long springs • Adding 2 very light short springs from the sliding crossbar with handles for hands combined with LE in arm-spring, long-spring crossover
Starting position	• Supine on table with feet in Y-loops • Hands holding vertical side poles, forearms parallel to ceiling, thumbs pointing down, wrists neither flexed nor extended • For crossover hold handles on very light short springs

Movement description
- Bilateral hip and knee flexion and extension
  - Repeat 8 times
- Abduction/external rotation/extension/adduction/flexion
  - Repeat 5 times in both directions
- Alternating flexion and extension with knees extended
  - Alternating flexion and extension with unilateral knee flexion and extension
  - Extend unilateral hip joint with knee extended; at end of extension flex knee and flex hip joint as knee extends
- Add arm springs for crossover
- Homologous
  - Shoulder flexion with hip extension
  - Shoulder extension with hip flexion
- Homolateral
  - Alternate right UE LE flexion and left UE LE extension
  - Reverse
- Contralateral
  - Alternate right UE flexion with left LE extension, right UE extension with left LE hip flexion

CUES
- Counteract pelvic rotation focusing on the mons pubis during LE flexion and extension
- Slight anterior pelvic rotation to counter a posterior rotation
- Slight posterior pelvic rotation to counter anterior rotation

Author note
Light long springs were initially required encouraging torso support while LE moves. Once embodied, added medium long springs to imprint newfound pelvifemoral movement. The long-spring crossover series integrated an organic developmental blueprint pattern of walking/gait patterning.

8. Press-Up with Handles Facing In on Wunda Chair

Derivative of J. H. Pilates Wunda Chair Press-Up with Handles Facing In, performed traditionally on High Back Chair (NPCE Study Guide 2021, p. 80)

Intent
- UE weight bearing with extended torso
- Retaining thoracic extension in elbow flexion
- Using posterior shoulder activations to bring head of humerus into socket with heart lifted

Gait reasoning	● Posterior shoulder connection to extend shoulder in gait arm swing
	● UE activation to decrease excessive anterior-posterior curves
Set-up	● 2 springs: one high at the front, one high at the back
Starting position	● Standing on front balls of feet, feet dorsiflexed and LE adducted
	● Hands in overhand grip on handles, externally rotated humerus, extended and adducted shoulder
	● Assistance to lift pedal and pitch body weight forwards and up
Movement description	● Inhale to elbow flexion and press pedal down
	● Exhale to lift heart and extend elbows
	● Retain thoracic integration and extension with hip extension on both inhale and exhale
	● 6–8 repetitions

CUES

- Maintain pressing through UE, especially on elbow bending and pedal lowering
- Keep heels heavy and ankles dorsiflexed with soft knees
- Initiate from the torso extension, not the legs
- Wide collar bones with scapula upward rotation

Author note

We approached this exercise in Session 11. Exploring thoracic extension, freeing the diaphragm, improving thoracic mobility, and all the previous prone and down stretch work prepared for this. On reflection, I could have introduced it sooner as the client's ICD/armpit had less discomfort and she would have benefited.

9. Achilles Stretch on Wunda Chair	Derivative of J. H. Pilates Achilles Stretch on Wunda Chair (NPCE Study Guide 2021, p. 79)
Intent	● To increase mobility at talus and subtalar joints
	● To feel forefoot and metatarsal heads
	● Calf pump to mobilize calf muscles as part of improving the cardiovascular venous return (McLeod and Pierce 2013)
Gait reasoning	● Ankle mobility for heel strike and rolling through the foot and toe-off in gait

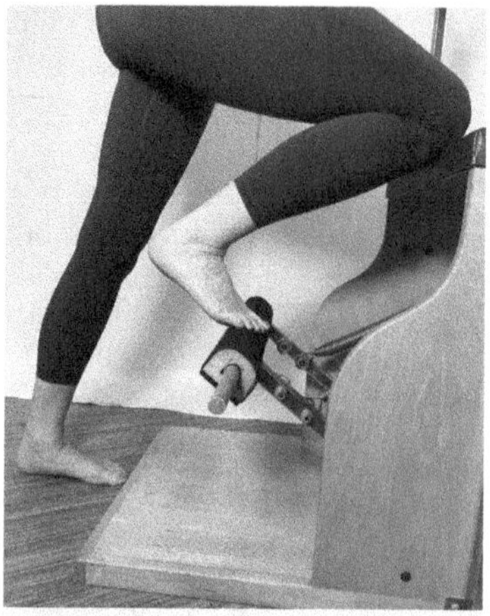

Chapter 13

Figure 13.9

Set-up	• 2 springs: one high at the front, one middle at the back
Starting position	• Standing, LE aligned and parallel • Working foot with ball of foot on pedal • Knee on edge of seat pad of Wunda Chair • Forearms resting on top of handles actively extending shoulder/pressing down
Movement description	• Plantar flex, pressing pedal down and keeping knee static, weight-bearing over 2nd toe • Dorsiflex as pedal brings front foot back up • 6–10 repetitions

CUES

- Return the pedal up as smoothly as possible to control the deceleration/eccentric work of the LE
- Reach the heel further behind you as the pedal lifts to gap the talus

Author note

On exhausted days we used the spikey balls to stand one foot on and massage the soles of the feet. Keeping the heel and ankle on the ground while the front foot was on the ball gave that similar sense of deceleration and prehensile foot positioning that is needed to mobilize the metatarsal heads to improve mobility through the bones of the feet.

The journey to Session 11

Session 4/12
Client self-report

- Fatigue scale 8
- Pain scale 3

Key changes observed

- Mild right pelvic rotation
- Difficulty weight bearing in quadruped due to fatigue
- Cue "Lean into the back of heart and open the front of heart" improved thoracic extension in Long Stretch on Universal Reformer

Reasoning behind choice of movements

- Decrease right pelvic rotation integrating it with movement sequence
- Ease neck and osteoarthritis discomfort
- Explore imagery of the heart gliding during thoracic flexion and extension
- Increase ROM shoulder flexion within comfortable ROM due to ICD

Session movement sequence

1. Standing left hip extension

2. Seated right hip joint external rotation/flexion

3. Hip joints coordination with balls

4. Roller: bridge with plantar flexion and dorsiflexion

5. Prone extension on roller progressions

6. Quadruped hover and plank

7. Standing plantar flexion and dorsiflexion series

8. Eve's Lunge on Universal Reformer, left side only

9. Ladder Barrel, right side only

10. Trapeze Table

- Supine upper arms and leg slides

11. Universal Reformer

- Chest Expansion: derivative seated on box
- Rowing: derivative seated on box
  - No flexion or extension, only UE and shoulder girdle movement
- Salute: derivative seated on box
- Shoulder abduction with elbow flexion seated on box
  - Move UE anteriorly, laterally, posteriorly
  - Repeat

12. Additional movements

- Trapeze Table
  - Seated with sling around thorax, springs on high eyelets, torso leans posteriorly into sling then returns to starting position
- Universal Reformer
  - Jackrabbit
  - Long Stretch
  - Upstretch in extension
- Wunda Chair
  - Step down with hands behind head heel raises

Chapter 13

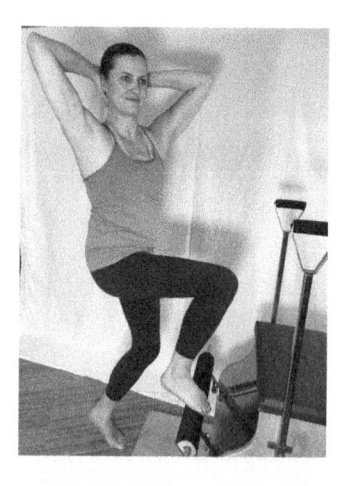

Figure 13.10

Session 5/12
Client self-report

- Fatigue scale 5
- Pain scale 6
- Cardiologist confirmed beta blocker medication no longer required. Client reports feeling energetically different having not taken meds for past 6 or 7 days. Client booked for osteopathy appointment after Pilates session to address cervical pain

Key changes observed

- Improved pelvic organization
- Improved verticality
- Decreased discomfort from ICD
- Reports "no low back and hip pain"
- Found UE exercises activated and improved extension

Reasoning behind choice of movements

- Improved proprioception of head, torso, shoulder girdle, and UE facilitated reduced head and neck discomfort

Session movement sequence

1. Hip joints coordination with balls

2. Breathing with weighted prop, supine and prone

3. Two progressions with band and chair

4. Roller: thoracic extension

5. Bridge with plantar flexion and dorsiflexion

6. Two arm progressions with band and chair

7. Prone extension on roller progressions

8. Trapeze Table

- Supine upper arms and leg slides, unilateral with cervical rotations
- Supine upper arms and leg slides, bilateral
- Long spring arm crossover series

9. Wunda Chair

- Forward Step Down, hands holding handles, hands behind head

10. Additional movements

- Quadruped hover and plank
- Standing plantar flexion and dorsiflexion series

470

Session 6/12
Client self-report

- Fatigue scale 2
- Pain scale 2
- Mild headache
- Discontinued heart medicines
- Neck discomfort

Key changes observed

- Improved anterior-posterior, transverse, coronal planes
- Reduced headache, less discomfort behind eyes
- Shoulder girdle and thoracic organization appears to be more comfortable, verticality improved
- Increased ROM of hip joints

Reasoning behind choice of movements

- Organize head and cervical region with UE and LE movements
- Increase awareness of shoulder girdle in seated position and with elbow flexion
- Improved hip congruency in quadruped weight bearing

Session movement sequence

1. Hip joints coordination with balls

2. Breathing with weighted prop, supine and prone

3. Prone extension on roller progressions

4. Two arm progressions with band and chair

5. Quadruped hover with forearm on mat and plank into Adho Mukha Svanasana (Downward Facing Dog)

6. Trapeze Table
- Supine scapular movement with alternate leg slides
- Push-through bar pull-down
  - Single arm and head turn to opposite direction of pulling arm and double arm pull-down with head turns
- Long leg springs: added Magician with alternating LE flexion and extension
- Swan

7. Additional movements

- Trapeze Table
  - Kneeling holding with roll-down bar
  - Elbow flexion and extension
  - With elbows extended increase knee flexion with midline organization of torso
- Universal Reformer
  - Long stretch and Jackrabbit combination

Session 7/12
Client self-report

- Fatigue scale 5
- Pain scale 2
- Limited ROM of neck
- Described "a feeling of held tension in upper body yet a heaviness with fatigue"

Key changes observed

- Improved pelvic organization
- Improved verticality
- Breathing appeared slower, and even rhythm giving the diaphragm an appearance of enhanced excursion improving standing organization
- Improved cervical movement strategy for rotation decreasing the compensatory strategy of rotation, side bend, lateral translation, and chin tuck

- Arm swing increased anteriorly and posteriorly facilitated by improved cervical strategy for rotation
- Pain free, less discomfort of ICD when thorax extended with UE abduction

Reasoning behind choice of movements

- Facilitate interoception of heart and lung movement through breathing
- UE movements stimulating parasympathetic system to decrease trauma response to ICD promoting a calmer state
- Focus on breathwork with UE weight bearing
- Self-awareness shifting fatigue feeling

Session movement sequence
1. Roller: thoracic extension

2. Roller: contralateral UE and LE

3. Prone extension on roller progressions

4. Quadruped hover, plank, and Mountain Climber

5. Supine head on Overball chin tucks, chin lifts, head and neck rotations

6. Trapeze Table

- Supine scapular movement with alternate leg slides

7. Mat

- Breathing with weighted prop, supine and prone
- Standing plantar flexion and dorsiflexion series, no UE overhead due to ICD

8. Universal Reformer

- Footwork series
  - Double leg press
  - Single leg press
  - Calf stretch
  - Running in place
- Down Stretch
- Jackrabbit into Long Stretch
- Chest Expansion: derivative seated on box
- Rowing: derivative seated on box
  - No flexion or extension, only UE and shoulder girdle movement

9. Additional movements

- Overball
  - Extend and flex thoracic region on ball, rotate side to side
- Foot massage on balls

Session 8/12
Client self-report

- "Felt achy after last session"
- Post-acupuncture treatment: much less heat at night and a reduced feeling of heart racing. Neck limited ROM with osteoarthritis discomfort
- Fatigue scale 0
- Pain scale 2

Key changes observed

- Pelvis appears in right rotation
- Torso left lateral flexion, so suggested alternating leading leg to get on and off turbo bike
- Observe improved thoracic extension
- Feet feel evenly loaded
- Awareness of thorax integrating with whole body

Reasoning behind choice of movements

- Improved pelvic organization
- Improved verticality

- Improved torso lateral flexion before movement sequence
- Ease neck, shoulder, and osteoarthritis discomfort
- Continue to explore heart focused movement during thoracic flexion and extension
- Increase ROM in shoulder flexion within range of ICD
- Build confidence by introducing jump board, hops, and jogs to improve adaptation strategies

Session movement sequence

1. Eve's Lunge on Universal Reformer, left side only

2. Seated right hip joint external rotation/flexion

3. Hip joints coordination with balls

4. Single leg bridge with both hands counter-pressure on right thigh

5. Roller: bridge with plantar flexion and dorsiflexion

6. Prone extension on roller progressions

7. Quadruped hover, plank, and Mountain Climber

8. Eve's Lunge on Universal Reformer, left side only

9. Ladder Barrel, right side only

10. Hip joints coordination with balls

11. Universal Reformer

- Single leg bridge (standing on left foot only) on mat and Universal Reformer
- Footwork series
- Single leg bridge, added knee extension

12. Additional movements

- Universal Reformer
  - Jump board, jumps, hops, contralateral patterning jogs
- Trapeze Table
  - Supine scapular movement
  - Swan
- Quadruped on mat into leg pull and Mountain Climber
- Squats
  - Holding door handle
  - Add plantar flexion with shoulder extension

Session 9/12
Client self-report

- Fatigue scale 0
- Pain scale 1
- Reports "stiffness in neck on right side especially. Feeling quite tall already. Noticing toes lifting on turbo bike when working out at home"
- Client feeling positive about how different she feels, loving the reduction in exaggerated anterior-posterior curves

Key changes observed

- Improved midline orientation
- Facilitate thoracic extension and shoulder flexion for ease in placing a coat on hook
- Breath pattern easier with expansive inhale into posterior thorax with softening heart on exhale
- A sense of energetic presence walking into studio and stance with grounded feet, and improved overall organization

Reasoning behind choice of movements

- The integration of helical gait pattern in sequences
- Improve venous return/secondary heart pump and lymphatic drainage through lower limb deceleration, foot pump, bridging

> **Author note**
> The pumping quality of the movement from the foot and ankle has been recognized as a secondary heart pump for encouraging venous return (McLeod and Pierce 2013).

Session movement sequence

1. Eve's Lunge on Universal Reformer, left side only

2. Seated right hip joint external rotation/flexion

3. Hip joints coordination with balls

4. Single leg bridge with both hands, counter-pressure on right thigh

5. Roller: bridge with plantar flexion and dorsiflexion

6. Prone extension on roller progressions

7. Quadruped hover, plank, and Mountain Climber

8. Eve's Lunge on Universal Reformer, left side only

9. Ladder Barrel, right side only

10. Footwork series

11. Single left leg bridge with both hands, counter-pressure on right thigh

12. Trapeze Table

- Push-Through Seated Front and circle Saw

13. Additional movements

- Universal Reformer
  - Jackrabbit
  - Long Stretch
  - Upstretch
- Trapeze Table
  - Magician
  - Arm springs and leg springs crossover, alternating homologous, homolateral, and contralateral
- Wunda Chair
  - Press-Up with Handles Facing In
  - Achilles stretch
  - Forward Step Down, hands holding handles, hands behind head
    - Pulse hands lightly holding handles

Session 10/12
Client self-report

- Fatigue scale 0
- Pain scale 0
- Lack of ROM in neck. Requested to review home program and next steps to keep pain free and moving well. Keen to exercise more

Key changes observed

- Improved pelvis organization and midline orientation
- Breathing awareness
- Improvement in daily activities, sleeping, and work environment
- Improved balance

- Increased confidence in bending, lifting, leg tracking, balance, and mind-body awareness
- No longer "feels twisted, painful, and stuck"

Reasoning behind choice of movements

- Clarify home program meets client's maintenance goals of optimal organization and pain free
- Include bone-loading exercises to counter hours of sitting at work and driving
- Include organ motility intended exercise selections for heart, lungs, liver, kidneys, blood, and lymph corresponding to thoracic extension
- Integrate helical cross-patterning of limbs with torso for gait patterning
- Neck articulations and headache-reducing exercises

Editor note

Neuromyofascial organization affects organ motility. When the connective tissue is dehydrated, lacking the ability to glide between levels, the biotensegrity balance between tension and compression is restricted. During breathing, the lungs have an excursion that moves through all dimensions, a spherical-like motion.

Organ motility is a normal intrinsic rhythm of an organ and movement that is inherent to the organ itself to allow for function. Motility can be reduced by an issue within the organ itself, such as inflammation, emotional concerns, or in relation to medication. Motility reduction may also be due to surrounding structures that have been binding an organ and impinging on its cellular motion (Barral Institute 2012).

Session movement sequence

1. Roller: Thoracic extension

2. Roller: Bridge with plantar flexion and dorsiflexion

3. Roller: Three movements

- Lateral thoracic flexion
- Arms with thoracic rotation
- Arm circles

4. Prone extension on roller progressions

5. Quadruped hover, plank, Mountain Climber, cycling pattern, weight transfers anteriorly and posteriorly

6. Trapeze Table

- Push-through bar unilateral with oppositional head rotations
- Push-through bar bilateral with alternating head rotations
  - Two arm progressions with band and chair
  - Long Leg Springs Series, all
  - Arm springs and leg springs, alternating homologous, homolateral, and contralateral
  - Swan

7. Additional movements

- Roller: contralateral UE and LE
- Supine, head on Overball: chin tucks, chin lifts, head/neck rotations, and spirals
- Side lying hip movements
  - Full range of flexion, abduction/external rotation/adduction/flexion abduction, flexion
  - Abduction
  - Extension with knee flexion holding foot
- Standing
  - Contralateral pattern of UE and LE

- Lunge: right foot anterior knee flexion, left foot posterior knee extension
- Left shoulder flexion with elbow extension
- Swing alternating lunges with contralateral UE flexion and extension
- Progress to adding heel raise/hop with hand weights
• Squats
  - Holding door handle
  - Holding hand weights with bilateral shoulder flexion and extension
  - Added plantar flexion with shoulder extension

References

Bainbridge Cohen, B. (2018) *Basic Neurocellular Patterns: Exploring Developmental Movement.* El Sobrante, CA: Burchfield Rose Publishers, p. 327. https://bonniebainbridgecohen.com/collections/books/products/basic-neurocellular-patterns. [Accessed October 3, 2023].

Barral Institute (2012) "Visceral motility testing." *Visceral Mobility and Motility Testing: Comprehensive Illustrated Collection of Visceral Motion.* [Standing Flip Chart]. Barral Productions, p. 1. barralinstitute.com.

Dommershuijsen, L. J., Isik, B. M., Darweesh, S. K. L., van der Geest, J. N., Ikram, M. K., and Ikram, M. A. (2019) "Unravelling the association between gait and mortality—one step at a time." *The Journals of Gerontology. Series A, Biological Sciences and Medical Sciences, 75,* 6, 1184–1190.

Guimarães, G. V., Carvalho, V. O., Bocchi, E. A., and d'Avila, V. M. (2012) "Pilates in heart failure patients: A randomized controlled pilot trial." *Cardiovascular Therapeutics, 30,* 6, 351–356.

McLeod, K. J. and Pierce, C. (2013) "Cardiomyopathy in women: Second heart failure." In: J. Milei and G. Ambrosio (Eds.) *Cardiomyopathies.* InTech. [Online]. Available at: www.intechopen.com/chapters/41976. [Accessed October 3, 2023].

NPCE Study Guide (National Pilates Certification Exam Study Guide) (2021) Miami, FL: National Pilates Certification Program, Inc.

Schleip, R. and Jaeger, H. (2012) "Interoception: A new correlate for intricate connections between fascial receptors, emotion, and self recognition." In: R. Schleip, T. W. Findley, L. Chaitow, and P. A. Huijing (Eds.) *Fascia: The Tensional Network of the Human Body: The Science and Clinical Applications in Manual and Movement Therapy.* Edinburgh: Churchill Livingstone, pp. 89–94.

Chapter 14

Pilates for Recovery from Ovarian Cancer Post-Surgery: Effect on Gait

Emilee Garfield

Ovarian cancer is the fifth most commonly occurring cancer in women (American Cancer Society 2023). There were 313,959 new cases worldwide in 2020 (Huang *et al.* 2022). The most well-established risk factors for ovarian cancer are unmodifiable factors including age, Caucasian race, Ashkenazi Jewish descent, BRCA1 or BRCA2 mutations, and a family history of breast or ovarian cancer. Furthermore, obesity, nulliparity, infertility, and endometriosis have also been associated with increased risk. By the time ovarian cancer is detected, it may have spread to other organs within the pelvis (Cannioto and Moysich 2015). The prognosis of ovarian cancer is usually poor, with a five-year survival rate of only 17 percent for a patient at an advanced stage (Huang *et al.* 2022).

Diagnosis

Ovarian cancer is often diagnosed at a late stage, making this malignancy the most lethal gynecological cancer (Huang *et al.* 2022). There is no screening test for ovarian cancer. A pap smear does not detect ovarian cancer. A genetic test will be conducted due to the unmodified risk for ovarian cancer being genetic. A pelvic exam, a rectovaginal examination, transvaginal ultrasound, biopsies, and CT or MRI scans are performed as well as the CA 125 blood test.

Key symptoms include bloating, constipation, low back pain, pelvic pain, painful sex, abnormal bleeding, and urinary tract infections.

Treatment

The treatment strategies for ovarian cancer depend on its pathological stages. Current treatment options are combining debulking surgery, a surgical technique to remove as much of the tumor as possible, drug treatment, and radiation therapy.

Surgery is considered the primary treatment option for most women with ovarian cancer. The surgery removes any cancer found in nearby organs and tissues. This can include the uterus, ovaries, fallopian tubes, and possibly parts of the bladder or liver.

Post-surgery leads to complications, such as infection, blood clots in the pelvis or legs, and damage to the bladder or bowel. Leg swelling or lower limb lymphedema may occur. Fluid buildup in the genital area is also common. The client may need to wear a colostomy bag to collect stools or a catheter to remove urine.

Chemotherapy is the most vital part of ovarian cancer treatment. Chemotherapeutic agents will be selected for treatment based on the stage of ovarian cancer.

Complications from chemotherapy

- Side effects include nausea, vomiting, loss of appetite, hair loss, mouth sores, rashes, fatigue, weakness, and pain
- Leukopenia: low white blood cell count, increasing the risk of infection
- Thrombocytopenia: low platelet counts that can lead to easy bruising or bleeding
- Kidney damage
- Neuropathy: nerve damage, numbness, tingling, or pain in the hands and feet
- Hearing loss: cisplatin (chemotherapy drug) can damage nerves to the ear affecting hearing loss
- Early menopause
- Bladder problems
- Ascites: collections of fluid in the abdominal cavity caused by cancer
- Pleural effusion: a build-up of fluid between the thin membranes that line the lungs and the inside of the chest cavity. It can cause breathing difficulties and other symptoms

Exercise guidelines

In 2019, the American College of Sports Medicine (ACSM) published three papers following an International Multidisciplinary Roundtable (Campbell *et al.* 2019) that reviewed and disseminated the scientific literature regarding the safety and efficacy of exercise training during and after cancer treatment. The guidelines (ACSM 2019) recommend an exercise program for cancer patients and survivors focusing on:

- Improving physical fitness
- Improving body image and body composition
- Enhancing overall quality of life
- Improving cardiorespiratory, endocrine, neurological, cognitive, psychosocial, and muscular outcomes
- Delaying or preventing cancer recurrence
- Decreasing and/or preventing long-term deleterious effects of cancer treatment
- Improving the ability to psychologically and physically withstand ongoing anxiety regarding the possibility of cancer recurrence and future treatments

To ensure the safety and efficacy of an exercise program, all cancer patients and survivors should receive medical evaluation for treatment-related conditions prior to beginning an exercise program (Cannioto and Moysich 2015).

Editor note

Adhesions are a complication of scarring, which is a result of a wound, such as a surgical incision in the skin. Adhesions are more amenable to change, for instance by manual therapy or even by movement (Guimberteau and Armstrong 2015).

The external appearance of a scar can be misleading because it does not always indicate the extent of the underlying tissue destruction. A breach in the cutaneous barrier and the brutal exposure of the subcutaneous world to the external environment upsets the fibrillar harmony. If the injury is not fatal, the damaged tissue will be repaired but not always to its exact former state, and usually with variations in the quality of the scar tissue.

Scar formation is not selective. It initially forms at the site of tissue damage. Subsequently, the repair process encompasses and incorporates any type of injured tissue into the same scar. This applies to all types of tissue, including the dermis, muscles, tendons, and bone.

The morphodynamic organization of the fibrillar collagen network creates tensional forces that influence the attempt to repair the damaged tissue. Everything depends on the nature of the initial trauma. The greater the tissue destruction, the less successful the repair will be, especially if different types of tissue are involved (Guimberteau and Armstrong 2015).

Extracellular matrix (ECM) is a three-dimensional structure and a vital participant in tissue activity and wound healing through connective tissue remodeling and reorganization. ECM comprises a complex assortment of proteins, including collagens, elastin, and smaller quantities of structural proteins (Diller and Tabor 2022; Xue and Jackson 2015).

The final stage of the healing process is remodeling. ECM type III collagen is replaced by a stronger fiber such as type I collagen; however, the type I collagen is aligned without a specific order which results in gaining of more strength but loss of elasticity (Pilat 2022). Scar tissue is helpful for healing, but it may cause pain and restrict movement.

Even though the biological repair process is one of the primary survival mechanisms, and the potential for satisfactory repair exists, it is not always completely successful. Initially, the same repair process applies to all tissue components and the scar tissue remains undifferentiated for several weeks. Subsequently, over time, a specific movement or function may be restored.

Client description: 42-year-old female, identifies as female; an advocate with the Nature Conservancy and with nonprofits coordinating a meditation center and researching how cannabis affects living with cancer

Dates of case report: Session 1: December 6, 2019; Session 12: February 2, 2020

Studio apparatus and props
Pilates equipment

- Universal Reformer
- Trapeze Table
- Ladder Barrel

Props used with equipment

- 2 balls, 9 in. (23 cm), three-quarters inflated
- Air cushion disc
- Magic Circle
- Foam roller
- Resistance band, light
- Small, firm ball 1.5 in. (40 mm) for feet
- Ball, 22 in. (55 cm)
- Pilates Arc
- Mat

Home program props

- Mat
- Magic Circle
- Foam roller
- SmartSpine™ globe

Methods and materials

Session 1/12
1. Health history interview

- 2015: diagnosed with stage 3C ovarian cancer
- Prior to being diagnosed client had symptoms of bloating, constipation, low back pain, repeated urinary tract infections, painful sex, fatigue, and abnormal bleeding

Chapter 14

- MRI, CT, and PET scans along with CA 125 blood test confirmed metastasized cancer throughout the abdominal wall cavity, including into the diaphragm and omentum and peritoneal area
- Client was treated with chemotherapy: carboplatin and taxol
- 2015, first surgery: went in for a surgery called a debulking surgery. Total hysterectomy, with the cervix, fallopian tubes, and ovaries removed. A section of the diaphragm was removed. Complete removal of the omentum, peritoneal lining, appendix, gallbladder, and 10 lymph nodes
- 2015: had nine cycles of chemotherapy. Each 3-week period is called a treatment cycle. Total rounds of weekly chemotherapy were 18 cycles
- Client was considered NED (no evidence of disease) for about 1 year and reported first recurrence in 2016
- Began drug called Avastin
- 2016: second abdominal surgery to remove tumors
- Experiences bowel obstruction from scar tissue around the small intestines and incision site
- At start date of this case report, 2019, client had third recurrence. Reinstitution of chemotherapy and immunotherapy drugs

2. Symptoms

- General fatigue
- Deconditioned, loss of muscle mass from lack of exercise; no physical movement for 6 months since last surgery
- Difficulty breathing when walking
- Diaphragm tightness and spasms, especially with flexion
- Depressed and anxious
- Neuropathy in toes; painful feet
- Movement restriction in hip joints, medial region of femur to pubis rami
- Lumbar region pain

3. Movement aids

- No movement aids

Final result of case report

The client was able to build confidence with less kinesiophobia from feeling safe in the Pilates environment. She increased walking endurance and improved body awareness. She reported decreased back pain. The client practices home program sequence (Session 3) to help with painful scar tissue of the abdominal region.

Session 2/12: Initial assessment

1. General observations of gait

- Gait asymmetries attributed to surgery and/or pain
- Torso presents in flexion due to post-surgical abdominal scar tissue
- Transverse plane asymmetries may be attributed to abdominal scar tissue and/or scoliosis
- Feet are stiff and not supple in gait—this may be attributed to chemotherapy induced neuropathy

2. Standing tests

- Full torso rotation
- Observations of inefficient side: right
  - Lacks thoracic rotation
  - Rotation primarily occurs at pelvifemoral joints
  - Lacks internal rotation of right femoral joint
  - Exaggerated right ankle inversion and left ankle eversion to facilitate rotation
- Hemipelvis inferior motion
- Observations of inefficient sides: both
  - Pelvis left rotation
  - Thorax translates right
- Hemipelvis superior motion
- Observations of inefficient sides: both
  - Right
    - Right innominate elevated in standing
    - Right hip joint limited abduction

Session 12/12: Post-assessment

1. General observations of gait

- Gait strategy improved orientating to the vertical axis, displaying more confidence
- Torso flexion less prominent
- Transverse plane asymmetries less pronounced
- Feet became more supple and able to roll from rear foot to forefoot

2. Standing tests

- Full torso rotation
- Observations of inefficient side: right
  - Improved thoracic rotation
  - Rotation is distributed between thoracic region and pelvis
  - Enhanced pelvis on femur relative to right femur internal rotation, left femur external rotation
  - Improved articulation of rear foot and forefoot, lessening the ankle inversion and eversion
- Hemipelvis inferior motion
- Observations of inefficient sides: both
  - No change

Editor note
There was no change due to the nature of the scar tissue. The author focused on the ability to organize the body for improved function through motor control and proprioception (see

Chapter 14

- ○ Left hip joint limited adduction
- ○ Right plantar flexion limited
- ○ Left dorsiflexion limited
- ■ Left
  - ○ Left innominate inferior in standing
  - ○ Left hip joint limited abduction
  - ○ Right hip joint limited adduction
  - ○ Left plantar flexion
  - ○ Right dorsiflexion limited

◆ Lateral pelvic shift

● Observations of inefficient sides: both
  - ■ Right
    - ○ Thorax excessively translates to the left
    - ○ Limited right femoral adduction
    - ○ Limited left femoral abduction
    - ○ Feet do not adapt well
  - ■ Left
    - ○ Thorax translates right
    - ○ Limited left femoral adduction
    - ○ Limited right femoral abduction
    - ○ Feet do not adapt well

3. Seated tests

◆ Thoracic rotation

● Observations of inefficient sides: both
  - ■ Right
    - ○ Right ischial tuberosity bears more weight than left
    - ○ Increases thoracic flexion with left rotation
    - ○ Protracts left scapula and retracted right scapula
  - ■ Left
    - ○ Right ischial tuberosity bears more weight than left
    - ○ Left thoracic rotation greater range than right
    - ○ Protracts right scapula and retracted left scapula

Editor note on adhesions and scar tissue at the beginning of this chapter).

◆ Hemipelvis superior motion

● Observations of inefficient sides: both
  - ■ No change

◆ Lateral pelvic shift

● Observations of inefficient sides: both
  - ■ Right
    - ○ Decreased left thoracic translation
    - ○ Limited right femoral adduction
    - ○ Limited left femoral abduction
    - ○ Feet adapted well
  - ■ Left
    - ○ Decreased right thorax translation
    - ○ Limited left femoral adduction
    - ○ Limited right femoral abduction
    - ○ Feet adapted well

3. Seated tests

◆ Thoracic rotation

● Observations of inefficient sides: both
  - ■ Right
    - ○ Conscious of sharing weight on both ischial tuberosities
    - ○ Decreased thoracic flexion and left rotation
    - ○ Improved shoulder girdle organization contributes to efficient scapulae thoracic contact
  - ■ Left
    - ○ Left thoracic rotation greater than right
    - ○ Improved shoulder girdle organization contributes to efficient scapulae thoracic contact

- ◆ Hip joint and knee flexion
- ● Observations of inefficient sides: both
  - ■ Right and left
    - ○ Right ischial tuberosity bears more weight than left
    - ○ Increases thoracic flexion

4. Sit and stand

- ◆ Lateral view

- ● To stand, shifts weight to right lower extremity (LE)
- ● Increases thoracic flexion
- ● Femoral adduction comprising knee tracking
- ● Unable to deaccelerate to sit
- ● Neuropathy affecting foot contact

- ◆ Anterior view

- ● Femoral adduction comprising knee tracking
- ● Feet pronate excessively

5. Standing balance

- ◆ Two-leg stance, eyes open

- ● 45 seconds

- ◆ One-leg stance, eyes open

- ● Left leg: 60 seconds, better balance than on right
- ● Right leg: 10 seconds

- ◆ One-leg stance, eyes closed

- ● Balance was a struggle and opened eyes after a few seconds

---

- ◆ Hip joint and knee flexion
- ● Observations of inefficient sides: both
  - ■ Right and left
    - ○ Conscious of sharing weight on both ischial tuberosities
    - ○ Decreased thoracic distortion

4. Sit and stand

- ◆ Lateral view

- ● In standing client is conscious of equalizing weight distribution on LE
- ● Improved torso organization in vertical axis
- ● Conscious awareness of hip-knee-ankle tracking
- ● Neuropathy present, improved foot-ankle articulation and contact

- ◆ Anterior view

- ● Conscious awareness of hip-knee-ankle tracking
- ● Neuropathy present, improved foot-ankle articulation and contact

5. Standing balance

- ◆ Two-leg stance, eyes open

- ● 60 seconds

- ◆ One-leg stance, eyes open

- ● Right leg: 60 seconds
- ● Left leg: 60 seconds

- ◆ One-leg stance, eyes closed

- ● Right leg: 30 seconds
- ● Left leg: 30 seconds

Chapter 14

Session 3/12: Home program

Fatigue scale	5
Pain scale	3
Client self-report	• Depressed from feeling body weakness and neuropathy in feet; complaining that her feet feel hot and achy; loss of balance; diaphragm feels tight all the time making it hard to take deep breaths. Excited to start program. Client has not participated in any physical exercise for 6 months
Key changes observed by author at end of Session 3/12	• Able to coordinate breathing • Understands the relationships between the thoracic diaphragm, and pelvic diaphragm for torso support • Improved body awareness around scar tissue and its effect on movement • Diaphragm spasms in flexion, limited any flexion movement
Reason behind choice of sequencing	• Foot, ankle, and LE exercises to lessen post-chemotherapy and surgery stiffness, neuropathy, and feeling of soreness • To promote LE circulation and bring awareness to the foundation of the feet • To facilitate hip joint articulation and glide • Supine work allows clients to feel safe • Help the client experience embodiment • Support the mental and physical recovery • Gentle torso extension promotes tissue reorganization and reduces spasms

Session movement sequence

1. Ankle pumps

Intent	• Stimulate blood flow and circulation • Nerve gliding of feet and LE • Facilitate joint articulation • Foster embodiment from sensory input of feet • To improve dorsiflexion and plantar flexion
Gait reasoning	• Proprioception • Sensory input from feet • Articulation of ankle joints • Foot patterning of heel strike to push-off in supine
Starting position	• Supine • Hip and knee extension on mat

| Movement description | • Dorsiflexion and plantar flexion
• 20 times slowly with the emphasis on heel strike |

Author note

Blood clots are a concern after surgery and treatment. Ankle dorsiflexion and plantar flexion movements influence venous return from the lower limbs and prevent deep vein thrombosis of the lower limbs (Pi *et al.* 2018). The ankle movements enhance sensory awareness of the feet and ankles. Rhythmic ankle dorsiflexion and plantar flexion create whole-body oscillation.

2. Leg slides (See Chapter 5 in Volume 1, Gentry, Leg slides)

| Intent | • Stimulate blood flow and circulation
• Increase venous return to reduce lower limb lymphedema
• Relieve pain
• Facilitate hip, knee, and ankle articulation |
| Gait reasoning | • Activate LE
• Increase range of motion (ROM) of knee
• Stimulate torso control with moving limb |
| Starting position | • Supine
• Hip and knee flexion
• Knee flexion approximately 45 degrees
• Feet on mat |
| Movement description | • Slide right foot extending hip and knee
• Slide right foot flexing hip and knee
• Return to starting position
• Repeat 10–20 times
• Repeat with left leg
• Repeat 10–20 times |

3. Pelvic clocks (Black 2022)

Author note

The pelvic clock for post-abdominal surgery may be beneficial by gently increasing movement of the lumbopelvic-femoral joints. It relieves discomfort in the low back, sacrum, and pelvis.

| Intent | • Facilitate lumbopelvic-femoral glide that is limited due to scar tissue restrictions
• Decrease back pain
• Improve proprioception of lumbopelvic-femoral glide for better execution of other exercises requiring this movement |

Gait reasoning	• Improve proprioceptive awareness of lumbopelvic-femoral glide in gait
	• Improve torso orientation to midline with femoral gliding during gait
	• Increase ability to rotate torso
Starting position	• Supine with pelvis in a relaxed sense
	• Hip and knee flexion with feet on mat
Movement description	• Imagine wearing a clock on the front of the pelvis
	• 12 is at navel, 6 at pubic symphysis
	• Move pelvis in clockwise direction
	• Pause at each point on the clock
	• Reverse direction

4. Wall squat

Intent	• Foot proprioception and sensory input
	• Increase load of LE
	• Challenge balance
	• Increase pelvifemoral articulation
Gait reasoning	• Bring awareness to sensory input of the feet and its relationship to load transfer in gait
	• Improve pelvifemoral articulation for stance and swing phases
Starting position	• Place ball against the wall
	• Lean torso on ball at thoracolumbar junction
	• Feet parallel, placed forward for 90 degrees hip and knee flexion
Movement description	• Flex at ankles, knees, and hip joints
	• Allow ball to glide down wall
	• Return to starting position by pushing through the feet
	• Extend hip joints and knees
	• Allow ball to glide up wall
	• Repeat 5 times and increase to 10 times

5. Single-leg balance swings

- Intent
  - Activate the standing, non-moving LE
  - Improve single-leg stance for balance
  - Challenge adaptability of ankle of standing LE
- Gait reasoning
  - Improve single-leg stance movement
  - Articulation of ankle, knee, hip joint for swing
  - Contralateral movement
- Starting position
  - Stand on mat with feet equally weighted in alignment of hip joints
  - Hold chair for balance if needed
- Movement description
  - Flex right hip joint and knee lifting foot off mat
  - Simultaneously flex left upper extremity (UE) with elbow extended
  - Swing right LE posteriorly extending right hip joint and allowing right knee to flex slightly
  - Right UE moves anteriorly for counterbalance
  - Feel right UE and LE moving away from each other
  - Press into left foot for activation
  - Return to starting position
  - Repeat 3–5 times on each leg

6. Modified Downward Dog

- Intent
  - Increase articulation of ankles, hip joints, and shoulder girdle
  - Closed kinematic chain torso activation from hands and feet
  - Organize the torso in relationship to limbs
- Gait reasoning
  - Midline organization
  - Improve dorsiflexion for stance
- Starting position
  - Quadruped position on mat
- Movement description
  - Lift flexed knees off the floor
  - Press hands into the floor
  - Increase flexion as the ischial tuberosities move posteriorly and superiorly
  - Extend the knees
  - Hold for 30–60 seconds
  - Repeat 3 times

Chapter 14

7. Variation of Downward Dog with ankle focus

Intent	• Increase articulation of ankles, hip joints, and shoulder girdle • Closed kinematic chain torso activation from hands and feet • Organize torso in relationship to limbs
Gait reasoning	• Ankle dorsiflexion and plantar flexion for transference of weight in gait cycle
Starting position	• Quadruped position on mat
Movement description	• Flex right knee • Extend left knee and press left heel into floor • Inhale and exhale holding for 30 seconds • Repeat with left knee flexed and right knee extended • 2 repetitions on each leg

8. Extension over ball

Intent	• Improve torso extension with emphasis on thoracic region • Gentle force vectors through abdominal scar tissue • Facilitating thoracic excursion promotes breathing efficiency (Iguchi *et al.* 2022)
Gait reasoning	• Increase ability to rotate thorax • Organize to midline orientation

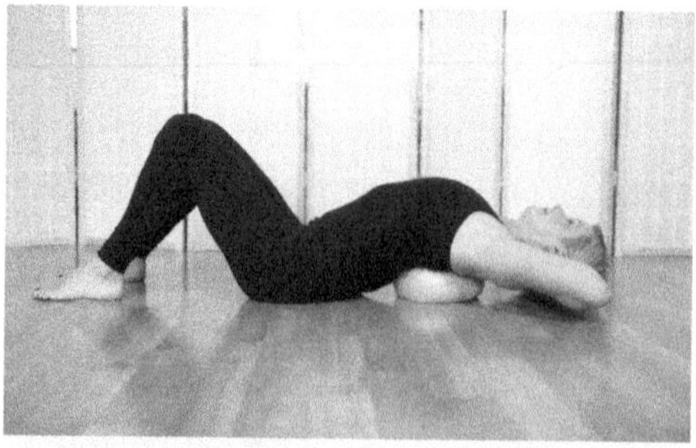

Figure 14.1

Starting position	• Seated with hip joints and knees flexed, feet on floor • Place 9 in. (23 cm) ball behind mid-thorax • Place second 9 in. ball between knees • Interlace fingers, place hands on occiput

Pilates for Recovery from Ovarian Cancer Post-Surgery: Effect on Gait

Movement description
- Extend torso over ball
- Breathe slowly expanding the thorax
- Breathe into the abdomen to focus on scar tissue and surrounding connective tissues
- Stay for 30 seconds to 1 minute

9. Roll-Up modified with 2 balls Derivative of J. H. Pilates Roll-Up (NPCE Study Guide 2021, p. 46)

Intent
- Increase torso articulation
- Gentle force vectors through abdominal scar tissue
- Coordinated sequencing of torso flexors and extensors

Gait reasoning
- Improve orientation of vertical axis for reciprocal motion of thorax and pelvic regions

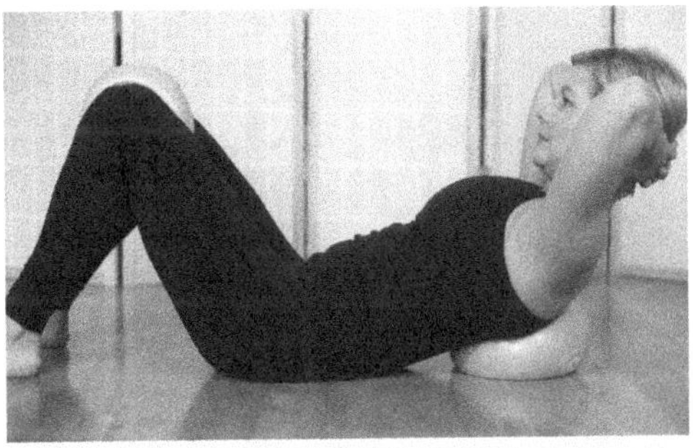

Figure 14.2

Starting position
- Seated with hip joints and knees flexed, feet on floor
- Place 9 in. (23 cm) ball behind mid-thorax
- Place second 9 in. ball between knees
- Interlace fingers, place hands on occiput

Movement description
- Lean back onto ball at mid-thorax
- Press thorax into ball as head and upper thorax move anteriorly into slight flexion
- Keep eyes gazing at ball between knees
- Hold for 4 counts
- On each exhale, feel anterior abdominal wall activation
- Lean back to extend over the ball
- Repeat 5 times

Author note
During my own recovery from ovarian cancer, I found this exercise helpful to feel the activation of the torso as if I was performing a plank. It is a safe way to rebuild a sustained torso activation necessary for gait and gave me a sense of regaining control of my body.

10. Bridge with ball

Intent
- Activate extensors
- Improve balance
- Challenge torso dynamic stability

Gait reasoning
- Activating extensors for push-off
- Organize to midline orientation

Starting position
- Supine
- Place 22 in. (55 cm) ball against wall for support
- Place feet together on ball with knee flexion
- Maintain LE adducted orientating midline

Movement description
- Keep ball still
- Press feet and heels into ball
- Extend hip joints elevating into bridge
- Slowly flex hip joints lowering to mat while keeping ball still
- Return to starting position
- Repeat 5–10 times
- Progress to moving ball away from wall

CUE
- The primary motion is pelvifemoral flexion and extension, not articulation of the torso

Author note
The activation of the LE in adducted position assists with activation of the LE to pelvic diaphragm continuously through the abdominal cavity. For the post-abdominal surgery client, this supports a felt sense of midline and sense of control and improves balance (proprioception and interoception) (Schleip and Stecco 2021).

11. Bilateral and unilateral extended bridge on ball

Intent
- Activate extensors
- Improve balance and coordination
- Challenges torso dynamic stability

Gait reasoning
- Activating extensors for push-off
- Orientation to midline
- LE deacceleration of swing phase prior to heel strike

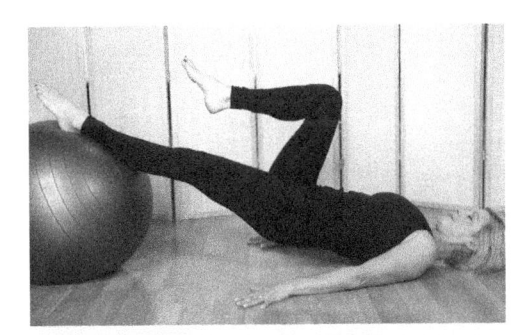

Figure 14.3

Starting position
- Supine on mat
- Place heels together on 22 in. (55 cm) ball with knees extended
- Maintain the LE adducted orientating midline

Movement description
- Flex knees and extend hip joints to pull ball and lift pelvis
- Extend hip joints and knees in bridge position
- Flex hip joints to lower pelvis to mat
- Repeat 5 times
- Flex knees and extend hip joints to pull ball and lift pelvis
- Extend hip joints and knees in bridge position
- Hold bridge position
- Flex right hip joint and knee
- Hold unilateral position
- Flex right hip joint to lower pelvis to mat
- Repeat 5 times
- Change sides
- Progress to a sustained elevated pelvis throughout exercise

12. Standing sagittal plane LE swing

Intent
- Challenge stance side
- Closed kinematic chain flexion and extension
- Increase endurance of standing on one leg

Gait reasoning
- Facilitates stance and swing motions

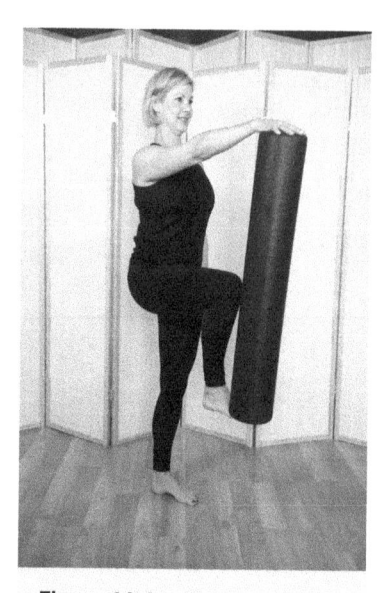

Figure 14.4

Starting position
- Standing
- Place foam roller on dorsum of right foot
- Right hand firmly pressing into foam roller
- Left UE by side

Movement description
- Press left foot into floor feeling tripod of the foot
- Slowly, flex at right hip joint and flex knee to 90 degrees
- Maintain contact of hand and foot with roller
- Slowly, extend hip joint and knee
- Repeat 10 times

Session 11/12: Studio session

Fatigue scale	1
Pain scale	3
Client self-report	• Reports ulcer is symptomatic • Experiences abdominal twitching and spasming with torso flexion • Neuropathy is inhibiting walking • Due to the recurrence, feeling depressed but determined to continue exercising
Key changes observed by author at end of Session 11/12	• Improved balance and coordination • Decreased pain • Improved single stance balance with oppositional LE swings
Reason behind choice of sequencing	• Basics of foundational Footwork • Work supine to lessen effort in gravity for movement reeducation • Relate Universal Reformer Footwork to extension and gait • Focus on dynamic stability • Challenge with unilateral movement

Session movement sequence

1. Footwork on Universal Reformer	Derivative of J. H. Pilates Footwork on Universal Reformer (NPCE Study Guide 2021, p. 52)
Intent	• Articulate ankles, knees, and hip joints in supine • Reorganization of gait patterning post-surgery • Basic Footwork is essential to increase awareness and control • Gentle force vectors from the feet through abdominal scar tissue
Gait reasoning	• Introduce LE patterning through sagittal plane • Increase pelvifemoral activation over knee dominance
Set-up	• Springs: 2 medium and 1 light • Footbar high
Starting position	• Supine • Bilateral mid-foot and rear foot on footbar • Resistance band around mid-femur

Author note
Feet sensitivity is present to anyone currently on chemotherapy and post-chemotherapy. Find the placement of the feet that is less sensitive.

Editor note
The use of the resistance band at mid-femur is to provide sensory feedback for ankle, knee, and hip joint tracking during Footwork. Extending the hips and knees, the band will be in contact without increasing tautness. The intention is to extend feeling the band on the posterior femur. During flexion, the band will be in contact with a slight tautness on the lateral side.

Movement description
- Gently roll plantar surface of feet on footbar if tolerable
- Change feet to cuboid contact
- Press feet into footbar to extend moving carriage away
- Maintain contact with resistance band without increased tautness
- 4 slow counts to fully extend LE
- Flex LE, slowly return carriage
- Maintain contact with resistance band adding a slight tautness
- 5–10 repetitions
- Repeat movement, changing feet positions
- Metatarsal arches on footbar parallel with small ball in between malleoli
- Metatarsal arches on footbar 35 degrees external rotation
- Cuboid contact, femurs abducted, externally rotated
- Metatarsal arches on footbar, hip joints abducted, externally rotated
- Metatarsal arches on footbar in parallel position
- Extend hip joints, knees, and ankles
- Maintain LE extension and dorsiflexion and plantar flexion of ankle joints
- Unilateral cuboid contact
- Change springs to 1 medium and 1 light, or 2 medium
- Unilateral metatarsal arch on footbar

Author note
Feet and LE can be sensitive and numb due to nerve damage caused by chemotherapy. Many cancer survivors feel weak and disembodied. They may feel embarrassed by their new normal. Encourage the client to focus on small action steps each time and be respectful and encouraging through positive feedback.

2. Straps: feet in loops on Universal Reformer	Derivative of J. H. Pilates Leg Springs Supine: Bicycle, Walking, Scissors, Circles (NPCE Study Guide 2021, pp. 67–68)
Intent	• Improve pelvifemoral relative movement • Facilitate femoral gliding in all planes • Enhance awareness of dynamic pelvic stability • Reduce lower limb lymphedema through elevation and movement • Balance activation of bilateral LE
Gait reasoning	• Coordination of pelvifemoral relative movement
Set-up	• Springs: 1 medium and 1 light, or 2 medium (see Author note) • Foot straps • Headrest up
Starting position	• Supine on carriage • Both feet in straps • Hip joints in flexion, abduction, and external rotation • Knee flexion • Feet in plantar flexion, right and left medial side of feet touching
Movement description	• Exhale to sense starting position • Inhale, extend and adduct LE with control • Exhale, return to starting position slowly • On the return, slight anterior rotation of pelvis to counter a posterior rotation • Repeat 5 times • Flex hips and extend knees • Adduct and externally rotate femur • Pull straps extending hips • Abduct hips in extended position • Abduct and flex hip joints • Adduct and flex hip joints • Repeat 3–5 times • Reverse direction

CUES
- Maintain LE within the frame of the Universal Reformer
- Avoid an anterior pelvic rotation at the end of the knee extension
- Avoid the tendency to go into posterior pelvic tilt from 110–125 degrees hip joints flexion

Chapter 14

Author note
An increase in load through springs may cause strain in the abdominal area and incite pain in clients post-surgery, for example after ostomy or hernia surgery. Choosing the best spring configuration is important (see Chapter 6).

Editor note
Ostomy surgery allows bodily waste to pass through a surgically created stoma on the abdomen into a prosthetic known as a pouch or ostomy bag on the outside of the body.

3. Supine arm series Derivative of J. H. Pilates Arm Springs: Circles Supine (NPCE Study Guide 2021, p. 69)

Intent
- Activate UE with torso dynamic stability

Gait reasoning
- Improved torso adaptability to UE movement for arm swing
- Increase proprioception of UE to torso

Set-up
- Medium spring
- Handles/loops

Starting position
- Supine
- Hold straps, shoulders in 90 degrees flexion with elbows extended
- 90 degrees hip joint flexion/abduction with knee flexion
- 1st metatarsophalangeal (MTP) joints together

Movement description
- Pulling the straps
  - Inhale, shoulder extension
  - Exhale, shoulder flexion
  - Repeat 5–10 times
  - Extension/abduction/horizontal adduction
  - Move in a slow tempo of 4 counts for each position
  - Return to starting position
  - Repeat 3–6 times

CUES
- The posterior surface of both scapulae and both innominates are equally weighted on the carriage
- Cue the rhythm of one UE repetition, requires 12 seconds to complete
- This facilitates the integration of torso and UE participation
- It is important for the client to feel the three-dimensional torso activation, not the UE effort

Author note
- When you control the tempo and calibrate the spring resistance appropriately for tissue integrity, it may promote remodeling of the adhesions (see Volume 1 Chapter 6) (see Editor note on adhesions and scarring at the beginning of this chapter)
- A 90 degrees hip joint flexion position may increase discomfort. Increase the hip joint flexion degree beyond 90 degrees and allow lower limb to hang

4. Single Leg Stretch on Universal Reformer

Derivative of J. H. Pilates Single Leg Stretch (NPCE Study Guide 2021, p. 46)

Intent
- Activate torso through limb resistance
- Improve torso dynamic stability and pelvic adaptability
- Gait reasoning
- Midline torso orientation with limb movement

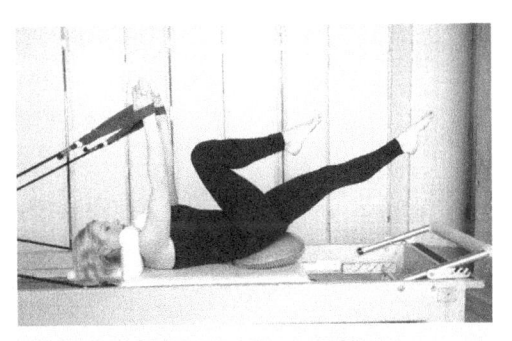

Figure 14.5

Set-up
- Medium spring
- Air cushion disc placed under pelvis
- Footbar high
- Headrest up

Editor note
The air cushion disc is an air-filled, soft, pliable PVC disc that allows the individual to adapt to weight shifts during a variety of movements. The air cushion disc provides sensory feedback to the client allowing the righting reflex response to organize to midline (see Editor note on air cushion disc, Chapter 7, Volume 1 in Chapter 21).

Chapter 14

Starting position
- Supine
- Hold straps, shoulders to 90 degrees flexion with elbows extended
- 90 degrees hip joint and knee flexion
- Head down

Movement description
- Extend bilateral shoulders and right hip joint and knee
- Maintain head down position
- Flex right hip joint and knee
- Repeat right side slowly 5 times
- Flex left hip joint and knee
- Repeat left side slowly 5 times
- Alternate right and left 5 times
- Return to starting position
- Place feet on footbar to rest

CUES
- Initiate with the pelvis sinking into the air cushion, with a slight posterior pelvic rotation to counter an anterior pelvic motion during LE movements
- Articulate the UE movement from scapulae to hands
- Visualize the thorax sinking into the scapulae and scapulae into the carriage

Author note
Abdominal surgery, chemotherapy, and radiation compromise connective tissue integrity. Scar tissue interferes with efficient force transmission. Unsupported cervical motion may increase intra-abdominal pressure (IAP) (see Chapter 10, Volume 1 Editor note). The increase in IAP may increase risk of a hernia post-surgery. Performing this exercise with the head down eliminates the possibility of increasing IAP. The head supported on the headrest promotes a sense of safety and accomplishment (Samimian *et al.* 2021).

5. Double Leg Stretch on Universal Reformer Derivative of J. H. Pilates Double Leg Stretch (NPCE Study Guide 2021, p. 47)

Intent
- Activate torso through limb resistance
- Improve torso dynamic stability and pelvic adaptability
- Articulation of bilateral LE flexion and extension

Gait reasoning
- Midline torso orientation with limb movement

Pilates for Recovery from Ovarian Cancer Post-Surgery: Effect on Gait

Set-up
- Medium spring
- Air cushion disc
- Footbar high
- Headrest up

Starting position
- Supine
- Hold straps, shoulders to 90 degrees flexion with elbows extended
- 90 degrees hip joint and knee flexion
- Head down

Movement description
- Extend bilateral shoulders and LE
- Maintain head down position
- Flex bilateral shoulders, LE to starting position
- Repeat slowly 5 times

CUES
- Initiate with the pelvis sinking into the air cushion disc, with a slight posterior pelvic rotation to counter an anterior pelvic motion during LE movements
- The degree of LE extension is relative to the ability to maintain the pelvis weighted into air cushion disc
- Articulate the UE movement from scapulae to hands
- Visualize the thorax sinking into the scapulae and scapulae into the carriage

6. Reverse Knee Stretch on Universal Reformer
Derivative of J. H. Pilates Knee Stretch Series: Kneeling, Round Back (NPCE Study Guide, p. 60)
(See Chapter 5 in Volume 1, Trier, Knee stretch variations)

Intent
- Improve flexion and extension articulation and activation
- Torso endurance in horizontal position
- Decrease posterior pelvic rotation for improved acetabular femoral relationship

Gait reasoning
- Ease in leg swing in sagittal plane
- Midline orientation during flexion and extension

Set-up
- Springs: 1 very light or 1 light

Starting position
- Quadruped position, feet toward footbar
- Knees touching shoulder stops
- Hands on sides of frame
- Shoulders in 110 degrees flexion, elbows extended
- Slightly pull the frame, moving the carriage to place hands under shoulders

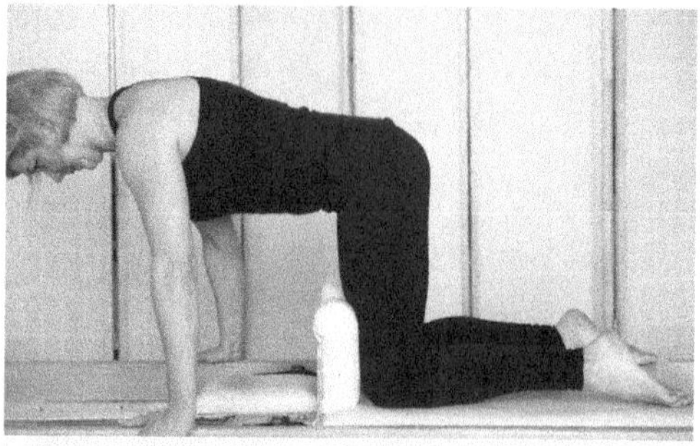

Chapter 14

Figure 14.6

Movement description
- Exhale, flex hip joints without changing torso organization, moving carriage toward hands
- LE extension moving carriage away from hands
- Eccentric control during extension returning carriage toward footbar
- Repeat 5 times

CUES
- Maintain torso organization
- Abdominal wall moves posteriorly on exhale
- Intend to maintain the abdominal wall posteriorly
- On exhale, the lowest ribs rotate anteriorly bringing the anterior ribs inferiorly and posterior ribs superiorly
- UE position remains under shoulders throughout movement

Author note
- There is a loss of sensation and proprioception of the pelvic area post-abdominal surgery
- This is an excellent exercise to restore proprioception and awareness of the breath relationship to the abdominal wall function

7. Teaser modified on Pilates Arc Derivative of J. H. Pilates Teaser on Universal Reformer (NPCE Study Guide 2021, p. 54)

Intent
- Challenge torso organization in an incline against resistance from UE

Gait reasoning
- Improve extension increasing midline orientation and vertical axis for rotation

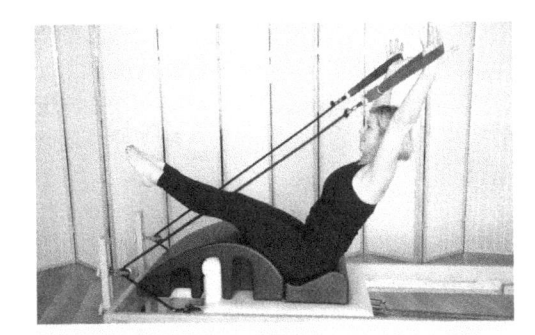

Pilates for Recovery from Ovarian Cancer Post-Surgery: Effect on Gait

Figure 14.7

Set-up	● Pilates Arc over the shoulder stops with seat area toward footbar
	● Springs: 1 very light or 1 light
	● Handles/loops
	● Strap length: longer straps allow for more back extension
Starting position	● Sit on seat facing straps
	● Hip joint and knee flexion
	● Torso upright
	● Holding straps with shoulder flexion and elbow extension
Movement description	● Variation 1
	■ Exhale, pull straps flexing the shoulders 170–180 degrees
	■ Unilateral knee extension
	■ Maintain torso upright organization
	■ Inhale, sternum posteriorly rotates extending the thorax
	■ Exhale, slowly extend shoulder to starting position
	■ Flex knee to starting position
	■ Repeat 5 times on both sides
	● Variation 2
	■ Exhale, pull straps flexing shoulders 170–180 degrees
	■ Bilateral knee extension
	■ Maintain torso upright organization
	■ Inhale, sternum posteriorly rotates extending thorax
	■ Exhale, slowly extend shoulder to starting position
	■ Flex knees to starting position
	■ Repeat 5 times both sides

- Variation 3: adding thoracic rotation
  - Lower right UE
  - Rotate thorax to right
  - Left UE remains flexed 170–180 degrees
  - Return to elevated UE position
  - Lower left UE
  - Rotate thorax to left
  - Right UE remains flexed 170–180 degrees
  - Return to elevated UE position
  - Repeat 3 times

CUES
- With each breath, focus on control of the whole body
- Use the inhale to prevent thoracic flexion
- Discontinue exercise if any abdominal or pelvic pain is present

8. Supine unilateral LE flexion with strap

Intent
- Motor control during LE flexion and extension
- Improve femoral glide in sagittal plane
- Activate torso through LE resistance
- Improve torso dynamic stability and pelvic adaptability

Gait reasoning
- Ease in leg swing in sagittal plane
- Midline orientation during flexion and extension

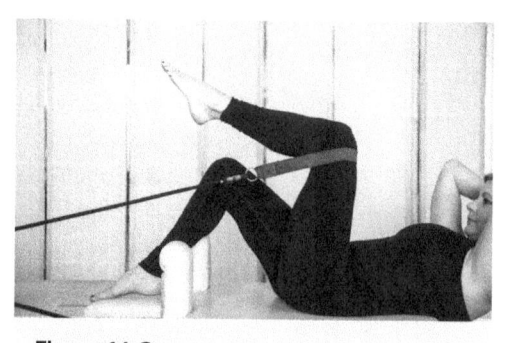

Figure 14.8

Set-up
- Springs: 1 very light or 1 light
- Foot strap

Pilates for Recovery from Ovarian Cancer Post-Surgery: Effect on Gait

Starting position
- Sit in middle of carriage facing shoulder stops
- Place feet on headrest
- Place foot strap above right knee
- Left foot on headrest
- Supine on carriage with right LE in 90 degrees flexion
- Interlace hands behind head fully supporting occiput
- Sink ribs into carriage
- Torso in small degree of flexion
- Maintain this position

Movement description
- Inhale, slowly extend right LE
- Exhale, slowly flex LE to 90–100 degrees
- Repeat 5 times
- Change to other side, repeat

CUES
- Gently press occiput into hands
- Use the exhale to allow the femoral head to glide posteriorly
- On the inhale focus on maintaining pelvic and lower rib contact on carriage

Author note
Practicing this movement in a single-leg action versus a double-leg action allows the individual to find the dynamic adaptation of the hip joint glide and pelvis response to a single-leg action.

9. Side lying hip joint variations

Intent
- Improve hip joint abduction and femoral medial glide
- Promote hip medial and lateral glide
- Activation of pelvifemoral neuromyofascia

Gait reasoning
- Improve balance
- Fall prevention strategy

Set-up
- Mat
- Head support: pillow or folded blanket

Starting position
- Lie on side with ankles, knees, pelvis, shoulders, and ears aligned
- Support head with pillow or folded blanket

Movement description
- Abduct right femur with knee extension
- Hold for 10 seconds
- Repeat 10 times on each side

Chapter 14

CUES
- Maintain the side contact points—ankle, pelvis, lower thorax, shoulders, and lateral head—throughout the movement
- Be conscious of femoral motion without pelvic hiking

Author note
- If any discomfort is experienced, stop this movement
- Anteriorly rotate the hemipelvis of the moving leg providing an optimal position to enhance medial femoral glide and posterior-lateral myofascia activation.

The journey to Session 11

Session 4/12
Client self-report

- Feels good
- Tightness in groin area and lumbar region
- Pain scale 4
- Fatigue scale 4

Key changes observed

- Increased feelings of excitement and hopefulness

Reasoning behind choice of movements

- Address connective tissue restrictions and scar adhesions in abdominal and pelvic regions

Session movement sequence
1. Extension over ball

2. Pelvic clocks

3. Modified Downward Dog

4. Side lying abduction with knee flexion

5. Supine: right abduction, knee flexion, ankle dorsiflexion with right ankle on left femur, change sides

6. Trapeze Table

- Thigh Stretch
- Unilateral LE series
- Roll-Up

7. Ladder Barrel

- Lateral flexion
- Standing hip joint flexion with knee extension
- Standing hip joint extension with knee flexion

Session 5/12
Client self-report

- Feels better mentally
- Experiencing stiffness in hip joints
- Fatigue scale 2
- Pain scale 1

Key changes observed

- Improved feet and knee alignment in squat
- Increased awareness of feet pronation
- Able to reorganize rear foot establishing a balance point on feet

Reasoning behind choice of movements

- Improve overall ability to move fully

Pilates for Recovery from Ovarian Cancer Post-Surgery: Effect on Gait

- Increase plantar flexion and dorsiflexion
- Increase torso range of movement in all directions

Session movement sequence
1. Ankle pumps using resistance band around feet

2. Pelvic clocks

3. Wall squat

4. Variation of Downward Dog-ankle focus

5. Standing sagittal plane LE swing

6. Universal Reformer

- Footwork
- Straps: feet in loops
- Supine arm work

7. Additional movement

- Supine unilateral hip joint flexion and knee extension using Magic Circle

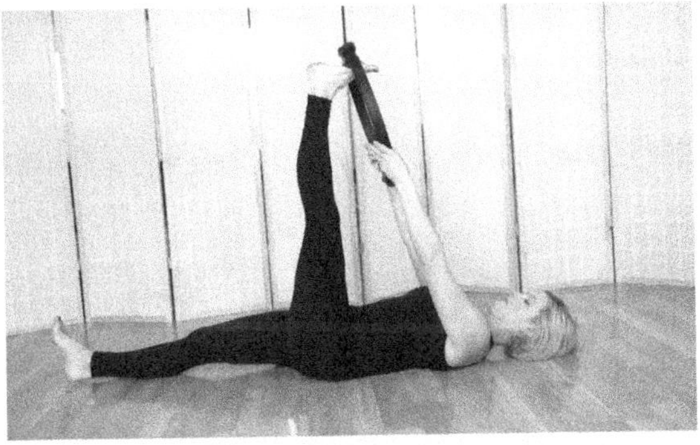

Figure 14.9

Session 6/12
Client self-report

- Feeling tight and restricted in diaphragm region where she had surgery
- Notices scar adhesions, desires to address the scarring
- States feet are numb and always in pain
- Pain scale 4
- Fatigue scale 2

Key changes observed

- Less fearful of movement
- Decrease in pain

Reasoning behind choice of movements

- Continue with mobility and articulation to alleviate discomfort and stiff feelings
- Improve stance balance
- Increase load from feet to torso
- Promote extension

Session movement sequence
1. Downward Dog

2. Extension over ball

3. Roll-Up modified with 2 balls

4. Universal Reformer

- Straps: feet in loops
- Supine arm work
- Seated chest expansion

5. Additional movement

- SmartSpine heat therapy for scar adhesions

Chapter 14

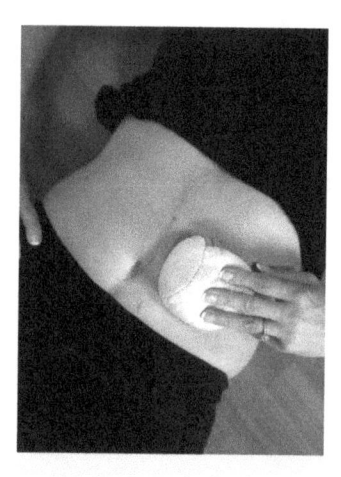

Figure 14.10

Author note
Heat in the therapeutic range with temperatures up to 104 degrees F (40 degrees C) contributes to relaxation of fascial stiffness in relation to myofascial dysfunction (Chaitow 2018). The *SmartSpine* system uses the fascial properties of thermoreception, interoception, and proprioception as an effective delivery system to increase movement potential as well as movement ease, improving the fascial hydrodynamic ability (Schleip and Stecco 2021).

Session 7/12
Client self-report

- Reports increase of energy and feeling a sense of improvement
- Pain scale 0
- Fatigue scale 1

Key changes observed

- Increased articulation and mobility in all planes of thoracic region

- During Footwork improved plantar flexion and dorsiflexion

Reasoning behind choice of movements

- Client is feeling embodied and confident
- Continue to increase awareness of body organization for improved gait
- Reduce lower limb lymphedema

Session movement sequence
1. Standing sagittal plane LE swing

2. Single-leg balance swings

- Roll-Up modified with 2 balls

3. Bicycle (on mat) with 9 in. (23 cm) stability ball under pelvis

4. Universal Reformer

- Straps: feet in loops
- Supine arm work
- Single Leg Stretch with air cushion disc
- Double Leg Stretch with air cushion disc

5. Additional movement

- Supine unilateral hip joint flexion and knee extension using Magic Circle

Session 8/12
Client self-report

- Fatigue scale 2
- Pain scale 3
- Reports feeling dizzy
- Neuropathy has increased, painful to stand
- Increased stress about tumor metastasis

Key changes observed

- Walking time increased
- Neuropathy challenging single-leg balance

Reasoning behind choice of movements

- Focus on grounding whole-body movement to support anxiety
- Chose to use SmartSpine to ease stiffness

Session movement sequence

1. Ankle pumps

2. Leg slides

3. Pelvic clocks

4. Wall squat

5. Supine: right femoral abduction, knee flexion, ankle dorsiflexion with right ankle on left femur, change sides

6. Trapeze Table used as a table to place SmartSpine

- SmartSpine
- Pelvic clocks
- Knee folds
- Supported hip flexion with knee extension
- Slow breathing

Session 9/12
Client self-report

- Feeling better, more energy
- Pain scale 0
- Fatigue scale 1

Key changes observed

- Overall improved body organization
- Increased energy

Reasoning behind choice of movements

- Continue building torso strength
- Improve single-leg stance balance
- Build confidence addressing kinesiophobia

Session movement sequence

1. Extension over ball

2. Roll-Up modified with 2 balls

3. Single-leg balance swings

4. Standing sagittal plane LE swing

5. Universal Reformer

- Supine arm series
- Single Leg Stretch
- Reverse Knee Stretch

6. Pilates Arc

- Modified Teaser

7. Additional movement

- Supine unilateral hip joint flexion and knee extension using Magic Circle

Session 10/12
Client self-report

- Feeling excited about moving again after a lapse of 6 months with no exercise
- Pain scale 0
- Fatigue scale 0

Key changes observed

- Improved overall body organization
- Smoother gait rhythm, no limp
- Stopped placing hands on abdomen as protection while standing or supine

Reasoning behind choice of movements

- Activate torso flexors without risk of herniation or strain
- Build confidence and self esteem
- Improve balance

Session movement sequence

1. Standing sagittal plane LE swing

2. Universal Reformer

- Supine arm series
- Single Leg Stretch
- Reverse Knee Stretch

3. Pilates Arc

- Modified Teaser

4. Additional movement

- Supine unilateral hip flexion and knee extension using Magic Circle

References

ACSM (American College of Sports Medicine) (2019) New infographic available: Exercise Guidelines for Cancer Patients and Survivors. November 27, 2019. "Effects of exercise on health-related outcomes in those with cancer." [Infographic]. www.acsm.org/news-detail/2019/11/27/new-infographic-available-exercise-guidelines-cancer-patients-survivors.

American Cancer Society (2023) Key statistics for ovarian cancer. October 3, 2023. www.cancer.org/cancer/ovarian-cancer/about/key-statistics.html. [Accessed October 29, 2023].

Black, M. (2022) *Centered: Organizing the Body through Kinesiology, Movement Theory and Pilates Techniques.* Edinburgh: Handspring Publishing, pp. 123–125.

Campbell, K. L., Winters-Stone, K. M., Wiskemann, J., May, A. M. et al. (2019) "Exercise guidelines for cancer survivors: Consensus statement from International Multidisciplinary Roundtable." *Medicine & Science in Sports & Exercise, 51,* 11, 2375–2390.

Cannioto, R. A. and Moysich, K. B. (2015) "Epithelial ovarian cancer and recreational physical activity: A review of the epidemiological literature and implications for exercise prescription." *Gynecologic Oncology, 137,* 3, 559–573.

Chaitow, L. (2018) "Removing obstacles to recovery: Therapeutic methods, mechanisms and fascia." In: L. Chaitow (Ed.) *Fascial Dysfunction: Manual Therapy Approaches.* 2nd Ed. Edinburgh: Handspring Publishing, p. 127.

Diller, R. B. and Tabor, A. J. (2022) "The role of the extracellular matrix (ECM) in wound healing: A review." *Biomimetics, 7,* 87. DOI: 10.3390/biomimetics7030087.

Guimberteau, J.-C. and Armstrong, C. (2015) *Architecture of Human Living Fascia: The Extracellular Matrix and Cells Revealed Through Endoscopy.* Edinburgh: Handspring Publishing, pp. 143–154.

Huang, J., Chan, W. C., Ngai, C. H., Lok, V. et al. (2022) On Behalf of NCD Global Health Research Group of Association of Pacific Rim Universities (APRU). "Worldwide burden, risk factors, and temporal trends of ovarian cancer: A global study." *Cancers (Basel), 14,* 9. DOI: 10.3390/cancers14092230.

Iguchi, N., Mano, T., Iwasa, N., Ozaki, M. et al. (2022) "Thoracic excursion is a biomarker for evaluating respiratory function in amyotrophic lateral sclerosis." *Frontiers in Neurology, 13,* 2022. DOI: 10.3389/fneur.2022.853469.

NPCE Study Guide (National Pilates Certification Exam Study Guide) (2021) Miami, FL: National Pilates Certification Program, Inc.

Pi, H., Ku, H., Zhao, T., Wang, J., and Fu, Y. (2018) "Influence of ankle active dorsiflexion movement guided by inspiration on the venous return from the lower limbs: A prospective study." *The Journal of Nursing Research, 26,* 2, 123–129.

Pilat, A. (2022) *Myofascial Induction: Volume 1—The Upper Body.* Edinburgh: Handspring Publishing, pp. 199–201.

Samimian, S., Ashrafi, S., Khaleghdoost Mohammadi, T., Yeganeh, M. R. et al. (2021) "The correlation between head of bed angle and intra-abdominal pressure of intubated patients; a pre-post clinical trial." *Archives of Academic Emergency Medicine, 9,* 1. DOI: 10.22037/aaem.v9i1.1065.

Schleip, R. and Stecco, C. (2021) "Fascia as a sensory organ." In: R. Schleip and J. Wilke (Eds.) *Fascia in Sport and Movement.* 2nd Ed. Edinburgh: Handspring Publishing, pp. 176–177.

Xue, M. and Jackson, C. J. (2015) "Extracellular matrix reorganization during wound healing and its impact on abnormal scarring." *Advances in Wound Care (New Rochelle), 4,* 3, 119–136.

Chapter 15

Pilates and Post-Robotic Nerve-Sparing Radical Prostatectomy: Effect on Gait

Dawn-Marie Ickes

In 2021, the American Cancer Society estimated that about one man in eight will be diagnosed with prostate cancer during their lifetime (Sung et al. 2021). Prostate cancer is more likely to develop in older men and in non-Hispanic Black men. About six cases in 10 are diagnosed in men who are 65 or older, and it is rare in men under 40. The average age of men at diagnosis is about 66. Prostate cancer is the second leading cause of cancer death behind lung cancer in American men. Most men diagnosed with prostate cancer do not die from it, and more than 3.1 million men in the United States are prostate cancer survivors. A prostatectomy—the complete removal of the prostate—helps eliminate the cancer; however, this procedure often causes other undesirable consequences, including incontinence. Incontinence after a prostatectomy is not experienced by everyone, but those who are affected may suffer from it for up to two years following surgery.

After a prostatectomy normal pelvic function is affected; this is known as pelvic floor dysfunction (PFD). There are three categories of PFD: weakness from underactivity; overactivity due to tightness or spasm; dyssynergia—abnormal coordination with inappropriate or poorly timed activations. A majority of post-prostatectomy men with stress urinary incontinence (SUI) have both overactivity and underactivity. Among other comorbid conditions associated with urinary incontinence after surgery, the literature identifies depression as the most debilitating mental health condition (Strojek et al. 2021).

One way to help reduce incontinence after surgery is to normalize pelvic diaphragm function through specific and variable training sequences (Hodges et al. 2020; Scott et al. 2020). The pelvic diaphragm is located at the base of the pelvis between the pubic bone and coccyx. Its structures consist of an intricate web of connective tissues that help support pelvic organs, help control bladder and bowel function, and are involved in sexual function.

In a study by Scott et al. (2020), 87 percent of the subjects showed significant improvement in incontinence symptoms following individualized physical training and movement reeducation. Besides improvements in incontinence, patients also showed a decrease in pain and improved mental health.

Movement contraindications

- No bearing down (Valsalva maneuver)
- No lifting more than 10 lb (4.5 kg) for 6 weeks
- No increase in intra-abdominal pressure (IAP) for 6 weeks
- No sexual activity for 4 to 6 weeks—requires MD clearance
- No running or jumping for 12 weeks

Chapter 15

Client description: 60-year-old individual, identifies as male; contractor

Dates of case report: Session 1: December 15, 2019; Session 12: March 2, 2020

Studio apparatus and props
Pilates equipment

- Universal Reformer

Props used with equipment

- Universal Reformer box
- Small 1 in. (2.5 cm) pads, 0.25 in. (62 mm) thick, for feet
- Weighted bamboo yoga block
- 9 in. (23 cm) diameter ball, three-quarters inflated
- 6 in. (15 cm) diameter ball, fully inflated
- Air cushion disc
- 26 in. (65 cm) ball
- 2 rotator discs

Home program props

- Wall space
- Heavy resistance band, 6 ft (1.8 m)
- Yoga block
- 9 in. (23 cm) diameter ball, three-quarters inflated
- 6 in. (15 cm) diameter ball, fully inflated
- Soft foam roller, 36 in. (92 cm) long, 6 in. (15 cm) in diameter
- Slider

Methods and materials

Session 1/12
1. Health history interview

- Client reports laparoscopic prostatectomy 2 weeks prior
- Cleared by MD for gentle exercise with precautions and contraindications
- No prior history of pelvic girdle pain, urinary incontinence, or balance issues
- Past orthopedic history of frozen shoulder with good resolution

2. Symptoms

- Deep ache in pelvis
- General fatigue
- Abdominal soreness at incisional sites
- SUI
- Low back tightness with mild ache
- Physical stress increases symptoms such as: standing up from couch; quick stepping after standing up; lifting grandchild—watches 3 times a week

3. Movement aids

- None

Final result of case report

The client was able to stand up quickly without leakage, lift 30 lb (13.5 kg), step reactively, and walk at a faster pace without leakage or dribbling. Discontinued use of adult protective briefs. The client was able to squat and lift grandchild (30 lb/13.5 kg) without incidence of SUI or pain.

Center of mass (COM) was restored to center one-third of weight-bearing circumference and weight-bearing balance between left and right improved to within 2 degrees or less.

Session 2/12: Initial assessment

1. General observations of gait

- Left transverse plane rotation
- Left ribcage shift
- Decreased stance time on right leg
- Decreased torso oppositional rotation, on right more than on left

2. Standing tests

- Full torso rotation
- Observations of inefficient side: right
  - Begins in left transverse plane rotation, decreased segmental movement through motion
  - Rotation occurs from T4–T7 only
  - Decreased pelvic rotation on the femurs
- Hemipelvis inferior motion
- Observations of inefficient side: left
  - Difficulty lowering left hemipelvis adapts with right transverse plane rotation
  - Decreased right lumbar lateral flexion
  - Lateral shift to right
- Hemipelvis superior motion
- Observations of inefficient side: right
  - Left side more efficient but decreased range
  - Lateral shift
  - Inability to shift pelvis without pelvic torsion

Session 12/12: Post-assessment

1. General observations of gait

- No transverse plane rotation noted statically or dynamically
- Ribcage midline centered
- Equal stance time, bilateral in loading
- Improved torso rotation

2. Standing tests

- Full torso rotation
- Observations of inefficient side: both
  - Segmental movement noted in rotation
  - Improved pelvic rotation on femurs
- Hemipelvis inferior motion
- Observations of inefficient side: both
  - Improved lowering of left hemipelvis
  - Pelvis maintains frontal plane alignment—no compensatory transverse plane rotation
  - Torso centered over pelvis
  - Slight lateral shift to right
- Hemipelvis superior motion
- Observations of inefficient side: right
  - Left biased but functional range
  - Slight lateral shift
  - Improved control of torso over pelvis
- Lateral pelvic shift
- Observations of inefficient side: both
  - No loss of balance

Chapter 15

- ◆ Lateral pelvic shift

- ● Observations of inefficient side: right
  - Loss of balance with sway to right
  - Thorax translates excessively to left
  - Feet not adapting
  - Limited in left femoral abduction and right adduction

3. Seated tests

- ◆ Thoracic rotation

- ● Observations of inefficient side: left
  - Weight shift to left ischial tuberosity
  - Complained of left tightness
  - Torso translated left through mid-thorax decreasing left thoracic rotation

- ◆ Hip flexion

- ● Observations of inefficient side: left
  - Experiences pinching with left hip flexion
  - Moderate limitation of motion

4. Sit and stand

- ◆ Lateral view

- ● Hip hinge with left weight shift
- ● Moves with care
- ● Appears anxious

- ◆ Anterior view

- ● Weight shift onto left lower extremity
- ● Complained of tissue adhesion pulling in abdomen with transition to stand but not reverse to sit

- ■ Thorax translates to the left within functional limit
- ■ Feet adaptations noted
- ■ COM stays centered between left and right until shift

3. Seated tests

- ◆ Thoracic rotation

- ● Observations of inefficient side: left
  - Decreased tightness
  - Weight shift to left ischial tuberosity reduced but present
  - Decreased torso translation through mid-thorax

- ◆ Hip flexion

- ● Observations of inefficient side: both
  - No pinching
  - Slight left thorax translation

4. Sit and stand

- ◆ Lateral view

- ● Hip hinge with even weight distribution
- ● Moves with ease
- ● Nose over toes without effort

- ◆ Anterior view

- ● Weight balanced over both feet
- ● No tissue adhesion pulling sensation

5. Standing balance

- ◆ Two-leg stance, eyes open
- 60 seconds
- ◆ One-leg stance, eyes open
- Left leg: 10 seconds
- Right leg: 5 seconds

5. Standing balance

- ◆ Two-leg stance, eyes open
- 60 seconds
- ◆ One-leg stance, eyes open
- Left leg: 30 seconds
- Right leg: 25 seconds

Session 3/12: Home program

Fatigue scale	6
Pain scale	4
Client self-report	• Awareness is different with standing and walking, able to get a sense of pelvis and hips and feel the difference between left and right
Key changes observed by author at end of Session 3/12	• Smoother transitions off and on table • Accurate physical response to verbal cues • Able to adjust his compensation to a more optimal movement with verbal or tactile cues
Reason behind choice of sequencing	• Standing work facilitates proprioception of feet to torso • Oppositional thoracic-pelvic patterning • Pelvic diaphragm reeducation • Addressing imbalances and awareness • Prone and quadruped positions for torso reeducation • Hip activation through closed kinematic chain

Session movement sequence

1. Standing on pencils (Black 2022)

Intent	• Sensory awareness of feet in standing • COM shift under talus • Optimal foot-ankle organization • Proper talus positioning • Torso activation in relation to weight-distribution changes • Reasoning related to gait • Train coordination for adaptability during gait • Increase sensory awareness of foot positioning with weight bearing • Sensory input to adapt to ground surfaces • Reset COM placement for single-leg balance at stance phase • Talar positional influence on hip centralization in acetabulum for optimal mobility • Intrinsic foot training for improved gait sequencing
Gait reasoning	• Stand with two pencils running diagonally from the base of big toe to lateral front edge of calcaneus • Stand with both feet in parallel bringing awareness to 1st to 5th metatarsal heads and medial and lateral borders of calcaneus

Starting position	● Seated on mat or on a chair with torso upright ● Legs can be in any comfortable position ● Place each hand on lower lateral ribcage
Movement description	● Stand and explore whole-body sensations while standing on pencils ● Remove the pencils ● Stand and feel how the weight is distributed ● Shift weight from heels to forefoot to find optimal foot-ankle organization ● Inhale during hip and knee flexion, activating the pelvic diaphragm ● Exhale during hip and knee extension, relaxing the pelvic diaphragm ● Repeat 5 times ● Switch the breath ● Repeat 5 times ● Exhale, flex hip and knee joints activating the pelvic diaphragm ● Inhale, extend hip and knee joints relaxing the pelvic diaphragm ● Repeat: 　■ Heels together in 45 degrees hip external rotation 　■ Wide stance, 45 degrees hip external rotation and abduction 　■ Parallel hip adduction and heels elevated

2. Windmill rotation with dowel

Intent	● Standing with even weight-bearing through rotational range of motion (ROM) ● Increase ability to rotate
Gait reasoning	● Proprioception of COM placement while rotating ● Sensory input adapting to ground surfaces ● Reset COM placement for double- and single-leg balance ● Preparation for oppositional thoracic rotation relationship to pelvis

Chapter 15

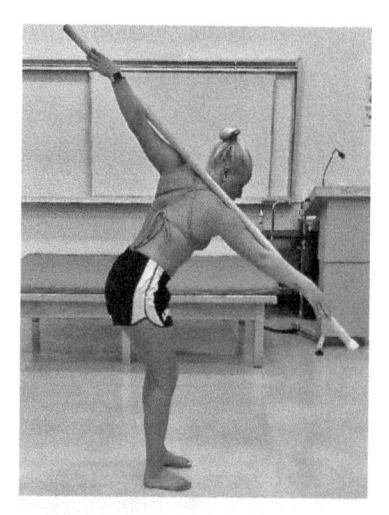

Figure 15.1

Starting position
- Stand with feet slightly wider apart than shoulder width, 7–10 degrees external rotation
- Place a dowel across upper thorax spanning arms
- Hold dowel
- Hinge from hips with torso at 45-degree angle relative to hips
- Feel optimal foot-ankle positioning
- Extend through crown of head

Movement description
- Inhale, and maintaining ischial tuberosities wide rotate to right
- Exhale, return to center
- Rotate to left
- Return to standing upright
- Repeat 5 sets

3. Ball-sit differentiation

Intent
- Introduce compression to the perineum
- Increase awareness of strategies for seated weight bearing
- Preparation for organization of pelvis in standing

Editor note
Tissue compression stimulates circulation and sensory input to reduce movement inhibition due to post-surgical pain. It is not recommended for a person who is not cleared by their medical doctor concerning healing and tissue health.

Gait reasoning	● Preparation for gait patterning ● Increase awareness of proximal initiation

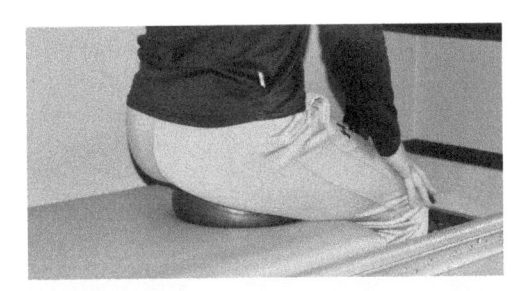

Figure 15.2

Starting position	● Sitting on a stool ● Perform 1 sustained 5 second activation of pelvic diaphragm without ball to establish a baseline comparison ● Place 9 in. (23 cm) diameter ball, three-quarters inflated, in center of triangle created by pubic bone and ischial tuberosities ● Identify strategy of weight bearing on ischial tuberosities ● Decrease asymmetry by adjusting weight through ischia ● Arms reach forward to challenge torso control
Movement description	● Sit on ball for 30 seconds monitoring breathing patterns, pain-free ● Stop early if painful or creates spasm ● To increase tolerance use softer ball or use hands to unload weight ● Remove ball and sit ● Ask client to notice the sensation without ball in sitting ● Practice breathing patterns with focus on sensations from the pelvic diaphragm up through the torso ● Sustain inhale breath for 6 seconds, exhalation for 6 seconds or longer, maintaining the sensation of pelvic diaphragm ● Follow 5 rapid rhythmic activations of pelvic diaphragm ● Repeat breath pattern and rapid rhythmic activation for 3 sets, progressing to 5 sets ● Encourage client to be aware of any changes of sensation ● Progress to 60 seconds ● Add torso rotation during sustained inhalation breathing pattern ● Repeat entire sequence replacing ball with soft foam roller

4. Wall squat with 9 in. (23 cm) ball

Intent
- Loading for synergistic activation and spontaneous neuro-myofascial response
- Increase connection to active and passive phases of the diaphragmic system
- Enhance diaphragmic system function during activities of daily living

Gait reasoning
- Proprioception
- Sensory input to adapt to ground surfaces
- Reset COM placement for double- and single-leg balance

Starting position
- Place ball against wall at lower thorax
- Squat down to 60 degrees hip flexion with both hands on posterior-lateral aspect of hips
- Feet are parallel with normal torso sagittal plane curves

Movement description
- Progression 1
  - In squat position, 5 rapid rhythmic activations of the pelvic diaphragm
  - Return to standing for 15 second rest
  - Repeat 10 times
- Progression 2
  - In squat position, hold a sustained activation of pelvic diaphragm for 5 seconds
  - Return to standing for 15 second rest
  - Repeat 10 times

5. Side lying hip abduction

Intent
- Increase activation of posterior-lateral hip in coordination with torso control
- Isometric activation of torso during active leg movement
- Activation of pelvic diaphragm in coordination with sustained torso position

Gait reasoning
- Improve load response and single-leg stance balance
- Enhance connection and awareness of pelvic diaphragm with hip rotation
- Practice coordinated length changes of external rotation of hip

Pilates and Post-Robotic Nerve-Sparing Radical Prostatectomy: Effect on Gait

Starting position
- Lie on left side on mat
- Support head with a small bolster or rolled towel
- Hips and knees in flexion with head, shoulders, pelvis, and heels aligned along back edge of mat
- Reach right ischium toward right heel to translate thorax to right to avoid collapsing left side into mat

Movement description
- Inhale, press feet together while abducting right hip
- Torso remains in side position, not rolling anteriorly or posteriorly
- Exhale, returning to starting position
- Relax but do not change position
- Repeat 10 times on each side
- Rest for 2 minutes
- Repeat with opposite breath patterning, 5 times on each side for 10 sets

6. Quadruped four-corner diagonal preparation

Intent
- Preparation for loading hip joint
- Increase and balance hip mobility focusing on abduction phase for medial-inferior capsule; adduction phase for superior-lateral capsule
- Motor control and function of pelvifemoral motion

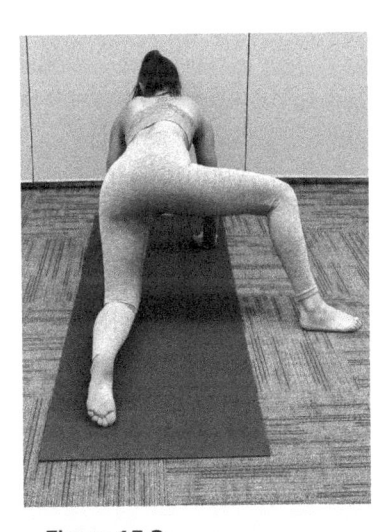

Figure 15.3

Chapter 15

Gait reasoning	• Improve hip joint mobility and reduce overactive tissue tensions that limit mobility
	• Vary the degrees of hip flexion in coordination with hip rotation to improve adaptation to ground forces
Starting position	• Quadruped position with slider under right foot
	• Maintain torso position while moving
Movement description	• Prepare by unweighting right hand and left knee 5 times to establish sensation of torso organization
	• Slide right foot posterior into hip extension with foot on slider
	• Slide right foot into hip and knee flexion starting position
	• Repeat 5 times
	• Repeat 5 times on left side

7. Quadruped four-corner diagonal

Intent	• Triplanar coordination relative to gait
	• Pelvis-femur differentiation
	• Integrated motion through varying degrees of flexion coupled with dynamic rotational movement
Gait reasoning	• Hip synergy for gait optimization
	• Proximal loading of hip for stance leg and multi-planar hip motions for swing phase
Starting position	• Quadruped position
	• Place slider under right foot, ankle dorsiflexed, metatarsals on slider, phalanges extended
	• Place slider under left hand, elbow extended
Movement description	• Inhale to prepare
	• Exhale, slide left hand superiorly and at the same time slide right slider posteriorly extending hip and knee
	• Inhale, left hand slides back to quadruped maintaining extended right lower extremity (LE)
	• Exhale, slide right LE from posterior to lateral abducting and externally rotating the hip and flex the knee to assume flat foot position on slider
	• Inhale, pause
	• Exhale, reverse movement returning to starting position
	• Observe for torso flexion, extension or rotating with unloading

8. **Lunge with 26 in. (65 cm) ball** (Black 2015, pp. 169-73)

Intent	• Increase hip extension
	• Optimize posterior hip recruitment
	• Mobility of pelvis in frontal and sagittal planes
Gait reasoning	• Proximal pelvic unleveling for gait pelvic patterning and torso adaptation
	• Extend the torso and hip for functional reorganization of torso to LE
	• Facilitate reciprocal motions in frontal plane while maintaining midline
	• Pre-loading of stance leg
Starting position	• Standing at a counter or behind a stable chair
	• Pitch torso 40–45 degrees from upright standing
	• Place right shin bone on top of ball, knee and hip flexed
	• Femoral joints balanced
	• Shift weight distribution from 50 percent on each leg to 25 percent on stance leg and 75 percent on ball
Movement description	• Inhale, flex left hip and knee, lowering body as ball rolls back simultaneously, extending right hip and increasing length tension at anterior hip
	• Exhale, maintaining torso position, assess levelness of pelvis and femoral joints
	• Inhale, lower the right hemipelvis inferiorly as the left hemipelvis responds superiorly
	• Exhale, level pelvis
	• Inhale, maintain position, assess levelness of pelvis
	• Exhale, return to initial starting position
	• Repeat 3 times on each side

9. **Prone extension**

Intent	• Mobility and activation of torso extension with rotation
	• Neuromyofascial activation of posterior LE coordinated with torso
Gait reasoning	• Economy of gait movement through reciprocal rotation and extensor activation

Chapter 15

Starting position	• Prone on mat
	• Forehead on stacked hands
	• Palms gently pressing hands into forehead for isometric engagement of upper extremity (UE) into torso
	• LE alignment connection at ankles with yoga block at medial heels for feedback
Movement description	• Inhale to prepare
	• Exhale, gently lift anterior abdominal wall away from the mat while sensing pelvis contact on the mat
	• Inhale, feeling the posterior thorax expansion with axial elongation through crown of head
	• Exhale, practice a 5 second sustained hold of pelvic diaphragm position
	• Repeat 5 times
	• Repeat, practice 5 rapid rhythmic activations of the pelvic diaphragm for 5 sets
	• Progression
	▪ Change UE to shoulder abduction with elbow flexion
	▪ Exhale, extend upper torso floating UE 1–2 in. (2.5–5 cm) off floor
	▪ Inhale, hold emphasizing axial elongation
	▪ Exhale, direct sternum to right maintaining lower ribs in contact with mat
	▪ Inhale, back to center in extension
	▪ Exhale, lower torso and head to starting position
	▪ Repeat 5 times in each direction
	• Progress to rotating right and left in extension before returning to starting position

10. Butterfly lift

Intent	• Moderate torso load training
	• Coordination of breath with movement
Gait reasoning	• Hip activation and adaptability
Starting position	• Supine on mat with knees flexed, heels in line with ischial tuberosities

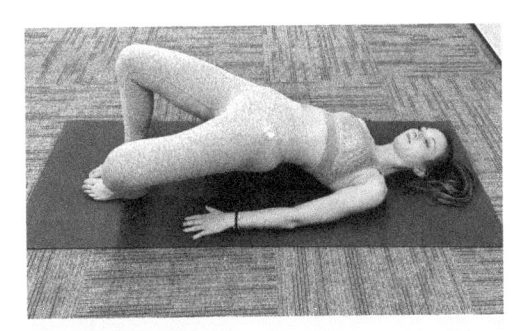

Pilates and Post-Robotic Nerve-Sparing Radical Prostatectomy: Effect on Gait

Figure 15.4

Movement description
- Inhale to prepare
- Exhale, reach both knees over toes, dorsiflexing ankles as hip joints extend
- Sequentially move through torso up to scapula into bridge position
- At the top of the bridge, pause
- Inhale, abduct right LE and return to center while maintaining torso control
- Exhale, pause, inhale, repeat on left side
- Exhale, articulate down to starting position
- Repeat 5 times
- Progress using resistance band around mid-thighs
- Increase challenge by lifting heels for decreased base of support
- Progress to bilateral hip abduction

11. Standing three-way hip with sliders

Intent
- Standing balance
- Activation of LE to hip to torso
- Proprioception with single-leg standing

Gait reasoning
- Hip motion for stance and swing phases
- Leg recruitment for improved stance phase
- Torso mobility for three-dimensional motions of torso

Starting position
- Stand holding on to the back of a chair or counter top
- Parallel stance with left foot metatarsals on a slider

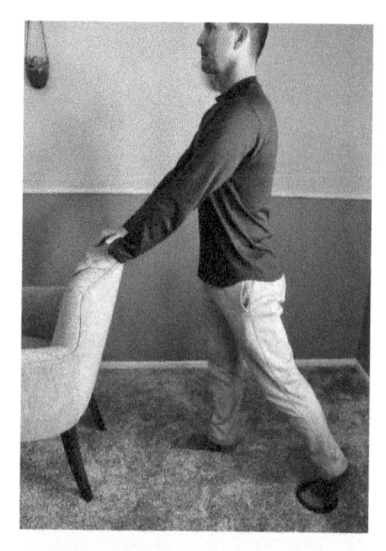

Figure 15.5

Movement description
- Progression 1
  - Maintain weight of standing leg through optimal foot-ankle organization
  - Inhale as right hip and knee extends sliding slider posterior
  - Exhale, return to starting stance position
  - Repeat 10 times
  - Repeat on other side
- Progression 2
  - Maintain weight of standing leg through optimal foot-ankle organization
  - Inhale as right hip abducts and right knee extends
  - Exhale, return to starting stance position
  - Repeat 10 times
  - Repeat on other side
- Progression 3
  - Maintain weight of standing leg through optimal foot-ankle organization
  - Inhale as right hip abducts and right knee extends circling LE in a semicircle
  - Exhale, return to starting stance position
  - Repeat 10 times
  - Reverse circle, repeat 10 times
  - Repeat on other side

12. Feet on wall: Hip abduction and external rotation

(See Chapter 5 in Volume 1, Eve Gentry, Wall: wall walks)

Intent	• Reduce hypertonicity of pelvic diaphragm to enhance femoral joint mobility
	• Decrease overactivity and hypomobility of LE to pelvis
Gait reasoning	• Improve pelvifemoral movement in three planes of motion
	• Coordinate activation and relaxation of diaphragm system with breathing
Starting position	• Supine with both feet on the wall, hips and knees flexed at 90/90, tibia parallel to floor
	• Reach arms posteriorly toward sitz bones
	• Be sure pelvis is not posteriorly rotated, COM at S2
Movement description	• Visualize a line from one ischial tuberosity to the other
	• Intentionally work to relax the muscles along this line for 30–45 seconds
	• Breathe slowly, 6 counts in and 6 counts out
	• As relaxation occurs, manually pull ischial tuberosities laterally
	• Inhale, bringing awareness to pelvic diaphragm
	• Exhale, activate the pelvic diaphragm without excessive tension
	• Gradually progress legs into more abduction, repeat sequence

Session 11/12: Studio Session

Fatigue scale	2
Pain scale	0–1
Client self-report	• Pain only noted once in past week after driving for 90 minutes in traffic. Described as mild heaviness, not really pain in peritoneal region. No episodes of leakage for 2 days after last visit
Key changes observed by author at end of Session 11/12	• Gait patterning improved, balanced right to left
	• Transverse plane motion increased
	• Improved awareness and motor control

Chapter 15

Reason behind choice of sequencing	• Progression builds confidence in awareness and proficiency for use with home program developing positive mindset • Deepening challenge of integrated movement

Session movement sequence

1. Spine Stretch Forward in well of Universal Reformer	Derivative of J. H. Pilates Spine Stretch (NPCE Study Guide 2021, p. 47)
Intent	• Sequential torso articulation • Scapulothoracic mobility • Proprioception and balanced weight bearing • Increase complexity by adding movement flow
Gait reasoning	• Improve sagittal plane movement to help decrease torso transverse plane rotation • Decrease rib shift • Improved COM and equal weight bearing

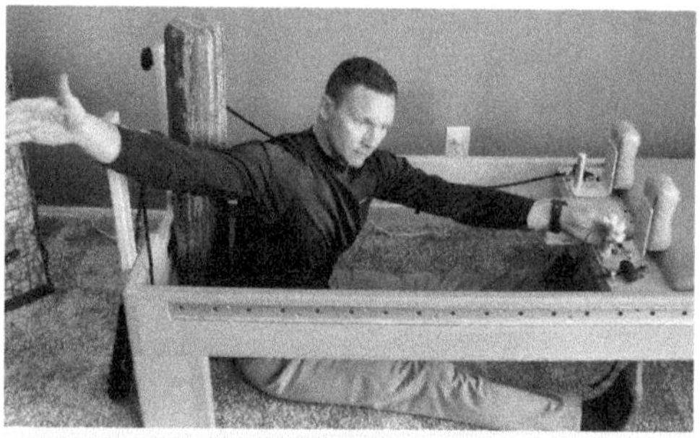

Figure 15.6

Set-up	• Springs: 1 light to 1 medium • Medium- to firm-density foam roller
Starting position	• Sitting upright between back frame of Universal Reformer and carriage, facing carriage • Place roller vertically between spine and frame • Legs extended, feet shoulder-width apart • Torso axial elongation • Shoulder flexion to 90 degrees, elbows extended, hands reaching toward Universal Reformer carriage

Movement description	- Inhale, feeling ischial tuberosities grounding inferiorly as crown of head moves in opposition, superiorly
- Exhale, draw anterior abdominal wall inward without going into flexion
- Flex from top of head articulating torso along roller
- Pause before pelvis moves posteriorly
- Maintain even weight bearing through ischial tuberosities
- In end range of flexion, shoulder, ears, and elbow are aligned
- Inhale, protract shoulders reaching toward shoulder stops
- Hold position
- Retract and protract scapulae repeating several times
- Inhale, segmentally extend torso to upright from pelvis to head without excessive abdominal doming
- Exhale at the top sensing ischial tuberosities grounding
- Repeat 5 times
	CUES
- At start sitting position shift weight right to left increasing awareness of weight distribution on the ischial tuberosities prior to initiating movement
- Lean into the roller segmentally to feel the articulation
	Author note
In the earlier sessions, this movement was a coordination challenge for the client and had a significant impact on his proprioception of force transmission from the ground and organizing the torso.
2. Footwork on Universal Reformer: Hip abduction and external rotation	Derivative of J. H. Pilates Footwork on Universal Reformer (NPCE Study Guide 2021, p. 52)
Intent	- Increase complexity of movement sequences
- LE to torso neuromyofascial training
- Motor control of femoral joints
Gait reasoning	- Increase proprioception by stimulating foot to hip patterns
- Coordinating breath and LE movements for IAP changes
- Eccentric diaphragmic challenge
Set-up	- 3 to 4 medium springs
Starting position	- Supine on carriage
- Feet wide on footbar, heels on bar
- Hips in flexion, abduction, and external rotation
- Knee flexion

Movement description
- Progression 1
  - Inhale, press feet into bar, extend hips and knees moving carriage away from footbar
  - Exhale slowly, return carriage home by flexing, externally rotating and abducting hips, knee flexion
  - Use the exhale to focus on sensations of diaphragmic redoming as carriage returns
  - Repeat 8–10 times with a 5 second count out and in, encouraging continuous movement
- Progression 2
  - Inhale, press on footbar and move carriage 1–2 inches off stoppers, hold position
  - 5 rapid rhythmic activations of pelvic diaphragm
  - Exhale, return to starting position
  - Repeat 5 times
- Progression 3
  - Inhale, press on footbar and move carriage 1–2 inches off stoppers, hold position
  - Sustain an activation of pelvic diaphragm for 5 seconds
  - Repeat 5 times
  - Reverse the breathing with entire series

3. Straps: feet in loops on Universal Reformer: Hip flexion, abduction, external rotation with knee flexion

Intent
- Reverse and add variability to typical activation of pelvic diaphragm
- Increase complexity of training
- Challenge adaptability to length-tension changes of medial LE

Gait reasoning
- Improved pelvifemoral motions in all three planes

Set-up
- Medium spring
- Rotator discs

Starting position
- Supine on carriage
- Both feet in straps
- Hips in flexion, abduction, and external rotation
- Knee flexion
- Feet plantar flexed with toes touching

Movement description	• Maintain LE within frame of Universal Reformer
• The positional mid-range is the optimal place to generate force from feet to hip joint
• Avoid anterior pelvic rotation at end of hip extension
• Avoid tendency to go into posterior pelvic tilt from 110–125 degrees hip flexion
• Sense weight at middle third of sacrum on carriage
• Teach client self-monitoring of abdominal wall
• Exhale to sense starting position
• Inhale, extend hips maintaining hip abduction and external rotation with knee flexion with toes touching
• Exhale, flex hips maintaining hip abduction and external rotation with knee flexion with toes touching
• Slight oppositional motion of pelvis anteriorly avoiding posterior pelvic rotation
• Repeat 5 times
• Reverse breathing, repeat 5 times
• Progress by decreasing spring tensions

CUE
- Maintain knees within the frame of the Universal Reformer

Author note
Watch for the tendency to go into posterior pelvic tilt from 110–125 degrees. Check hips during hip flexion phase.

4. Pelvic power lift on Universal Reformer	Derivative of J. H. Pilates Spine Stretch (NPCE Study Guide 2021, p. 47)
Intent	• Neuromyofascial connectivity from loading of feet through LE and torso
• Dynamic activation of LE, especially pelvifemoral movements
Gait reasoning	• Increase ability to flex and extend hip with femoral joint centralized
• Torso organization toward midline during hip movement
Set-up	• Springs fully loaded so carriage does not move
• Medium, 9 in. (23 cm), soft ball
Starting position	• Supine on carriage with feet on footbar
• Feet aligned in parallel on footbar
• Arms by sides pressing into carriage

Chapter 15

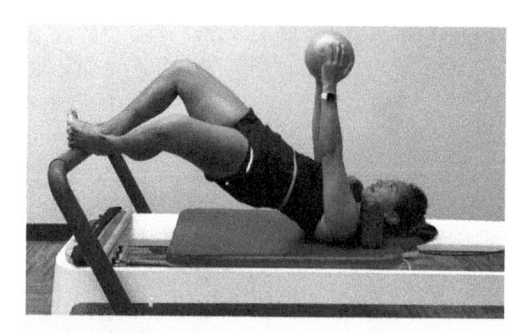

Figure 15.7

Movement description
- Inhale, sense torso weight on carriage
- Exhale, bridging up to mid-thorax focusing on sustained activation of pelvic diaphragm for 3–5 seconds
- Inhale, pause with hips lifted and in line with midline of torso
- Exhale, perform 5 rapid rhythmic activations of pelvic diaphragm
- Inhale, pause
- Exhale, return to starting position articulating from hip joints first
- Repeat 5 times
- Progress to single-leg extension
- Place ball at mid-point of femurs above knee
- Exhale into bridge, hold
- Inhale, extend right knee, foot off footbar, hold
- Exhale with 5 rapid rhythmic activations of pelvic diaphragm
- Inhale, return to starting position
- Repeat on other side
- Repeat sequence 5 times
- Repeat sequence adding 5 quick adduction presses on ball with 5 rapid rhythmic activations of pelvic diaphragm
- Repeat 3 times

CUE
- The bridge position is maintained, no dropping or rotating of torso during 5 rapid rhythmic activations of pelvic diaphragm

5. Butterfly lift on Universal Reformer

Intent
- Developing and enhancing neuromuscular connectivity by using gravity to assist both sustained and rapid rhythmic activations
- Coordinate both types of activations with hip movement

Gait reasoning
- Ability to adapt to ground forces
- Balance weight transference right to left

Set-up
- Springs, 2 medium and 1 heavy
- 9 in. (23 cm) diameter ball, three-quarters inflated, for biofeedback of pelvis-thorax relationship for optimal infra-sternal angle (ISA)

Starting position
- Supine on carriage
- Place ball under sacrum
- Feet aligned in parallel on footbar
- Arms pressing into carriage

Movement description
- Inhale, sense torso and feet
- Exhale, articulate into bridge to mid-thorax focusing on sustained activation of pelvic diaphragm for 3–5 seconds
- Inhale, right LE abducts maintaining control of the pelvis
- Exhale, return right LE to midline
- Inhale, repeat on left LE
- Exhale, return to starting position articulating from hip joints
- Repeat 5 times
- Remove ball, sense the ISA
- Repeat without ball 5 times
- Progress to adding resistance band around mid-thigh

CUES
- Maintain height of torso which may limit hip extension
- Synergistic activation of anterior and posterior torso to decrease strain in posterior torso
- Sense activation from medial ankle superiorly to pubic symphysis

Chapter 15

6. Prone extension on Universal Reformer long box

Intent
- Endurance of torso extension
- Proprioception of torso extension prior to standing

Gait reasoning
- Proprioception learning, prone to be transposed to standing
- Extensors activity for propulsion phase

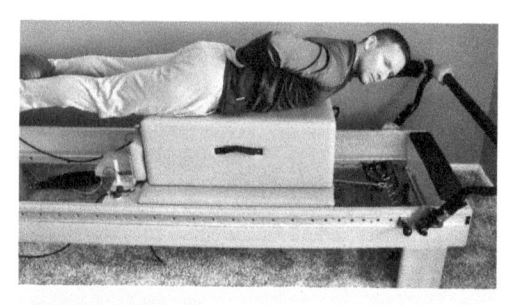

Figure 15.8

Set-up
- Long box set-up on Universal Reformer
- Full spring load for progression 1
- 2 medium springs for bilateral UE
- Medium spring for unilateral UE

Starting position
- Prone on box facing front
- Mid-chest at long edge of box
- Head in line with torso
- Hands holding footbar

Movement description
- Inhale to prepare, feel anterior torso on box
- Exhale, gently activate anterior abdominal wall away from box maintaining anterior pelvis contact on box
- Inhale, feel breath expand posterior torso with axial elongation
- Exhale for 5 seconds with sustained activation of anterior abdominal wall sensing pelvic diaphragm connection
- Repeat 5 times
- Repeat sequence changing activation to 5 rapid activations of pelvic diaphragm
- Repeat 5 times
- Progress to adding small degree of torso extension

Author note
Exhalation during extension of the torso may be cued to draw the lower thoracic volume toward the pelvis. As the thorax approximates the pelvis, the anterior and lateral abdominal myofascial tissues tension the thoracolumbar fascia (TLF) for support.

Editor note
The TLF is a three-dimensional girdling structure, consisting of several aponeurotic and fascial layers, that separates the paraspinal muscles from the muscles of the posterior abdominal wall. The thoracolumbar composite assists in maintaining the integrity of the lower lumbar region and the sacroiliac joint. The latissimus dorsi, gluteus maximus, and abdominal muscles, primarily the transversus abdominis, attach to the TLF. Tension applied by these muscles can be transmitted through the TLF to beneficially stiffen the lumbar region, creating stability and increasing force closure of the sacroiliac joint (Larkam 2017).

7. Standing Splits: Side on Universal Reformer

Derivative of J. H. Pilates Splits: Side on Universal Reformer (NPCE Study Guide 2021, p. 61)

Intent
- Lateral movement challenge with resistance
- Medial and lateral motion of hip joint
- Increase movement complexity by adding synergistic continuous movement

Gait reasoning
- Balanced and controlled movement for lateral adaptation
- Dynamic whole-body coordination

Set-up
- Medium spring
- Rotator discs
- Extended platform

Starting position
- Stand sideways right foot on frame, left foot on edge of carriage
- UE abducted, elbows extended

Chapter 15

Movement description
- Inhale, ground into foot position to prepare
- Exhale, press carriage out abducting LE with control
- Inhale, pause in abduction without allowing any movement of carriage
- Exhale, activate anterior abdominal wall
- Adducting LE, move carriage inward to starting position
- Repeat 5 times
- Progress by decreasing spring tension
- Repeat 5 times
- Progress by adding rotator discs under each foot maintaining parallel LE during movement

Author note

Lateral movements, as in Splits: Side, challenge balance and the ability of the body to adapt to the carriage motion. The pushing and pulling of the carriage from the LE enhances femoral spin medially and laterally activating the pelvifemoral neuromyofascia of the hip, which is necessary for single-leg stance during gait.

8. Eve's Lunge on Universal Reformer

(See Chapter 5 in Volume 1, Gentry, Eve's Lunge)

Intent
- Torso adaptability with controlled mobility
- Increase movement complexity by adding synergistic continuous movement

Gait reasoning
- Improve torso adaptability during all phases of gait
- Train hip medial motion during hip extension

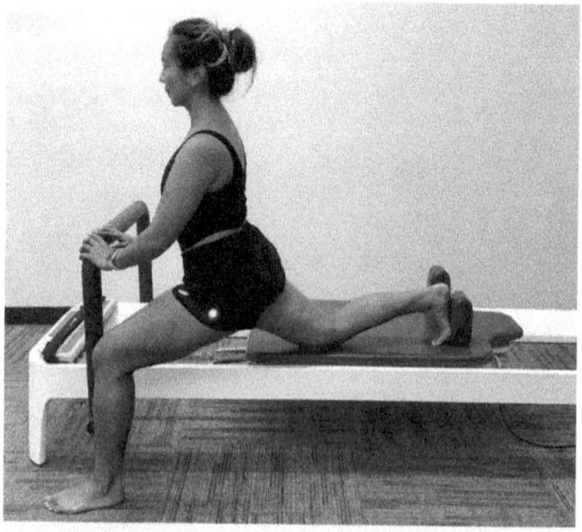

Figure 15.9

Set-up	● Medium spring
Starting position	● Stand in lunge position facing footbar ● Left knee resting on carriage with metatarsals and heel against shoulder stop, phalanges extended on carriage ● Right hip and knee flexion with foot placed at front leg of Universal Reformer ● Torso in an incline axial elongation with hands on footbar, elbows extended
Movement description	● Inhale, ground into left foot to prepare with 60–75 percent weight into carriage ● Exhale, press carriage back extending left hip while flexing right hip and knee ● Torso lowers ● Inhale, pause, noting balance of pelvis, add 5 fast pelvic diaphragm pulses ● Exhale, control carriage in toward starting position, focus on gentle anterior abdominal activation with axial elongation ● Repeat 5 times ● Progress to Eve's Lunge sequence ■ Inhale, press carriage out adding torso extension ■ Exhale, flexion from head through mid-thorax as carriage returns ■ Repeat 5 times

CUES
- Use manual cueing to enhance awareness and provide feedback to client
- During carriage movement, cue lower ring of ribcage to ensure no increase in ISA, or rotation in the transverse plane

Author note
For clients, pelvic proprioception in all three planes can be difficult to sense. In cueing, focus on sagittal plane awareness first, then transverse plane, and lastly frontal plane.

Chapter 15

9. Mermaid on Universal Reformer

Derivative of J.H. Pilates Mermaid on Universal Reformer (NPCE Study Guide 2021, p. 64)

Intent
- Increased thoracic movement in rotation and lateral flexion
- Abdominal coordinated activation during rotation
- Mobility with balanced weight bearing in variable hip positions
- Lateral torso mobility through UE

Gait reasoning
- Improve torso movement limitations seen in assessment
- Breath coordination with movement
- Midline awareness: anterior to posterior, left to right, normalizing ISA

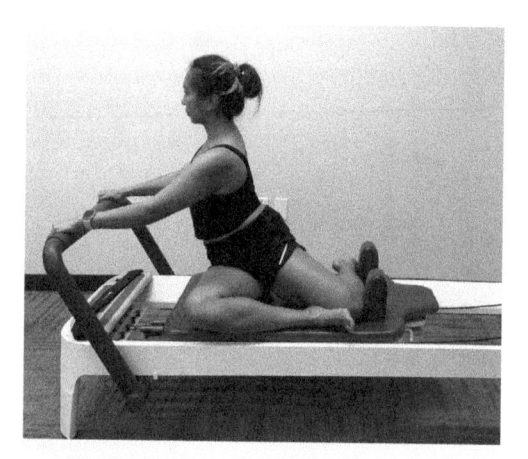

Figure 15.10

Set-up
- Medium spring

Starting position
- Sit sideways on carriage with knees bent, left leg positioned with shin flush against shoulder stops, right heel in contact with left knee creating a triangle position
- Place right hand on footbar in front of shoulder approximately 30 degrees from frontal plane

Movement description
- Inhale, with right hand press carriage away from footbar as left UE reaches overhead with right lateral torso flexion
- Exhale, return to starting position, reestablish sitz bones evenly weighted on carriage
- Inhale, reverse lateral flexion to left by reaching right UE toward the ceiling as right arm rests on shoulder stop
- Repeat 3 times
- Repeat pressing carriage out and lateral torso flexion, hold
- Rotate torso toward the floor bringing left hand to footbar, unweight right hand to reposition toward far side of footbar
- Inhale, breathe into sides of ribs deepening hip flexion
- Exhale, derotate, reposition support arm in center of footbar maintaining lateral torso flexion
- Inhale, return to starting position
- Repeat once in deepened hip flexion in the well, exhale, pause
- Inhale, pressing through hand, lifting upper torso into extension, broadening shoulders, opening across chest
- Exhale, return to deep flexion facing the well, derotate, follow return sequence to starting position
- Progress to deepened hip flexion position, use the exhale reaching arm under side of torso in rotation while pressing away
- Inhale, returning from rotation facing the well
- Exhale, derotate out of position, bring carriage in returning to starting position

CUES
- Try gentle anterior-posterior motion of the pelvis to increase mobility and congruency with surface of carriage
- Reach in opposition of support arm and opposite hip while pressing carriage out

Author note
Rotation and counter-rotation have a multitude of benefits for improving gait patterning such as bringing awareness to rotation, interoception of oppositional thorax and pelvis rotation, and UE relationship to rotational patterning of torso.

Chapter 15

The journey to Session 11

Session 4/12
Client self-report

- Workout type of soreness
- Dull ache at underside of pelvis, sense of a "void"
- Fatigue scale 4–5
- Pain scale 2

Key changes observed

- Weight shift to left appears less
- Weight shift into toes less pronounced with Footwork
- Improved ability for rapid activations and sustaining activation of 5 seconds
- Aware of body "twist"

Reasoning behind choice of movements

- Starting in standing for proprioceptive connections of feet
- Developing awareness
- Triplanar motion to enhance gait patterning

Session movement sequence
1. Mermaid on 26 in. (65 cm) ball added

2. Quadruped exercise, fine-tuned

3. Universal Reformer

- Spine Stretch Forward at footbar to long box
- Footwork with standard breathing
- Straps: feet in loops
    - Parallel and external rotation with hip and knee flexion
- Prone with long box
- Pelvic power lift
- Seated hover
    - Sit on front carriage edge, no springs, with feet on floor
    - Activate as if standing up
    - Hover feeling for posterior hip activation

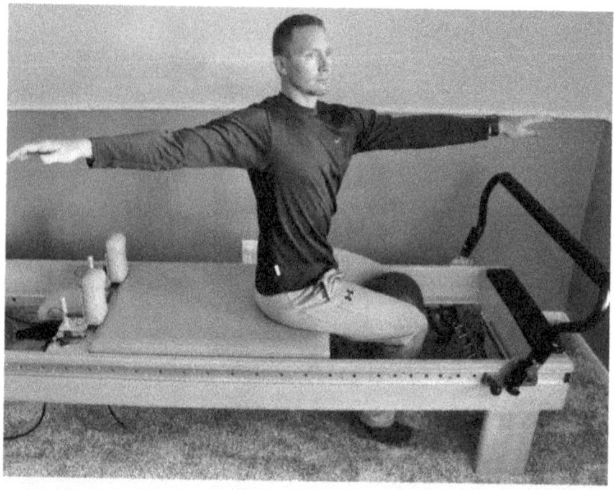

Figure 15.11

- Eve's Lunge
- Mermaid, lateral flexion only

Session 5/12
Client self-report

- Felt soreness on right internal oblique, more than on left, lower abdominal area
- Tightness of posterior LE
- Fatigue scale 4
- Pain scale 2

Key changes observed

- Subject did not practice home program prior to the session, pelvic motions appeared stiff, incongruent
- Rib shift and left hemipelvis superior motion observable
- Overall stiffness especially in hip joints, needed hip prop for Mermaid
- As the session progressed hip mobility improved

538

Reasoning behind choice of movements

- Bring sensory input for balance
- Posterior hip and foot intrinsic work for gait propulsion

Session movement sequence
1. Universal Reformer

- Spine Stretch Forward at footbar to long box
- Footwork
- Straps: feet in loops
  - Parallel, external rotation with hip and knee flexion, 18 in. (46 cm)
- Prone extension with long box
- Pelvic power lift
- Butterfly lift
- Seated hover
  - Added 2 lb (0.90 kg) weights at 90 degrees of shoulder flexion
- Eve's Lunge
- Mermaid
  - Lateral flexion only
  - Added lateral flexion away from footbar

2. Additional movement

- Increased complexity of straps: feet in loops, hover, and Mermaid

Session 6/12
Client self-report

- Driving a lot for work this week, 90 minute commute, one way
- Fatigue scale 4
- Pain scale 2

Key changes observed

- Overall stiffness especially in hip joints, needed hip prop for Mermaid
- Rotation quality is diminished to left

Reasoning behind choice of movements

- Working torso functionality for rotational load transition in gait
- Practice to enhance adapting to loading
- Decrease excessive thoracic translation
- Improve oppositional rotation of thorax and pelvis
- Continue activating and proprioception of the foot

Session movement sequence
1. Quadruped sequence progressed for hip external rotation/internal rotation

2. Side lying hip abduction: breath pattern reversal

3. Progressed 26 in. (65 cm) ball lunge to standing hip extension with slider

4. Resistance band ribcage facilitation as home program preparation

5. Universal Reformer

- Spine Stretch Forward at footbar to long box
- Footwork: hip abduction and external rotation
- Straps: feet in loops
  - Parallel, external rotation with hip and knee flexion, 18 in. (46 cm), internal rotation
- Prone extension with long box
- Pelvic power lift
- Butterfly lift
- Seated hover
  - Roller under feet, knees 120 degrees extension
  - Move carriage toward roller to 90 degrees knee flexion
- Eve's Lunge
  - Reverse breath patterns

Chapter 15

- Mermaid
    - Addition of rotation

6. Additional movement

- Used resistance band and in lateral flexion to enhance awareness for ribcage expansion

Session 7/12
Client self-report

- Good home program this week, feeling stronger, fewer episodes of leakage, noting aversion to drinking water
- Fatigue scale 3
- Pain scale 1

Key changes observed

- Improved precision of exercises
- Integrated awareness of whole-body during movement appears improved
- Improved symmetry with loading in gait
- Client reports ability to "feel" pelvis more centered while walking
- Torso adapts well with addition of rotation component

Reasoning behind choice of movements

- Hip abduction with external rotation: Footwork and the addition of feet on wall: hip abduction and external rotation brings input from feet to torso
- Spine Stretch from wall for feedback with segmental articulation
- Increased movement complexity with LE activation coupled with rotation in sitting

Session movement sequence
1. Universal Reformer

- Spine Stretch Forward in well
- Footwork with reverse breathing, hip abduction and external rotation
- Straps: feet in loops
    - Parallel, external rotation with hip and knee flexion, 18 in. (46 cm), internal rotation
- Pelvic power lift
- Butterfly lift
- Prone extension on long box
- Seated hover
    - Roller under feet
    - Move carriage to 90 degrees knee flexion, hold
    - Rotate torso right, center
    - Return to starting position
    - Repeat with left rotation
- Eve's Lunge
    - Reversed breathing patterns
- Mermaid
    - Lateral flexion and rotation

2. Additional movements

- Rotation added to seated hover for coordinating rotation with torso and hip patterning
- Progressed in session to coordinating both movements simultaneously

Session 8/12
Client self-report

- To improve driving tolerance, agreed to add stretch breaks when driving for more than 1 hour
- Diaphragm exercises are getting easier, especially rapid articulations
- Fatigue scale 3
- Pain scale 0

Key changes observed

- Good coordination of reversed breathing
- Able to maintain torso position with bridging when adding complexity

Reasoning behind choice of movements

- Hip abduction enhanced with feet on wall: hip abduction and external rotation
- Coordination of hip movements

Session movement sequence

1. Prone torso rotation to pelvic extension added

2. Universal Reformer

- Spine Stretch Forward in well
- Footwork with reversed breathing, hip abduction and external rotation
- Straps: feet in loops
  - Parallel, external rotation with hip and knee flexion, 18 in. (46 cm) boxes, internal rotation, wide V
- Pelvic power lift
- Butterfly lift
- Prone extension on long box, added rotation
- Seated hover
  - Roller under feet
  - Move carriage to 90 degrees knee flexion, hold
  - Rotate torso right, center
  - Return to starting position
  - Repeat with left rotation
- Eve's Lunge
- Mermaid
  - Lateral flexion and rotation

3. Additional movements

- Hip abduction/adduction component
- Rotation complexity in prone extension

Session 9/12
Client self-report

- Not thinking about leakage or limiting drinking water at all—pleased with progress; notes skipped a few home program days—was feeling good, did not notice any ramifications
- Fatigue scale 2
- Pain scale 0

Key changes observed

- Ability to move continuously with hip motions in all planes
- Improved coordination in walking and torso rotation symmetry noted with loading response left and right

Reasoning behind choice of movements

- Continue developing confidence and motor control of the new available movement of pelvifemoral and torso articulation

Session movement sequence

1. Spine Stretch from wall with addition of foam roller and Half Saw

2. Universal Reformer

- Spine Stretch Forward in well
- Footwork with reversed breathing, hip abduction and external rotation
- Straps: feet in loops
  - Parallel, external rotation with hip and knee flexion, 18 in. (46 cm), internal rotation, wide V
- Pelvic power lift
- Butterfly lift
- Prone extension on long box, added rotation
- Seated hover
  - Roller under feet
  - Move carriage to 90 degrees knee flexion, hold
  - Rotate torso right, center

- Return to starting position
- Repeat with left rotation, added hemipelvis superior motion
- Standing Splits: Side
- Eve's Lunge
- Mermaid
  - Lateral flexion and rotation

3. Additional movement

- Adding rotation in variable positions between flexion and extension

Session 10/12
Client self-report

- Increased stress/load at work—lifting more, feeling tired but demands have increased; feels he is adjusting well
- Fatigue scale 2
- Pain scale 0

Key changes observed

- Overall reciprocal gait patterning improved
- Fluid movement

Reasoning behind choice of movements

- Increasing challenge and load in sitting for better attenuation of load in rotation with functional movement patterns

Session movement sequence
1. Seated hover on chair with roller, torso rotation, with and without hemipelvis superior motion

2. Universal Reformer

- Spine Stretch Forward in well
- Footwork with reversed breathing, hip abduction and external rotation
- Straps: feet in loops
  - Parallel, external rotation with hip and knee flexion, 18 in. (46 cm), internal rotation, wide V
- Pelvic power lift
- Butterfly lift
- Prone extension on long box, added rotation
- Seated hover
  - Roller under feet
  - Move carriage to 90 degrees knee flexion, hold
  - Rotate torso right, center
  - Return to starting position
  - Repeat with left rotation, with and without hemipelvis superior motion
- Standing Splits: Side
- Eve's Lunge
- Mermaid
  - Lateral flexion and rotation

References

Black, M. (2015) *1st edition, Centered: Organizing the Body through Kinesiology, Movement Theory and Pilates Techniques*. 2nd Ed. Edinburgh: Handspring Publishing.

Black, M. (2022) *Centered: Organizing the Body through Kinesiology, Movement Theory and Pilates Techniques*. 2nd Ed. Edinburgh: Handspring Publishing, pp. 24–25.

Hodges, P. W., Stafford, R. E., Hall, L., Neumann, P. *et al.* (2020) "Reconsideration of pelvic floor muscle training to prevent and treat incontinence after radical prostatectomy." *Urologic Oncology: Seminars and Original Investigations, 38,* 5, 354–371.

Larkam, E. (2017) *Fascia in Motion: Fascia-Focused Movement for Pilates*. Edinburgh: Handspring Publishing, pp. 40–41.

NPCE Study Guide (National Pilates Certification Exam Study Guide) (2021) Miami, FL: National Pilates Certification Program, Inc.

Scott, K. M., Gosai, E., Bradley, M. H., Walton, S. *et al.* (2020) "Individualized pelvic physical therapy for the treatment of post-prostatectomy stress urinary incontinence and pelvic pain." *International Urology and Nephrology, 52,* 4, 655–659.

Strojek, K., Weber-Rajek, M., Strączyńska, A., Piekorz, Z. *et al.* (2021) "Randomized-controlled trial examining the effect of pelvic floor muscle training in the treatment of stress urinary incontinence in men after a laparoscopic radical prostatectomy pilot study." *Journal of Clinical Medicine, 10,* 13. DOI: 10.3390/jcm10132946.

Sung, H., Ferlay, J., Siegel, R. L., Laversanne, M. *et al.* (2021) "Global cancer statistics 2020: GLOBOCAN estimates of incidence and mortality worldwide for 36 cancers in 185 countries." *CA: A Cancer Journal for Clinicians, 71,* 3, 209–249.

Abbreviations

ABLR	active bent leg raise	NCPT	National Certified Pilates Teacher
ADLs	activities of daily living	NPCP	National Pilates Certification Program
ASIS	anterior superior iliac spine	OA	occipitoatlantal
ASLR	active straight leg raise	PEM	post-exertional malaise
COM	center of mass	PESE	post-exertional symptom exacerbation
CT	cervicothoracic; computed tomography	PET	positron emission tomography
DIP	distal interphalangeal	PFD	pelvic floor dysfunction
DRA	diastasis recti abdominis, diastasis rectus abdominis	PIP	proximal interphalangeal
FABER	flexion, abduction, external rotation	POTS	postural orthostatic tachycardia syndrome
FAI	femoral acetabular impingement	PT	physical therapist; physical therapy
GHJ	glenohumeral joint	ROM	range of motion
GT	greater trochanter	SCAN	somato (body)-cognitive (mind) action network
IAP	intra-abdominal pressure	SCM	sternocleidomastoid
ILA	inferior lateral angle	SIJ	sacroiliac joint
IRD	inter-rectus distance	SUI	stress urinary incontinence
ISA	infrasternal angle	TLF	thoracolumbar fascia
LA	linea alba	TLJ	thoracolumbar junction
LBP	low back pain	TrA	transversus abdominis
LE	lower extremity, lower extremities	TRX	total resistance exercise
ME/CFS	myalgic encephalomyelitis/chronic fatigue syndrome	UE	upper extremity, upper extremities
MRI	magnetic resonance imaging	UI	urinary incontinence
MTP	metatarsophalangeal	US	ultrasound

Glossary

abduction
the action of moving a limb away from the midline

activation
a stimulation of the neuromyofascial system for movement

adaptation
malleability and efficient response of the neuromyofascial system to changing conditions. Types of adaptation include fascial remodeling and reflexive responses

adduction
the action of moving a limb toward the midline

anterior
in front of or the front surface of the body

articulation
an action of creating movement through a region with anatomical congruity of the articulator surfaces and the ligaments, muscles, and fascia that support it

attenuating
refers to the reduction of magnitude of forces

auxetic
the property of a material that increases in width when "stretched." It does not narrow, become thinner and/or longer. See **stretch**

biotensegrity
a new paradigm for considering the balance of forces in a biological structure. Applied biotensegrity is an awareness of how the principles of biotensegrity are used in movement and by manual practitioners

breathe into a body area
to describe direction of the breath toward an area, stimulating activation or expansion in that region. Three-dimensional breathing is the torso's capacity to respond during inhalation in all planes of motion

clam
side lying hip joint abduction with knee flexion

closed kinematic chain
"closed kinematic chains" in biology, including human anatomy, are the coupling of multiple parts into continuous mechanical loops allowing the structure to self-regulate complex movements at all scales

compression
a force that presses or pushes together

connective tissue
provides support and framework for the body consisting of fibrous proteins and non-fibrous ground substance in varying proportions depending on their functions. This includes the tissues of muscles, fascia, fat, cartilage, bones, and blood

diaphragms
connective tissue structures at the level of the eyes (cranial diaphragm), the ring above the clavicle and shoulder girdle (thoracic outlet), the respiratory diaphragm, and the pelvic diaphragm. When these structures are activated in integrated movement they support comprehensive, whole-body movement

disassociate
a term used for intent and reasoning about treatment. To disassociate is to emphasize the articulation required for a movement task. See **articulation**

Glossary

dorsiflexion
moving the dorsal surface (top) of the foot toward the shin. The articulation of the ankle occurs at the tibial talus region, the talocrural joint

elasticity
the tendency of a material to "bounce back" to its original shape after a deformation

ethmoid bone
one of the eight bones of the cranium. It is situated at the roof of the nasal cavity and between the two orbital cavities

external (lateral) rotation
the joint action of moving away from the center relative to the classical anatomical position

FABER
flexion, abduction, external rotation. These three movements combined result in a clinical pain provocation test to assist in diagnosis of pathologies at the hip, lumbar, and sacroiliac region

fascia
matrix of fibers secreted by cells that encompasses cellular structure

fascial glide
fascia facilitates movement by allowing gliding around the structures it surrounds; the ability of fascial planes and muscles to glide on each other or against other tissues

force
an effort or exertion of power

glenohumeral
the region between the scapula (shoulder blade) and the humerus (arm bone); the glenoid is the articular surface of the scapula where the head of the humerus joins forming the glenohumeral joint

ground reaction force
force exerted by the ground on a body in contact with it

hemipelvis
one half of the pelvic bone (innominate), including all the associated tissues

hip joint
the anatomical term for hip joint is "acetabulofemoral joint." The common name and most widely used term is "hip joint." The term acetabulofemoral refers to the virtual space between the head of the femur and the acetabulum of the pelvis

hip quadrant test
a physical examination test used to assess hip joint mobility and identify any restrictions in the hip joint's range of motion

idiopathic
relating to or denoting any disease or condition for which the cause is unknown

iliac crest
the superior aspect of the iliac bones that form part of the pelvis

inferior
a structure that is below another structure or directed downward

internal (medial) rotation
the joint action of moving toward the center relative to the classical anatomical position

interoception
the collection of senses signaling the internal state of the body, both conscious and unconscious; the capacity to perceive and integrate body signals generating affective states

ischial tuberosity of the ischium
one of the bilateral "sitting" bones that form part of the pelvis

kinematics
the geometry of motion

kinetics
relating to or resulting from motion

lateral
to the side of, or away from, the middle of the body

lever model
the mechanistic idea of the body as a collection of levers and pulleys operating in a uniplanar, binary, linear hierarchy

medial
toward the middle or center

menisci
Greek *meniskos*, "crescent"-shaped fibrous cartilages or "discs" that partially line a joint cavity

motor control
the process that initiates, directs, and grades purposeful movement for performing a skillful task

myofascia
"myo" refers to muscle tissue; "fascia" refers to connective tissue

parallel
a position of the legs where the second toe of each foot lines up with the mid-patella and the hip joint

pelvic list
a small degree of inferior movement of the hemipelvis

pelvifemoral
movement of the pelvis relative to the femur

plantar flexion
moving the plantar surface of the foot toward the shin. The articulation of the ankle occurs at the tibial talus region, the talocrural joint

posterior
behind or the back surface of the body

powerhouse
the cylinder of strength between the top of the pelvis and the bottom of the ribs. J. H. Pilates encouraged activation of this region to initiate all Pilates exercises (Larkam 2017)

pronation
anatomical term for rotating the distal aspects of the limbs so the plantar/palmar surface presents inferiorly; medial rotation

proprioception
the perception of the position of the body and forces acting on it

proximal
an indication of a part of a limb that is closer to the torso

reflexive stability
a motor response of the neuromyofascial system based on sensory input to a force or demand placed upon the body

sacroiliac
the region on either side of the sacrum next to the iliac bones of the pelvis

scapulohumeral rhythm
biomotion of the shoulder describing the movement of the scapula in coordination with the humerus

spiral
the spiral is a line curving continuously away from a central point

stiffness
there are distinct uses of this word with different connotations. One is a felt sense of the tissue's resistance to movement. Stiffness is a resistance to deformation. Elasticity does not just refer to the amount we can stretch. Tissue stiffness refers to the ability or capacity to restore a change in shape. In material science, stiff springs can have more elasticity than weaker springs because they store more energy and rebound more efficiently

strategies for motor control
each person has their own established motor strategies developed over a lifetime. They provide the capacity to perform a task, process sensory input, interpret dynamic activity, and respond to unpredictable, unexpected, and challenging movement

Glossary

stretch
according to Jan Wilke, PhD, co-editor of *Fascia in Sport and Movement*: "The initially observed length changes during a stretch do not lead to a significant increase in strain because the collagen fibers, which are slightly wavy at rest, straighten" (Wilke 2021)

superior
a structure that is situated above another structure or directed upwards

supination
anatomical term for rotating the distal aspects of limbs so the palmar/plantar surface presents superiorly; lateral rotation

synergistic
the combining of two or more forces so that the result is more than the sum of the original two

tensegrity
tension + integrity—a term popularized by Buckminster Fuller to describe the concept of floating compression previously proposed by sculptor Kenneth Snelson

tension
a force of pulling apart

thoracolumbar
the region of the back between the thoracic (ribcage) and lumbar vertebrae

tissue
specialized regions of cellular organization between the level of the cell and the organ

translation
a term from spinal biomechanics. The ability to rotate around one axis and translate along another axis in a three-dimensional space

vector
a line that has magnitude and direction

vertical axis
the intersection of the three cardinal planes organizing around the midline of the body

vestibular
describes parts of the inner ear that control balance